# Gilbert Guide

From our family to yours,

Jill René Gilbert
Jason Gilbert
Harvey Gilbert, MD
Deanne Gilbert

# gilbert GUIDE

THE *only* INSIDER'S GUIDE TO THE BEST LONG-TERM CARE FACILITIES AND SERVICES

SENIOR CARE

The information in this guide is based on Gilbert Guide's independent research. Gilbert Guide, Inc. does not have any financial or personal interests in any of the facilities, services or resources listed in this guide.

# CREDITS



Published by Gilbert Guide, Inc., San Francisco, California
www.gilbertguide.com

Library of Congress Control Number: 2004117732

ISBN 978-0-9764346-2-8

#### GILBERT GUIDE, INC.

| | |
|---|---|
| President and CEO | Jill René Gilbert |
| COO and CFO | Jason Gilbert |
| Medical and Policies Director | Harvey A. Gilbert, MD |
| VP Programs and Marketing | Caitlin Morgan |
| Editorial and Content Manager | Nikki Jong |
| Copywriters | Jacqueline Esai |
| | Joanna Leon Guerrero |
| DFW Office Manager | Steven Lee Harris |
| Designer | Angie Gubler |
| Production | Yvonne Sartain |

#### SPECIAL SALES

Gilbert Guide publications are available at special bulk discounts for sales promotions or premiums. Special editions including personalized covers, excerpts of existing guides and corporate imprints can be created in large quantities for individual needs. For more information, please visit our website www.gilbertguide.com or email us at sales@gilbertguide.com.



Printed in the United States of America

First Edition

Care
Managers
Discharge Planners
nurses

WE DEDICATE THIS BOOK TO ALL CAREGIVERS
AND THE PEOPLE WHO SERVE THEM.

Counselors
Social Workers
doctors
Caregivers

# THANKS

Gilbert Guide is indebted to the following people for their dedication, input, expertise and creativity—not to mention elbow grease:

**JASON GILBERT** is the piece that completes the puzzle. His extensive business knowledge and keen sense for applying it have resulted in countless innovative ways of elevating the company to new levels. I feel so privileged to have the opportunity to build this company with Jason, who is not only my brother but is also my dear friend.

**NIKKI JONG'S** passion for perfection and amazing attention to detail ensures that Gilbert Guide meets the highest standard of quality and clarity. She embraces this work as if it were her life's mission. Nikki's friendship, dedication and work ethic goes far beyond the norm—her involvement will continue to shape Gilbert Guide for years to come.

**CAITLIN MORGAN**, an integral member of our Gilbert Guide team. Her total dedication to the field of long-term care and her belief in the positive influence and far-reaching scope of this project helps provide a clear vision for the company's growth.

**ANGIE GUBLER**, whose awesome creativity brings to life a fresh and innovative design that has far exceeded my expectations.

**OUR SURVEY TEAM**, for bringing their extensive knowledge and expertise to the process. Their eyes and ears help us bring our readers only the best.

**JACQUELINE ESAI AND JOANNA LEON GUERRERO**, whose tireless creativity make our *Portraits* jump off the page and come to life.

**STEVEN LEE HARRIS**, for hitting every curve ball thrown his way. His positive, can-do attitude have helped make our Dallas-Fort Worth guide the best resource for our readers.

**KAY PAGGI**, not only for stepping in at the eleventh hour and helping us get to press, but also for her complete commitment to the well-being of seniors and their caregivers.

**AARON VANCE**, for spearheading the extensive focus groups that helped guide our company's path.

Most importantly, I would like to thank my parents, **DR. HARVEY** and **DEANNE GILBERT**. Their infinite love and support have helped us create a viable and amazing company, and brought our dream to fruition, by allowing us to touch the lives of our many readers in an unforgettable way.

Jill René Gilbert
President and CEO, Gilbert Guide, Inc.

# WHAT MAKES US DIFFERENT

## GILBERT GUIDE IS THE ULTIMATE GUIDEBOOK TO FINDING THE BEST IN LONG-TERM CARE

### WE'RE COMPREHENSIVE AND SPECIFIC

When we set out to write a guide that would give caregivers the information they needed to make good decisions about local long-term care, we first looked at what was already out there. A number of good resources addressed state or national audiences, but few were comprehensive enough to help caregivers select the best local facilities, resources and services for their client or loved one. None of them adequately addressed all the questions caregivers really need answered.

### WE LISTENED TO YOUR NEEDS

We gathered focus groups comprised of professionals—hospital discharge planners, social workers, geriatricians, social services directors and geriatric care managers. We also recruited focus groups of informal caregivers—one group just starting to look for long-term care, and another who had already been through the process. Together, we formulated a comprehensive list of questions that caregivers need answered.

### WE ASKED THE EXPERTS

We put together a team of experts to ask the questions generated in our focus groups. Our knowledgeable representatives—including RNs, social workers, geriatric care managers and professional caregivers—visited, toured, explored and inquired about every facility in the guide. We collated and reviewed the information they gathered and put it into this practical and accessible guide—handcrafted to suit your needs.

### WE PROVIDE PERSONAL AND PROFESSIONAL INSIGHTS TO HELP YOU MAKE THE RIGHT DECISIONS FOR YOUR NEEDS

The resources in Gilbert Guide are the very best long-term care facilities, resources and services in your area. We made sure you'll have the essential facts and details about each facility at your fingertips. And we took it one step further: we asked our eyewitness experts to write narratives that give you an accurate picture of what each facility is really like. This unique blend of personal perspective and professional observation, resulting in a complete *Portrait,* tells you just what you want—and need—to know.

## WHAT YOU NEED TO KNOW BEFORE READING THIS BOOK

**Q**. I noticed that some of the facilities in my area are not listed in Gilbert Guide. Why?

**A**. There are several reasons why a facility may not be listed in the book:

- It did not meet the standards and criteria that we outline in chapter 1.
- It declined to participate in our survey process.
- It is not licensed by the government agency that regulates that particular type of facility. A few examples include Medicare and State Departments of Health and Social Services.

  *Note*: We always review new facilities, but only those that are licensed and have their doors open for business at the time when we collect our information.

**Q**. Can I trust your recommendations and skip doing my own research?

**A**. You may absolutely trust our recommendations; however, be aware that things change over time—and that prices, management and services may have undergone changes since this book was printed. Use Gilbert Guide to create your personal shortlist of facility favorites and schedule an appointment to view the facilities and verify these details.

# TABLE OF CONTENTS

# WELCOME TO GILBERT GUIDE,

## THE ONLY COMPREHENSIVE GUIDE TO LOCAL LONG-TERM CARE THAT COMBINES EXPERTISE WITH PERSONAL INSIGHT.

### EXPERTISE AND PERSONAL INSIGHT MEAN THE RIGHT CHOICE FOR YOU

When you're making choices about long-term care, the right decisions are the ones that best fit your individual needs. And the best way to make sure you meet those needs is to base your decisions on reliable information. That's why we made it our goal to educate and empower caregivers so that you can make informed choices.

### THE SHORTEST ROUTE TO THE BEST OPTIONS

We designed Gilbert Guide to give you the shortest route to finding the best options in long-term care: from the first stages, to end-of-life care and each level in between. Whether you're just beginning your search or you've already started looking, you'll find solid, dependable information about the best options in your area.

### MEETING YOUR UNIQUE NEEDS

No one's needs are just like yours. Many factors—including income levels, geographic requirements, language needs and health concerns—make each situation unique. One person may only have transportation needs, a second may need in-home care or skilled nursing care, while a third may need a parent to be cared for in another city. We've taken all these factors into consideration in compiling our data and we've done the legwork for you.

#### SAVING TIME AND GETTING IT RIGHT

The one thing that all caregivers seem to have in common is their limited time. Because we've already done the research, Gilbert Guide cuts your search time in half. We list only the very best facilities, resources and services in your area so you can quickly compile a shortlist of the ones that best meet your needs—without having to call every facility in the phone book and ask the same questions over and over. By the time you draft your shortlist, you'll be a well-informed consumer.

#### WELCOME TO OUR TEAM!

We consider you a vital part of our team. Even though using the information in Gilbert Guide will shorten your search considerably, it's still very important to do your own research on the list you've compiled. Before you choose a facility, it is absolutely necessary to make a personal visit so you can form your own impressions of the environment and management. When selecting in-home care, it's also crucial to make sure you address the most important issues affecting the person who will be receiving care. We encourage you to call the agencies directly and schedule interviews whenever possible.

We've done the best job we can to ensure you are choosing from quality resources. The last step—making the right choice for you—is yours to take.

—THE GILBERT GUIDE TEAM

# CATEGORIES OF CARE

- What is Long-term Care?
- Categories of Care
- Our Standards and Criteria
- Gilbert Guide Symbols and Ratings

## WHAT IS LONG-TERM CARE?

Long-term care covers a broad spectrum of services, some of which you may be surprised to learn about. Although it is often thought to serve only individuals who require skilled care, it frequently begins much sooner than that. *Long-term care begins when a previously independent individual can no longer perform the same activities that he or she once could.*

Long-term care encompasses: custodial care, which includes assistance with activities of daily living such as grocery shopping, bathing or driving; skilled care, either in a nursing facility or at home, such as rehabilitation after surgery or an illness; care for cognitive impairments such as Alzheimer's or other forms of dementia; and palliative care for individuals who can no longer benefit from regular medical treatment.

---

## CARE ASSESSMENT

*What It Is*

A care assessment is a comprehensive evaluation that identifies the care needs of an individual. The objective of an assessment is to draft a plan of care, which is based on the health, social, emotional and physical needs of that person. There are two sources for obtaining a care assessment: case managers and geriatric care managers.

Case managers and geriatric care managers are trained to recognize telltale signs in your loved one that indicate specific needs—signs that are clear to trained professionals, but which you may not be able to recognize yourself. A care assessment ensures that you will be focused on what to look for. In the long run, this will prevent frustrating wrong turns, save you time and money, and ensure that your loved one receives the appropriate care.

**Getting a professional care assessment up front is one of the strongest recommendations Gilbert Guide can make. The average cost of an assessment runs between $300-$700. Care managers usually charge by the hour, and the cost of an individual assessment depends on the amount of time it takes to conduct.**

### CASE MANAGERS

*What They Do*

Case managers, usually found through social service agencies or community organizations, are professional advocates for those who require care. While geriatric care managers serve the elderly and their families, case managers serve a population that is usually defined by disability rather than age. Trained in any number of fields related to long-term care, a case manager acts as a guide, primarily identifying problems and offering solutions.

*What to Expect*

Case managers begin the process by conducting a comprehensive care assessment of the individual to determine his or her needs. Case managers often work with other long-term care professionals to coordinate as few or as many services as are necessary to meet the specific needs of your loved one. The services a case manager provides include screening, arranging and monitoring the services your loved one requires; preserving financial resources by helping you avoid inappropriate placements and duplicated services; intervening in a crisis; counseling and supporting; educating and advocating; and much more. The case manager will continue to monitor care on an ongoing basis and will modify the care plan when appropriate.

Individuals who meet eligibility requirements may qualify for free case management services through federal, state or county programs such as Medicaid. Low-cost case management can sometimes be arranged through hospitals, mental health programs, home health agencies, social service agencies and other health-related programs.

*Our Standards and Criteria*

The case managers recommended by Gilbert Guide are pre-screened through the agencies that employ them. You will find these agencies listed in Helpful Organizations.

### GERIATRIC CARE MANAGERS (GCM)

*What They Do*

A GCM is a professional advocate who helps your loved one and you lead the highest possible quality of life. Trained in any of a number of fields related to long-term care, the GCM acts as your guide, primarily identifying problems and offering solutions.

*What to Expect*

GCMs begin the process by conducting a comprehensive care assessment of the older individual to determine his or her needs. GCMs often work with other long-term care professionals to coordinate as few or as many services as are necessary to meet the specific needs of your loved one. The services a GCM provides include screening, arranging and monitoring the services your loved one requires; preserving financial resources by helping you avoid inappropriate placements and duplicated services; intervening in a crisis; counseling and supporting; educating and advocating; and much more. The GCM will continue to monitor care on an ongoing basis and will modify the care plan when appropriate.

*Our Standards and Criteria*

Many of the GCMs recommended by Gilbert Guide are members of the National Association of Professional Geriatric Care Managers—the most widely recognized and respected organization of professional GCMs. The national association sets high standards of practice for its members, some of which are outlined below. A complete list of practice standards can be found at **www.caremanager.org.** Every GCM recommended by Gilbert Guide, regardless of membership status, follows these standards:

- Has at least a bachelor's degree in a field related to long-term care, which may include social work, counseling, nursing or gerontology. Many have specialized advanced degrees.
- Has a minimum of 2 years of experience as a professional GCM.
- Recognizes the older individual as the primary client, but acknowledges a larger "client system," which may include family members or other informal caregivers.
- Respects the client's right to privacy, as well as the client system's right to privacy.
- Clearly defines confidentiality limitations.
- Has a working knowledge of employment practice laws.
- Practices within his or her personal knowledge and capabilities when accepting fiduciary responsibilities for the client.
- Participates in continuing education programs to enhance professional growth.
- Discusses all fees for care management services, with the individual responsible for payment, before the services are rendered.
- Provides full disclosure regarding business, professional or personal relationships with any recommended business, agency or institution.

Every GCM listed in this guide performs these services:

- Conducts a comprehensive client assessment, evaluating the individual's levels of functioning, as well as health, emotional, financial and legal needs.
- Performs a home safety check, makes recommendations and orchestrates the necessary changes.
- Screens, arranges and monitors in-home care.
- Assists with client's financial and legal issues.
- Offers cost-effective solutions to client needs.
- Is available for emergencies.
- Works with doctors and other health care professionals to implement the care plan.
- Makes home visits and provides telephone reassurance to client.
- Provides regular updates to family members and involved health care professionals.
- Acts as a liaison for families who live remotely.
- Recommends, arranges and facilitates activities that promote increased socialization and/or intellectual stimulation.
- Prepares the home when a client returns from a hospital stay.
- Evaluates alternative living arrangements.

## IN-HOME CARE/PAS

*What It Is*

In-home care is non-medical care provided in the client's home. It includes custodial care and assistance with activities of daily living such as eating, bathing and providing medication reminders. In-home care workers are professionally trained caregivers who provide companionship and are responsible for maintaining a safe environment for the person receiving care. In Texas, in-home care is referred to as PAS (personal assistance service) and in-home care agencies are licensed as such.

There are three sources for obtaining in-home care: full-service agencies, referral agencies and private hire caregivers.

### IN-HOME CARE AGENCIES

*What to Expect*

In-home care can be arranged without a physician's order. In-home care is different from home health care, in that caregivers do not provide nursing care—for example, while they may provide medication reminders, they are not allowed to administer medication. Neither are caregivers housecleaners; although some light housekeeping may be necessary and appropriate, heavy housecleaning is normally not expected. In-home caregivers may provide care within a facility setting; check with the agency you have chosen to verify whether it offers this service.

*Our Standards and Criteria*

Many of the in-home care agencies Gilbert Guide recommends are members of the National Private Duty Association (NPDA), an organization whose standards of practice are highly regarded within the industry. A complete list of practice standards can be found at **www.privatedutyhomecare.org.** Each of the in-home care agencies listed in Gilbert Guide implements the following standards regarding all caregivers:

- Conducts a criminal background check
- Provides worker's compensation insurance
- Maintains professional liability insurance or bond
- Covers all payroll taxes
- Provides ongoing supervision
- Provides caregiver training

The NPDA is a fairly new organization, and while Gilbert Guide recognizes its potential to be a leading force in the industry, we also recognize that as the organization continues to build its membership, many reputable in-home care agencies are not currently members.

# Categories of Care

Every caregiver employed by an in-home care agency listed in this guide performs the following duties:

- Conducts a care assessment and creates a care plan
- Assists clients in bathing, grooming, dressing and using the toilet
- Provides transportation
- Tracks medication and provides reminders
- Prepares meals
- Performs light housekeeping tasks
- Provides laundry service
- Runs errands and does grocery shopping
- Helps with bill paying and record keeping

## REFERRAL AGENCIES

*What to Expect*

These agencies refer caregivers to the client, but they are not considered the caregiver's employer. Once the referral has been made, the relationship ends. The client becomes the employer and is responsible for scheduling, training, supervising and paying the caregiver directly. Caregivers who are referred for employment by a referral agency are not independent contractors; therefore, the client is also responsible for payroll taxes and carrying worker's compensation insurance.

*Why We Don't List Referral Agencies*

The guidelines for caregivers who are referred through an agency are set by the individual agencies and are not standardized, thus making it impossible to assess the quality of care except on a caregiver-by-caregiver basis. In addition, there is no ongoing relationship between caregivers and the referral agencies—it is simply an issue of placement—thus, it is the client who assumes the responsibilities associated with the employer-employee relationship. Gilbert Guide therefore provides listings only of reputable agencies that screen, train, supervise and employ their caregivers.

## PRIVATE HIRE CAREGIVERS

*What to Expect*

Caregivers who do not work through an agency are known as "private hire" caregivers. The client is the employer and is responsible for paying the caregiver directly. The client is also responsible for meeting all federal and state payroll requirements, carrying worker's compensation insurance, screening, supervising, training and assuming all professional liabilities associated with an employer-employee relationship.

*Why We Don't List Private Hire Caregivers*

There are no standardized guidelines for private hire caregivers, thus making it impossible to assess the quality of care except on a caregiver-by-caregiver basis. Gilbert Guide therefore provides listings only of reputable agencies—not individuals—that screen, train, supervise and employ their caregivers.

## HOME HEALTH CARE

*What It Is*

Home health care agencies provide in-home skilled nursing and other health care services, such as physical and occupational therapy. Home health care agencies are licensed by the state, but must adhere to federal regulations as well.

*What to Expect*

Home health care must be prescribed by a physician. Registered Nurses (RNs), Licensed Practical Nurses (LPNs) and Licensed Vocational Nurses (LVNs) provide the care, sometimes in conjunction with other health professionals. These providers may also enlist the assistance of a home health aide who can help with personal care such as bathing and using the toilet. Home health aides can also administer medication under the supervision of a nurse.

*Why We Don't List Home Health Agencies*

Gilbert Guide does not list home health care agencies because the physicians who prescribe home health care usually have established relationships with the providers, and it is simply a matter of placement. It is generally not a matter of choice for the patient.

## ADULT DAY CARE (ADC)

*What It Is*

Adult day care provides a safe and caring setting for adults. Adult day facilities are licensed by the Texas Department of Social Services. Programs are structured and designed, often through the development of a personal care plan, to cover the daily individual needs of each participant, including a variety of social and supportive services. Participants may be physically, mentally, or functionally impaired, or they may simply need companionship or supervision during part of the day.

*What to Expect*

Adult day care is based primarily around participants' social needs. Most programs offer meals and some provide transportation. A variety of activities are offered with the purpose of providing stimulation and socialization for participants. The programming often includes mentally stimulating activities such as word association, trivia questions and crossword puzzles; physically stimulating activities include exercise and dance.

*Our Standards and Criteria*

Gilbert Guide evaluates adult day care facilities on several criteria. First, we inspect the quality of the programs, making sure activities are suited to the participants' needs, interests and personal levels of functioning. We also consider the quality of the staff, including the care provided and interaction with participants. Finally, we evaluate the facilities on appearance and cleanliness. The facilities listed in Gilbert Guide reflect the highest level of quality in each of these areas. In addition to these criteria, we also make observations about the following:

- Staff-to-client ratio
- Administration and staff friendliness
- Activities and services provided
- Staff engagement and interaction with participants
- Staff response to participants' needs
- Clients' participation in activities and interaction with others
- Facility condition and smell
- Facility aesthetics
- Overall ambience
- Food and dietary needs addressed
- Family involvement in care plan

---

## ADULT DAY HEALTH CARE (ADHC)

*What It Is*

Like adult day care, adult day health care provides a safe, caring setting for adults who require supervision or care during the day; these facilities are also licensed by the Texas Department of Social Services. Adult day health programs are designed for individuals who require some health care. These programs offer medical services, such as rehabilitation, therapy, nursing care and special nutrition. The programs are structured and designed, often through the development of a personal care plan, to cover the daily individual needs of each participant.

*What to Expect*

Adult day health care is primarily based on participants' health care needs. Most programs offer meals and some provide transportation. The activities and programming reflect the diverse needs of participants and their levels of functioning. Common activities include current events classes, arts and crafts, music, mind-stimulating games, and exercise, as appropriate to each individual.

*Our Standards and Criteria*

Gilbert Guide evaluates adult day care facilities based on several criteria. First, we inspect the quality of the programs, making sure the scheduled activities are suited to participants' needs, interests and personal levels of functioning. We also consider the quality of the staff, including the care provided and interaction with participants. Finally, we evaluate the facilities on appearance and cleanliness. The facilities listed in Gilbert Guide reflect the highest level of quality in each of these areas. In addition to these criteria, we also make observations about the following:

- Staff-to-client ratio
- Administration and staff friendliness
- Activities and services provided
- Staff engagement and interaction with participants
- Staff response to participants' needs
- Clients' participation in activities and interaction with others
- Facility condition and smell
- Facility aesthetics
- Overall ambience
- Food and dietary needs addressed
- Family involvement in care plan

## CONTINUING CARE RETIREMENT COMMUNITIES (CCRCs)

### *What They Are*

A CCRC, also referred to as a *life-care community*, combines residential accommodations with health services. The purpose of a CCRC is to allow residents to receive the appropriate care across a continuum, from independent living to assisted living and skilled nursing care, as their needs change, without having to leave the community. This ensures that residents will be cared for through end-of-life.

### *What to Expect*

CCRCs usually charge residents an entrance fee as well as a monthly payment. The entrance fee may include the cost of purchasing a unit, or it may be a one-time fee in order to join the community. The CCRC provides housing and defined long-term care services for the life of the resident. Residents may select different options, which are noted in their contracts.

### *Our Standards and Criteria*

CCRCs, because of their dual nature, are evaluated using the same criteria that we use for assisted living facilities, as well as the criteria we use to evaluate skilled nursing facilities. Please refer to the Assisted Living Facilities and Skilled Nursing Facilities sections below for a definitive list of our standards and criteria.

## ASSISTED LIVING FACILITIES

*What They Are*

Assisted living is a general term used to describe residential facilities that provide care for individuals who cannot live independently, but do not require twenty-four hour skilled nursing care. These facilities are licensed and inspected by the Texas Department of Social Services and they must meet care and safety standards set by the state. Assisted living typically serves individuals age sixty and older, although younger persons with similar needs may be served as well. Some assisted living facilities offer Alzheimer's and dementia care. The facilities that specialize in Alzheimer's and dementia care are denoted by A/D.

There are two types of assisted living facilities:

LARGE-SCALE ASSISTED LIVING FACILITIES may have both shared and private rooms, as well as private apartments.

BOARD AND CARE HOMES are smaller-scale assisted living facilities, housed in a private residential home setting. They typically do not offer Alzheimer's or dementia care.

*What to Expect*

Assisted living facilities provide room and board, some housekeeping, social activities, supervision and assistance with basic activities like personal hygiene, dressing, eating and walking. Facility staff either provides or arranges transportation for residents. Most facilities offer three meals per day, as well as snacks in between meals.

Assisted living facilities are considered non-medical facilities and are not required to have nurses, certified nursing assistants or doctors on staff, although many of the facilities listed in Gilbert Guide do have medical staff either on-site or on call. Medications can be stored and distributed for residents to self-administer.

Assisted living staff members who provide hands-on care must have criminal record clearance.

*Our Standards and Criteria*

Gilbert Guide reviews facilities with capacities of fourteen persons or more. Following are some of the areas that we observe in our evaluation of each facility:

- Facility Aesthetics
  *Parking availability*
  *Neighborhood safety and appearance*
  *Exterior appearance*
  *Interior entrance appearance*
  *Appearance of residents' rooms/apartments*

*Appearance of dining area(s)*
*Appearance of common areas*
*Appearance of outdoor gardens/patios*
*Overall facility ambience*

- Facility Condition & Safety
  *State of repair*
  *Clear signage*
  *Hallways clear of obstacles*
  *Adequate lighting*
  *Overall temperature*
  *Odor throughout facility*
  *Odor throughout residents' rooms/apartments*
  *Overall state of cleanliness*

- Administration & Staff
  *Appearance*
  *Camaraderie*
  *Interaction with residents*
  *Familiarity with residents*
  *Willingness to help residents*
  *Friendliness and attitude toward residents*
  *Attitude toward families*
  *Ongoing training*
  *Turnover*

- Residents
  *Overall appearance and hygiene*
  *Overall energy level and mood*
  *Interaction with one another*

- Dietary & Food Selection
  *Menu variety*
  *Food availability and snacks provided*
  *Meal presentation*

- Activities
  *Creative variety of activities and field trips scheduled*
  *Appropriate for residents' interests and abilities*
  *Staff encouragement of residents' participation*
  *Residents' participation in activities*
  *Transportation provided for shopping and appointments*

- Alzheimer's & Dementia Capabilities
  *Proper lighting (bright, even and warm)*
  *Proper carpet and flooring (no busy patterns)*
  *Specialized activities that reflect residents' routines and skills*
  *Structured routine for residents*
  *Locked facility and proper security provided to prevent wandering*
  *Specialized staff training for dementia*
  *Residents' participation in activities*
  *Staff encouragement of residents' participation*
  *Staff-to-resident ratio*

---

## SKILLED NURSING FACILITIES (SNFs)

*What They Are*

Skilled nursing facilities, or SNFs (pronounced "sniffs"), are also known as *nursing homes* or *convalescent homes*. SNFs are live-in facilities, licensed and regulated by the Texas Department of Health Services, that provide medical treatment prescribed by a physician. These facilities cater to several types of patients: some patients require short-term rehab while recovering from surgery; others require long-term skilled nursing and medical supervision. In addition, some SNFs offer specialized care programs for Alzheimer's or other illnesses, or short-term respite care for frail or disabled persons when a family member requires a rest from providing care in the home. The facilities that specialize in Alzheimer's and dementia care are denoted by **A/D**.

*What to Expect*

SNFs provide twenty-four hour skilled nursing care; rehabilitation services such as physical, speech and occupational therapy; assistance with personal care activities such as eating, walking, bathing and using the toilet; coordinated management of patient care; social services; and activities.

*Our Standards and Criteria*

Gilbert Guide reviews only standalone SNFs—many hospitals have SNF wings, but those facilities generally only accept patients who have been discharged directly from that particular hospital.

Two other factors we consider are deficiencies and citations. SNFs are inspected at least every twelve to fifteen months. When a SNF fails to meet state and federal minimum standards for care, a deficiency is issued. A citation is issued when a SNF is fined for noncompliance with the state minimum standards. There are different levels of deficiencies—ranging from minor, which do not pose harm to residents, to major, which poses or causes harm to residents. It is important to keep in mind that most facilities receive some deficiencies and/or citations. Because of this, while Gilbert Guide has considered these in making our evaluations, they were not the sole basis of our determinations.

Following are some of the additional areas we observe in our evaluation of each facility:

- Facility Aesthetics
  *Parking availability*
  *Neighborhood safety and appearance*
  *Exterior appearance*
  *Interior entrance appearance*
  *Appearance of residents' rooms*
  *Appearance of dining area(s)*
  *Adequate seating in halls and common areas*
  *Appearance of outdoor gardens/patios*
  *Overall facility ambience*

- Facility Condition & Safety
  *State of repair*
  *Flooring condition*
  *Clear signage*
  *Hallways clear of obstacles*
  *Adequate lighting*
  *Overall temperature*
  *Odor throughout facility*
  *Odor throughout residents' rooms/apartments*
  *Overall state of cleanliness*
  *Condition of mobility aids, such as walkers and wheelchairs*

- Administration & Staff
  *Appearance*
  *Camaraderie*
  *Interaction with residents*
  *Familiarity with residents*
  *Attentiveness to residents*
  *Friendliness and attitude toward residents*
  *Attitude toward families*
  *Ongoing training*
  *Turnover*

- Residents
  *Overall appearance and hygiene*
  *Overall energy level and mood*
  *Interaction with staff and one another*

- Activities
  *Creative variety of activities scheduled*
  *Activities appropriate for residents' interests and abilities*
  *Staff encouragement of residents' participation*
  *Residents' participation in activities*

- Dietary & Food Selection
  *Menu variety*
  *Food availability and snacks provided*
  *Meal presentation*

- Access to Medical Care
  *Proximity to emergency care*
  *Transportation provided to off-site medical care*

- Alzheimer's & Dementia Capabilities
  *Proper lighting (bright, even and warm)*
  *Proper carpet and flooring (no busy patterns)*
  *Specialized activities that reflect residents' routines and skills*
  *Structured routine for residents*
  *Locked facility and proper security provided to prevent wandering*
  *Specialized staff training for dementia*
  *Residents' participation in activities*
  *Staff encouragement of residents' participation*
  *Staff-to-resident ratio*

## ADVANCE CARE PLANNING, PALLIATIVE AND HOSPICE CARE

Advance care planning is an essential step in making care decisions for yourself. The sections below describe how to take this step.

Understanding the difference between hospice and palliative care can be confusing. Basically, hospice is a form of palliative care that is offered in the last months of a person's life. However, unlike hospice, palliative care is not limited to care at the end of life; it can actually be provided to a person that has years to live.

The National Hospice and Palliative Care Organization (NHPCO) is the largest nonprofit membership organization representing hospice and palliative care programs and professionals in the U.S. A wealth of information can be found at **www.nhpco.org**.

## ADVANCE CARE PLANNING

### *What It Is*

Advance care planning means making decisions about the care you would want to receive should you become unable to speak for yourself. These are your decisions to make, and they are based on your personal values and preferences.

### *What is Involved*

Advance care planning involves communicating your wishes to loved ones and health care providers to guide and comfort them if something should happen to you. Establishing advance directives is an important part of advance care planning. Advance directives are legal documents that offer directions for your health care should you become unable to speak for yourself. A living will, one type of advance directive, provides directions to health care providers on the treatment you want (and do not want) if you are faced with an end-of-life situation. A health care power of attorney or durable power of attorney is another type of advance directive that appoints a person of your choice to speak on your behalf, should you become unable to do so.

State-specific advance directives, brochures about advance directives and other information about advance care planning can be found at **www.nhpco.org.**

## PALLIATIVE CARE

### *What It Is*

To *palliate* means to ease discomfort by treating the symptoms of an illness. Palliative care promotes the patient's comfort by addressing any issues causing physical or emotional pain or suffering. A team of people work together to provide palliative care, with the common goals of improving the quality of a life for the person who is seriously ill and supporting that person's loved ones.

### *What to Expect*

Palliative care may be provided by your physician or a team that might include a physician, a nurse, a social worker or other health care professional. Palliative care may include a monthly visit to your physician, or it may includeweekly home visits from a nurse and a social worker to and help manage your symptoms.

Unlike hospice, there is not a package benefit for palliative care, so it is important to determine what services are offered and who is responsible for the payment of those services.

## HOSPICE

### *What It Is*

Also known as end-of-life care, hospice is palliative care designed to help the patient through the last stages of a terminal illness. The goal is to keep pain and suffering to a minimum, not to cure the illness—by this point, the patient's doctor has determined that the patient can no longer benefit from regular medical treatment. Although hospice care is usually administered in the patient's residence, it can also take place in a hospice facility. When necessary, hospice services can be called into assisted living facilities and SNFs, as long as those facilities carry a hospice waiver.

### *What to Expect*

Hospice agencies provide many services, some of which include: nursing; physical, occupational and speech therapies; medical social services; home health aide assistance; medical supplies and appliances; drugs for symptom control and pain relief; physician services; psychological, spiritual, and nutritional counseling; group and bereavement counseling; caregiver support groups; and grief support.

### *Our Standards and Criteria*

In addition to providing the services listed above, every hospice agency we list meets the following standards:

- Licensed by the Texas Department of Health Services
- Medicare certified
- Caregivers are trained, supervised and monitored
- On-call supervisor 24 hours/day

## GILBERT GUIDE SYMBOLS AND RATINGS

Assisted living facilities and SNFs that specialize in Alzheimer's and dementia care are denoted by A/D.

Additional costs are denoted by ($).

Within a few of the facility listings you will find some shorthand symbols. This is what they denote:

(AL) Assisted Living
(ALZ) Alzheimer's
(IND) Independent Living
(SNF) Skilled Nursing

Within each facility listing, you will find ratings on our standards and criteria. Here is how it breaks down:

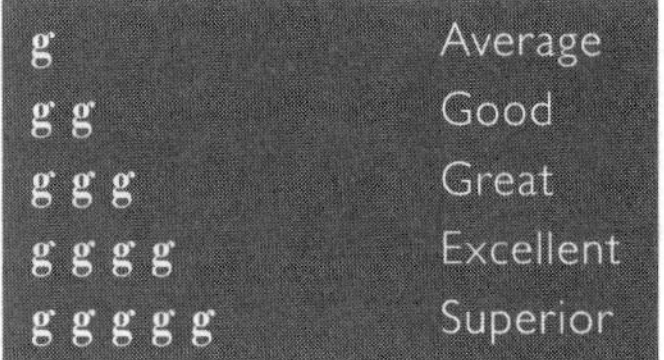

| | |
|---|---|
| g | Average |
| g g | Good |
| g g g | Great |
| g g g g | Excellent |
| g g g g g | Superior |

# WHO PAYS FOR WHAT?

- Planning and Financing Long-term Care
- Types of Coverage
- What's Covered
- Coverage At-a-Glance

## PLANNING AND FINANCING LONG-TERM CARE

Planning for long-term care is complicated. Each person's needs are unique; therefore, the cost of long-term care varies greatly. Some social and physical assistance is available for free or at a low cost, while very expensive nursing home or home health services can cost upwards of $200 per day.

There are many different ways to finance long-term care. You will probably need to use a combination of payment sources, which may include Medicare, Medicaid, long-term care insurance and other programs, in addition to your own resources.

It is essential to consult a professional such as an elder law attorney, financial planner or an accountant when planning for long-term care; this person should be well-versed in estate planning, public programs like Medicaid, and the issues and needs of older persons. These long-term care professionals often work as a team. Gilbert Guide recommends getting a second opinion before making any final decision on financial matters.

### TYPES OF COVERAGE

#### MEDICARE

Medicare is the federally administered health insurance program for people sixty-five years of age and older, certain disabled people under sixty-five years of age, and people with end-stage renal disease. Medicare is divided into two parts, known simply as Part A and Part B. The benefits associated with Part A are automatic once an individual turns sixty-five. Part B requires a monthly premium.

Part A—Hospital Insurance

- *Inpatient hospital care*
- *SNF care*
- *Hospice care*
- *Home health care (with certain restrictions)*

Part B—Medical Insurance

- *Doctors*
- *Services*
- *Outpatient hospital care*
- *Durable medical equipment, such as wheelchairs and hospital beds*
- *Additional medical services not covered by Part A*

*Eligibility and Qualifications*

Medicare is provided when Social Security benefits begin, unless the individual is under sixty-five years of age and disabled or has end-stage renal disease, in which case it is provided at that time.

### MEDIGAP

Medigap, also known as Medicare Supplemental Insurance, is a health insurance policy sold by private insurance companies that fills the gaps that Medicare fails to cover, such as coinsurance, co-payments and deductibles. There are ten distinct Medigap policies. All ten are regulated by the federal and state governments.

Medigap covers the following, depending on the policy:

- SNF stays
- Blood (first 3 pints annually)
- Medicare Part A coinsurance and hospital benefits
- Medicare Part B annual deductible
- Medicare Part B co-payments
- Excess doctor charges
- Foreign travel emergencies
- Routine checkups
- At-home recovery

Medigap coverage is renewed annually and requires a monthly premium. There are several important considerations when shopping for Medigap. First, a number of insurance companies offer policies with identical benefits, but at different rates. Second, not every company offers all ten policies. Finally, the policies themselves differ in coverage. Make sure you carefully consider which is the best policy for your needs—if you are married, you and your spouse must purchase separate policies.

*Eligibility and Qualifications*

- Must be a recipient of both Medicare Part A and Medicare Part B
- Cannot be a Medicaid recipient

### MANAGED CARE (HMO)

Managed care policies were originally designed to provide all the medical services and supplies offered by Medicare, plus additional benefits such as prescription drug, vision and hearing coverage, as well as enhanced SNF coverage. However, few insurance companies still provide these types of policies. Most policies require individuals to sign over their Medicare benefits and pay a monthly premium in return for full coverage by the HMO's doctors, hospitals and services.

There is a yearly out-of-pocket limit with Managed Care. Once you reach that limit, the HMO is financially responsible for all services except prescription drug co-payments and durable medical equipment.

NOTE: *HMO insurance companies only guarantee the policy for a year at a time. Each year, the insurance company decides whether or not to continue offering the policy. If the company opts to discontinue it, it is required to notify the policyholder ninety days before coverage ends and to provide information about purchasing a Medigap policy in the policyholder's area. Most people who already have Medigap coverage do not need to purchase a Managed Care policy.*

*Eligibility and Qualifications*

Coverage is available to:

- Individuals 65 years of age or older
- Individuals entitled to Medicare Part A and enrolled in Medicare Part B
- Individuals who reside at home or in an assisted living facility
- Individuals who reside in the insurance company's service area

Coverage not available to:

- Individuals with end-stage renal disease
- Individuals who reside in an institutional setting such as a SNF

**MEDICAID**

Medicaid is a federally aided, state-operated program that provides medical benefits for certain low-income individuals who have few resources. Medicaid is administered by the county.

Medicaid is not tied to Social Security benefits. The program provides 100% coverage of most medical expenses and does not require payment of premiums or deductibles. In addition, health care providers who accept Medicaid cannot bill for any additional charges (as they can with Medicare).

*Eligibility and Qualifications*

Medicaid qualifications vary from state to state. *Medicaid Asset Limitations* are based on whether the individual is single, or married with an at-home spouse. Meeting these limitations is the most difficult criteria when applying for Medicaid.

Single, unmarried individuals cannot have *countable assets** that exceed a certain amount. Additionally, those individuals cannot have an income that exceeds a specified amount per month. Similarly, married persons with an at-home spouse cannot have *combined* countable assets* that exceed a certain amount per month. However, the Medicaid applicant is allowed to keep a specified amount of income per month. Please refer to the Medicaid website at www.cms.hhs.gov for the current limitations.

*Countable Assets are defined as:

- Checking accounts, savings accounts and CDs
- Investment accounts, including mutual funds, stock and bonds
- Credit union accounts
- Certain life insurance policies, based on amount of face value

- Annuities that have not annuitized (beneficiary not yet receiving payments)
- Automobiles, if more than one is currently registered
- Second homes and non-business properties
- Revocable trust accounts
- Promissory notes

Exempt Assets are defined as:

- Primary residence, if applicant is married with an at-home spouse, or if applicant intends to return to home
- Property used in business or trade
- Pre-need burial expenses
- Certain life insurance policies, based on amount of face value
- IRAs
- Pensions
- Annuities, if the beneficiary is receiving payments

**LONG-TERM CARE INSURANCE (LTCI)**

Private insurance companies sell LTCI policies to offset the costs of long-term care. LTCI, like all insurance policies, requires premiums to help recipients avoid paying large sums later on in the event of an illness or a catastrophic event. Premiums are based on the individual's age at the time of purchase and are usually locked in for the life of the policy.

LTCI covers the following, depending on the policy you choose:

- SNF care
- Care in an assisted living facility
- Home health care
- Adult day health care

Buying a LTCI policy allows the policyholder to choose from many options, such as the amount of the daily benefit, the number of years the policy will pay benefits, and, after the applicant qualifies for a policy, the number of days or months before the policy will begin paying benefits.

It's very important to evaluate policies carefully to see which one offers the benefits you require with a premium that fits your budget. Policies differ in their benefits, contract conditions, deductibles and premiums. It is also important to take into account the rising cost of health care. Be sure the LTCI policy provides inflation protection for benefits to increase as health care costs continue to rise.

Policies are generally labeled according to the place in which benefits are paid.

- HOMECARE ONLY policies pay for care at home and in an adult day care or adult day health care facility—make sure the policy includes both types of day care.

- FACILITY ONLY policies pay for care in a SNF and in an assisted living facility.
- COMPREHENSIVE policies pay for care in a SNF, assisted living facility, adult day care or adult day health care facility, and at home.

Since LTCI claims are often paid many years after the purchase of the policy, it is imperative to check the following:

- Financial strength of the company. The industry's major rating services are A.M. Best, (**www.ambest.com**), Duff and Phelps (**www.dufflc.com**), Moody's (**www.moodys.com**), Standard and Poor's (**www.standardandpoors.com**) and Weiss Ratings (**www.weissratings.com**).
- Reputation and claims-paying history of the company.

Call the Texas Department of Insurance at (800) 252-3439 for information on specific private insurance companies.

*Eligibility and Qualifications*

- Applicant must be healthy at the time of application
- Each insurance company has individual requirements and/or limitations

### VETERANS BENEFITS

The Department of Veterans Affairs (VA) offers a benefits package that provides hospital and outpatient medical care and treatment. VA's priority system ensures that veterans with service-connected disabilities and those below the low-income threshold are granted top priority for receiving care. There is no monthly premium required for VA care. However, depending on the veteran's situation, co-payments may be required.

The Uniform Benefits Package available to all enrolled veterans includes:

- Inpatient hospital care
- Ambulatory care
- Emergency care in a VA facility
- Home health care
- Respite care
- Hospice care
- Prescription drugs, pharmaceuticals and durable medical equipment, such as wheelchairs and hospital beds
- Adult day health care

Although many veterans qualify for free health care services based on a compensable service-connected condition or other qualifying factor, most are required to complete an annual financial assessment to determine if they qualify for free services. Veterans whose household income and net worth exceed the established threshold must agree to co-payments to become eligible for VA health care services. The financial assessment determines the enrollment priority group and the co-payments, if any, that apply.

Call VA Health Care at (877) 222-VETS or visit the VA website at www.va.gov for more information.

*Eligibility and Qualifications*

- Veteran must be enrolled in the VA health care system
- Most veterans required to report household income and net worth annually

## WHAT'S COVERED

### SKILLED NURSING FACILITIES

#### MEDICARE

*What It Covers*

- First 20 days in a Medicare-approved SNF
- Days 21–100: Medicare beneficiary pays a specified amount per day; Medicare pays balance of covered charges**
- Doctors' visits
- Nursing care
- Semi-private room rates
- All meals (including special diets)
- Physical, occupational and speech therapies
- Lab and X-ray services
- Prosthetic devices
- Prescription drugs
- Some medical supplies and equipment

*Conditions and Limitations*

There are strict limitations to Medicare coverage in SNFs.

- Beneficiary must be in hospital for 3 consecutive days, not counting day of discharge
- Must be admitted to SNF within 30 days of hospital discharge
- Services must be related to condition that was treated in hospital
- Must require daily skilled nursing or rehabilitation services
- Must be determined that services can only be provided on an inpatient basis
- Doctor must specify need for daily skilled care services; and
- Doctor must re-certify need 14 days after admission and every 30 days thereafter
- Medicare must review and approve continued need for skilled care services
- SNF stay must be 100 days or less; and
- Medicare must approve the length of stay (100 days are not automatically granted)

After Medicare coverage stops, your options are LTCI, Medicaid and/or Private Payment.

**MEDIGAP**

*What It Covers*

Eight of the ten Medigap policies cover days 21–100 skilled nursing coinsurance.

**MANAGED CARE**

*What It Covers*

Managed Care policies cover everything that Medicare covers (see Medicare section above), The co-payment, however, for days 21–100, is about half the cost. In addition, no prior hospital stay is required.

*Conditions and Limitations*

- SNF must be Medicare-certified; and
- Resident must get authorization from the insurance company for services

**MEDICAID**

*What It Covers*

- All costs of skilled nursing services and medical equipment that a doctor deems necessary
- To hold a bed for 15 days if a resident requires temporary hospital care
- For leaves of absence of up to 18 days per year for visits with family or friends

**LTCI**

*What It Covers*

Facility Only and Comprehensive policies pay benefits in a SNF, but the amount of coverage depends on the individual policy.

**VETERANS BENEFITS**

*What It Covers*

VA provides skilled nursing care to eligible veterans through VA SNFs and *Community Contract* SNFs. Veterans who do not meet the conditions and limitations outlined below may still be eligible for care in a SNF, when space and resources are available.

*Conditions and Limitations*

- Veteran must meet the eligibility criteria for VA benefits, and
- Require skilled nursing care for a service-connected condition; or
- Have a service-connected disability rating of 70% or more; or
- Have a service-connected disability rating of 60% and be considered unemployable
- SNF care for non-service connected veterans is limited to six months

## HOME HEALTH AND IN-HOME CARE

### MEDICARE

*What It Covers*

Medicare is the principal provider of home health care in the U.S. Medicare covers a substantial part of home health care.

Your doctor must prescribe the following services and equipment for coverage:

- Part-time or intermittent nursing care provided by or under the supervision of an RN; up to 35 hours per week combined skilled nursing and home health aide services
- Physical, occupational and speech therapies
- Medical social services as directed by a physician
- Home health aides providing personal care services (must be administered at the same time as skilled services)
- Prescribed medical supplies
- Durable medical equipment, such as wheelchairs, hospital beds and oxygen pumps (covered at 80% of the Medicare-approved amount)

*Conditions and Limitations*

- Physician must determine need for home health care and prescribe care plan
- Beneficiary must be homebound
- Beneficiary must require intermittent skilled nursing care, physical, occupational or speech therapies
- Services must be received from a Medicare-certified home health agency

Medicare does not cover in-home care.

### MEDIGAP

*What It Covers*

Four Medigap policies have a benefit that covers home health and in-home care. The coverage varies according to the policy you choose. The benefits may include assistance with daily living activities such as bathing, grooming, medication monitoring, meal preparation, light housekeeping, laundry, errands, grocery shopping and transportation.

*Conditions and Limitations*

In order to be eligible for these benefits, the individual must currently be receiving Medicare-covered skilled home health care.

### MANAGED CARE

*What It Covers*

Utilizing its own network of doctors, hospitals and services, Managed Care policies cover everything that Medicare covers (see Medicare section above), in terms of home health care. You must get authorization from the insurance company before receiving services.

Managed Care policies do not cover in-home care.

**MEDICAID**

*What It Covers*

Medicaid pays for all skilled nursing services at home, including medical equipment that a doctor deems necessary, as long as it is less expensive than living in a SNF.

Medicaid does not cover in-home care.

**LTCI**

*What It Covers*

Homecare Only and Comprehensive policies pay home health care and in-home care benefits, but the amount of coverage depends on the individual policy.

*Conditions and Limitations*

Policies differ on conditions required to qualify for home health care and in-home care benefits. Each policy has a cap on the number of visits. Older policies require a prior hospital stay or time in a SNF; the newer policies require that beneficiaries be physically or cognitively impaired.

**VETERANS BENEFITS**

*What It Covers*

Home health care is provided by the VA or through contract agencies to veterans with chronic conditions. The services include skilled nursing, physical and occupational therapies and social services.

Veterans Benefits do not cover in-home care.

*Conditions and Limitations*

- Veteran must meet eligibility criteria for VA benefits, and
- Be homebound, and
- Demonstrate need for home health care

## ASSISTED LIVING FACILITIES

**MEDICARE, MEDIGAP, MANAGED CARE, MEDICAID**

Medicare, Medigap, Managed Care and Medicaid do not cover care in assisted living facilities.

**LTCI**

*What It Covers*

Facility Only and Comprehensive policies pay benefits in an assisted living facility, but the amount of coverage depends on the individual policy.

#### VETERANS BENEFITS

*What It Covers*

Veterans Benefits refers to care in an assisted living facility as *Community Residential Care.* The program provides health care supervision to eligible veterans who are unable to live independently and do not have anyone to provide the required supervision and care. The veteran must be able to function with minimal assistance.

*Conditions and Limitations*

- Veteran must meet eligibility criteria for VA benefits, and
- Demonstrate need for this type of care

### ADULT DAY CARE

Adult day care services are usually a private-pay option. However, some day care centers offer need-based scholarships and others have a sliding scale.

#### MEDICARE, MEDIGAP, MANAGED CARE, MEDICAID, VETERANS BENEFITS

Medicare, Medigap, Managed Care, Medicaid and Veterans Benefits do not cover adult day care.

#### LTCI

*What It Covers*

Homecare Only and Comprehensive policies pay benefits in an adult day care facility, but the amount of coverage depends on the individual policy.

### ADULT DAY HEALTH CARE

Adult day health care centers provide many health and social services for a set daily fee. Many centers have sliding scales.

#### MEDICARE, MEDIGAP, MANAGED CARE

Medicare, Medigap, and Managed Care do not cover care adult day health care.

#### MEDICAID

*What It Covers*

Medicaid usually covers all adult day health services.

*Conditions and Limitations*

In some instances, Medicaid approves coverage for fewer days per week than an individual requires. If, for example, Medicaid approves only three days per week, but the individual requires five days, then the individual is financially responsible for the two additional days of attendance.

#### LTCI

*What It Covers*

Homecare Only and Comprehensive policies pay benefits in an adult day health care facility, but the amount of coverage depends on the individual policy.

#### VETERANS BENEFITS

*What It Covers*

Veterans Benefits cover adult day health care services.

*Conditions and Limitations*

- Veteran must meet eligibility criteria for VA benefits, and
- Demonstrate need for this type of care

## GERIATRIC CARE MANAGER

#### MEDICARE, MEDIGAP, MANAGED CARE, MEDICAID, LTCI

Medicare, Medigap, Managed Care, Medicaid and LTCI do not cover geriatric care management.

#### VETERANS BENEFITS

*What It Covers*

While Veterans Benefits do not cover GCMs, they do cover *Geriatric Evaluation and Management* (GEM), a similar service that includes a comprehensive assessment of the veteran's physical, medical and emotional needs. The objective of the assessment is to build a customized plan of care that may include a combination of treatment, rehabilitation and social services.

*Conditions and Limitations*

The Veteran must meet the eligibility criteria for VA benefits.

## HOSPICE

#### MEDICARE

*What It Covers*

Medicare is the principal provider of hospice care in the U.S. Medicare Part A only pays for hospice care provided by a Medicare-certified program. All of the hospice agencies listed in Gilbert Guide are Medicare-certified.

There is usually a 210-day cap on Medicare-covered hospice care. The 210 days are split into two ninety-day periods, followed by a thirty-day period. Each period may be extended when a doctor recertifies that the patient's condition remains terminal. In some circumstances, coverage may be extended indefinitely.

Medicare pays for most hospice services, including:

- Nursing services
- Durable medical equipment, such as wheelchairs and walkers
- Medical supplies
- Prescribed drugs
- Short-term hospital care, including respite care
- Home health aide and housekeeping services
- Physical, occupational and speech therapies
- Social worker services
- Nutritional counseling
- Grief counseling for patient and family

*Conditions and Limitations*

- Doctor and hospice medical director must verify that the patient has a terminal illness and probably has less than six months to live; and
- Patient must sign a statement choosing hospice care instead of standard Medicare-covered benefits (Medicare will continue to cover health problems unrelated to terminal illness)

IMPORTANT NOTE: *Hospice agencies sometimes charge more than Medicare pays. In these instances, the patient is responsible for the balance. Before providing care, the hospice must advise the patient how much of the bill Medicare will pay and inform the patient, in writing, of any items or services not covered. The bill is sent directly to Medicare.*

The patient may be charged for:

- Treatments designed to cure a terminal illness
- Treatment or services not related to comfort care, and
- Room and board (except respite care)

### MEDIGAP

Medigap does not cover hospice care.

### MANAGED CARE

*What It Covers*

Managed Care policies cover everything that Medicare covers (see Medicare section above).

*Conditions and Limitations*

Most policies only cover hospice care and services provided by Medicare-certified hospice agencies that are designated by the individual insurance company.

**MEDICAID**

*What It Covers*

- RN visits for pain management and symptom control
- 24-hour on call RN
- Medical social work visits
- Certified home health aide visits
- Chaplain visits
- Trained volunteer visits for support, companionship and errands
- Bereavement support for 13 months following the death of a loved one
- Authorized medications
- Durable medical supplies and equipment
- Coordination of hospital or nursing home admissions
- Respite care (limited to a 5-day stay)
- Hospital inpatient admission for symptom control

*Conditions and Limitations*

Before Medicaid will approve coverage for hospice care, you must:

- Receive a doctor's certification that the individual has a terminal illness and probably has less than 6 months to live, and
- Sign a statement choosing hospice care instead of standard Medicare-covered benefits (Medicare will continue to cover health problems unrelated to terminal illness)

NOTE: *Medicaid only pays for hospice care provided by a Medicare-certified agency.*

**LTCI**

*What It Covers*

Homecare Only and Comprehensive policies usually cover costs of hospice care, while Facility Only policies generally do not.

*Conditions and Limitations*

Policies vary. Because of potential limitations on hospice care coverage, it is important to carefully compare policies when selecting long-term care insurance.

**VETERANS BENEFITS**

*What It Covers*

Veterans Benefits cover hospice care.

*Conditions and Limitations*

- Veteran must meet eligibility criteria for VA benefits; and
- Demonstrate need for this type of care

## COVERAGE AT-A-GLANCE

**TYPES OF COVERAGE**

| CATEGORIES OF CARE | MEDICARE | MEDIGAP | MANAGED CARE (HMO) | MEDICAID | LTCI | VETERANS |
|---|---|---|---|---|---|---|
| Skilled Nursing Facility | ● | ● | ● | ● | ● | ● |
| Home Health Care | ● | ● | ● | ● | ● | ● |
| Homecare | | ● | | | ● | |
| Assisted Living Facility | | | | | ● | ● |
| Adult Day Care | | | | | ● | |
| Adult Day Health Care | | | | ● | ● | ● |
| Care Management | | | | | | ● |
| Hospice | ● | | ● | ● | ● | ● |

● *Denotes where some level of coverage is provided*

# DALLAS

ASSISTED LIVING FACILITIES

## Alterra Sterling House of Cedar Hill

602 East Beltline
Cedar Hill, TX 75104

(972) 291-5000
www.assisted.com

### GILBERT GUIDE OBSERVATIONS

| | | | |
|---|---|---|---|
| Administration & Staff | g g g | Residents | g g g |
| Facility Aesthetics | g g g | Dietary & Food Selection | g g g |
| Facility Condition & Safety | g g g | Activities | g g g |

### DETAILS

Year Built: 1997
Current Mgmt. Since: 1997
No. of Floors: 1
Resident Capacity: 60

### SPECIAL

Mild dementia care provided
Diets Accommodated: Diabetic, Low-fat, Low-salt
Proximity to Emergency Svcs.: Under 8 miles
Nearby shopping and entertainment
Pets allowed

### STAFF

Nurse/LVN/LPN: On-call 24/7
Caregiver Training: Dementia, Ethics, Family communication, Grief, Patient transfers, Stress management, Transition issues, Validation therapy
Criminal Background Check: Yes
Principal Staff Language(s): English
Other Staff Language(s): Spanish

### FACILITY FEATURES

Activities/Recreation
Beauty/Barber Shop ($)
Chapel Services
Facility Parking
Guest Meals ($)
Outside Patio/Gardens
Pharmaceutical Service ($)
Private Dining Room
Separate Therapy Room
Transportation
24-hour Security

### ROOM FEATURES

Cable TV Ready ($)
Emergency Call System
Grab Bars
Kitchenette
Private Bathrooms
Telephone Ready ($)
Temperature Controls

### COSTS

PRICES MAY INCREASE. PLEASE CALL FOR MOST CURRENT INFORMATION.

| | |
|---|---|
| Studio Apt. | $1,995/month |
| One Bedroom Apt. | $2,395–$2,595/month |
| Costs of Care | Up to $2,500/month based on individual need |
| Rate Increase | Annually; usually 1–5% |
| Reimbursement | LTCI, Private pay |

| | |
|---|---|
| Entrance Fee | $1,000 |
| Pet Deposit | $350 |

**PORTRAIT**

Alterra Sterling House residents enjoy a packed calendar of diverse activities that includes aromatherapy, bingo, movie nights, poetry recitals, religious services, spelling bees and performances by musical guests. When we arrived for our tour, a group of residents had gathered for an outing—the air buzzed with excitement! Residents and staff interact in a comfortable, friendly manner. Staff members were quick to wish each resident a good day or offer assistance. A number of residents took advantage of the agreeable weather by gardening or relaxing outside. The building's exterior is a sturdy combination of stone, brick and wood.

We observed residents socializing throughout the common areas, which are attractively decorated with a mix of solid and floral patterns. Tasteful window treatments and paintings of landscapes and flowers beautify the rooms. Meals are served restaurant-style in the dining room, where dark wooden tables and chairs host residents. The menu lists hearty meals such as chicken fried steak, mashed potatoes and mixed vegetables. Residents enjoy alternate options at each meal as well as snacks throughout the day. Expansive windows and brass and glass fixtures spread light throughout the home. Handrails offer support in the expansive hallways, which are ornamented with vases and landscapes. Residents' personalities are stamped on their rooms, which feature neutral-colored walls and carpets that accommodate a variety of personal styles.

## ALTERRA STERLING HOUSE OF DENTON

2525 Hinkle Drive
Denton, TX 76201

(940) 566-7054
www.assisted.com

---

**GILBERT GUIDE OBSERVATIONS**

| | | | |
|---|---|---|---|
| Administration & Staff | g g g g | Residents | g g g g |
| Facility Aesthetics | g g g g | Dietary & Food Selection | g g g |
| Facility Condition & Safety | g g g g g | Activities | g g g |

**DETAILS**

Year Built: 1992
Year Remodeled: Ongoing
Current Mgmt. Since: Unknown
No. of Floors: 1
Resident Capacity: 122

**SPECIAL**

Diets Accommodated: Diabetic, Low-fat, Low-salt, Renal
Proximity to Emergency Svcs.: Under 8 miles
Nearby shopping and entertainment
Pets allowed

ALTERRA STERLING HOUSE OF DENTON (CONTINUED)

**STAFF**

Nurse/LVN/LPN: On-call 24/7
Caregiver Training: Dementia, Ethics
Criminal Background Check: Yes
Principal Staff Language(s): English
Other Staff Language(s): Spanish

**FACILITY FEATURES**

Beauty/Barber Shop
Facility Parking
Outside Patio/Gardens
Private Dining Room
Transportation to MD Appointments, Personal Outings ($), Scheduled Outings
24-hour Security

**ROOM FEATURES**

Cable TV Ready ($)
Emergency Call System
Furnished
Grab Bars
Kitchenette
Private Bathrooms
Telephone Ready ($)
Temperature Controls

**COSTS**

PRICES MAY INCREASE. PLEASE CALL FOR MOST CURRENT INFORMATION.

| | |
|---|---|
| Studio Apt. | $2,240/month |
| One Bedroom Apt. | $2,520–$2,785/month<br>Double occupancy add $600/month |
| Costs of Care | Included in monthly rate |
| Rate Increase | Annually; usually 2% |
| Reimbursement | LTCI, Private pay |
| Entrance Fee | $700 |
| Pet Deposit | $250 |

**PORTRAIT**

Alterra Sterling House is located in a residential area on Hinkle Street. The building, surrounded by neatly groomed lawns, boasts ample parking. Two plush seating areas furnished with contemporary coffee tables, chairs and couches are located in the lobby. The common area, reminiscent of a hotel lobby, is homey nonetheless. We observed residents gathering around the fireplace, talking and reading their morning newspapers.

Individual "suites," as the residents call them, are moderately sized. Residents furnish and decorate to suit their tastes. The newly furnished dining room is also used for special programs, meetings and family gatherings. The kitchen staff prepares three nutritious meals a day. Hallways are spacious and neat. One staff member commented on how the residents regularly walk the halls of the U-shaped building for exercise. The shape of the building provides a semi-enclosed atrium. Residents exit the building through French doors and step onto a tiled deck with white wicker furniture, where they can enjoy the sunlight streaming in from the surrounding windows.

The staff wears casual attire—knit skirts and khakis, which is a nice change from the standard scrubs—to complement the homey atmosphere. Management and staff encourage participation from residents and their loved ones. Alterra's Family Connection is a special program that fosters open communication between families and staff. Another special feature is Alterra's Wellness Center, a hub for health care management. Residents and their families are encouraged to meet with the staff case manager, who is an RN, to learn about topics such as pain control, stress reduction and how to get a good night's sleep. Alterra residents appeared active in every corner of the building. Although the building is large, the environment is cozy due to constant interaction between residents and staff.

## Alterra Sterling House of Desoto

747 West Pleasant Run
Desoto, TX 75115

(972) 274-1700
www.assisted.com

---

**GILBERT GUIDE OBSERVATIONS**

| | | | |
|---|---|---|---|
| Administration & Staff | g g g | Residents | g g g |
| Facility Aesthetics | g g g g | Dietary & Food Selection | g g g |
| Facility Condition & Safety | g g g | Activities | g g g |

### DETAILS

Year Built: 1997
Current Mgmt. Since: 1997
No. of Floors: 1
Resident Capacity: 60

### SPECIAL

Mild dementia care provided
Diets Accommodated: Diabetic, Low-fat, Low-salt
Proximity to Emergency Svcs.: 9–15 Miles
Nearby shopping and entertainment
Pets allowed

### STAFF

Nurse/LVN/LPN: On-call 24/7
Caregiver Training: Dementia, Ethics, Family communication, Grief, Patient transfers, Stress management, Transition issues, Validation therapy
Criminal Background Check: Yes
Principal Staff Language(s): English
Other Staff Language(s): Spanish

### FACILITY FEATURES

Activities/Recreation
Beauty/Barber Shop ($)
Chapel Services
Facility Parking
Guest Meals ($)
Outside Patio/Gardens
Pharmaceutical Service ($)

### ROOM FEATURES

Cable TV Ready ($)
Emergency Call System
Grab Bars
Kitchenette
Private Bathrooms
Telephone Ready ($)
Temperature Controls

ALTERRA STERLING HOUSE OF DESOTO (CONTINUED)

**FACILITY FEATURES (CONTINUED)**

Private Dining Room
Room Service ($)
Transportation
24-hour Security

## COSTS

PRICES MAY INCREASE. PLEASE CALL FOR MOST CURRENT INFORMATION.

| | |
|---|---|
| Studio Apt. | $1,995/month |
| One Bedroom Apt. | $2,395–$2,595/month<br>Double occupancy add $600/month |
| Respite Stays | $95/day for private room |
| Costs of Care | Based on individual need |
| Rate Increase | Annually; usually 1–3% |
| Reimbursement | LTCI, Private pay |
| Entrance Fee | $1,000 |
| Pet Deposit | $250 |

## PORTRAIT

Alterra Sterling House of DeSoto and its grounds are surrounded by an undeveloped tract of wooded land, in utter peace and quiet. The facility resembles a large family home, with an inviting porch that leads to the white stone and brick exterior. Neat landscaping surrounds the home. Shade trees and comfortable seating make socializing in the outdoor area popular among residents, who also enjoy manicures, sewing, board games, arts and crafts, movie nights, happy hour and religious services. As we arrived for our tour, a lively group of residents prepared to go shopping. Cheerful residents mingled in small groups throughout the home. Staff members were friendly and enthusiastic as they went about their work.

The furnishings in the common areas feature a mix of solids and floral patterns. A fireplace creates a dramatic focal point in one of the common rooms, furnished with dark wood tables and armoires. Immaculate earth-toned carpet runs throughout the building. The library provides residents with a tranquil spot for reading or quiet contemplation. The home is brightened by natural and fluorescent light as well as brass and frosted glass fixtures. Painted landscapes hang on the pale walls of the broad hallways. Residents furnish the moderately sized rooms, which feature neutral-colored walls and carpet that complement a variety of décor. Wide chairs provide residents with comfortable seating as they take their meals at the matching dark wooden tables in the spacious dining area. The menu on the day of our visit announced a meal of beef stew, salad, baked apples and peach pie. Snacks are available all day long.

## Alterra Sterling House of Lancaster

2400 Pleasant Run Road
Lancaster, TX 75146

(972) 274-5000, (972) 269-7480
www.assisted.com

### GILBERT GUIDE OBSERVATIONS

| | | | |
|---|---|---|---|
| Administration & Staff | g g g | Residents | g g g |
| Facility Aesthetics | g g g | Dietary & Food Selection | g g g |
| Facility Condition & Safety | g g g | Activities | g g g |

### DETAILS

Year Built: 1997
Year Remodeled: Ongoing
Current Mgmt. Since: 1997
No. of Floors: 1
Resident Capacity: 50

### SPECIAL

Mild dementia care provided
Diets Accommodated: Diabetic, Low-salt
Proximity to Emergency Svcs.: Under 8 miles
Nearby shopping and entertainment
Pet visits allowed

### STAFF

Nurse/LVN/LPN: 40 hours/week, On-call 24/7
Caregiver Training: Dementia, Ethics, Grief, Stress management, Transition issues
Criminal Background Check: Yes
Principal Staff Language(s): English

### FACILITY FEATURES

Activities/Recreation
Beauty/Barber Shop ($)
Chapel Services
Computer/Internet Access
Facility Parking
Guest Meals ($)
Outside Patio/Gardens
Overnight Guest Room ($)
Pharmaceutical Service
Private Dining Room
Room Service ($)
Transportation to MD Appointments, Personal Outings
24-hour Security

### ROOM FEATURES

Cable TV Ready
Emergency Call System
Grab Bars
Kitchenette
Private Bathrooms
Telephone Ready
Temperature Controls

### COSTS

PRICES MAY INCREASE. PLEASE CALL FOR MOST CURRENT INFORMATION.

| | |
|---|---|
| One Bedroom Apt. | $1,995–$2,595/month<br>Double occupancy add $600/month |
| Respite Stays | Call for private room rates |
| Costs of Care | Included in monthly rate |
| Rate Increase | Annually; usually 1–5% |

ALTERRA STERLING HOUSE OF LANCASTER (CONTINUED)

| | |
|---|---|
| Reimbursement | LTCI, Private pay |
| Entrance Fee | $1,000 |

**PORTRAIT**

Alterra at Lancaster is situated on bustling West Pleasant Run Road. Green landscaped grounds of various shrubs and shade trees front this brick ranch home. The interior is lined with green carpeting and wallpapered in neutral tones. A group of residents basked in the sunlight and visited with each other in a comfortable seating area in the entrance when we visited.

Residents' rooms are snug, but have extra storage space. Each walk-in closet holds a safe. Personal furnishings and decorations are strongly encouraged. The kitchen staff prepares traditional Southern meals such as chicken fried steak, mashed potatoes and corn. Residents who prefer lighter fare order from an alternative menu. Watching programs on the big-screen TV in the movie room is a popular activity. Alterra boasts two patio areas. Residents enjoy feeding a family of rabbits on the smaller patio. The larger area is furnished with comfortable lounge furniture and used frequently on breezy afternoons. The well-maintained grounds provide enough shade and sunlight to accommodate personal preferences. The spacious hallways have several seating areas. A hodgepodge of artwork adorns the walls. Soft artificial light supplements the plentiful sunlight throughout the facility.

The residents and staff at Alterra have created a familial atmosphere. Residents busy themselves with a variety of activities including bingo, dominoes, word searches, evening social hour and field trips to Wal-Mart. Local Girl Scouts frequently join residents for scheduled activities. Two daughters of a former resident entertain the residents with sing-alongs at the piano. Even though their mother currently resides elsewhere, both women volunteer their services because they believe in the care and service that Alterra staff and management provides for their residents.

## ALTERRA STERLING HOUSE OF MANSFIELD

1771 Country Club Drive
Mansfield, TX 76063

(817) 477-0600
www.assisted.com

---

**GILBERT GUIDE OBSERVATIONS**

| | | | |
|---|---|---|---|
| Administration & Staff | g g g | Residents | g g g |
| Facility Aesthetics | g g g | Dietary & Food Selection | g g g |
| Facility Condition & Safety | g g g | Activities | g g g |

## DETAILS

Year Built: 1996
Year Remodeled: 2003
Current Mgmt. Since: 2000
No. of Floors: 1
Resident Capacity: 32

## SPECIAL

Mild dementia care provided
Diets Accommodated: Diabetic, Low-fat, Low-salt
Proximity to Emergency Svcs.: Under 8 miles
Nearby shopping and entertainment
Some pets allowed

## STAFF

Nurse/LVN/LPN: 40 hours/week, On-call 24/7
Caregiver Training: Dementia, Ethics, Family communication, Grief, Patient transfers, Stress management, Transition issues, Validation therapy
Criminal Background Check: Yes
Principal Staff Language(s): English
Other Staff Language(s): Spanish

## FACILITY FEATURES

Activities/Recreation
Beauty/Barber Shop ($)
Facility Parking
Guest Meals ($)
Outside Patio/Gardens
Pharmaceutical Service
Private Dining Room
Separate Therapy Room
Transportation

## ROOM FEATURES

Cable TV Ready ($)
Emergency Call System
Kitchenette
Private Bathrooms
Telephone Ready ($)
Temperature Controls

## COSTS

PRICES MAY INCREASE. PLEASE CALL FOR MOST CURRENT INFORMATION.

| | |
|---|---|
| Studio Apt. | $1,995/month |
| One Bedroom Apt. | $2395–$2,595/month |
| Costs of Care | $200–$1,300/month based on individual need |
| Rate Increase | Annually; usually 3.5% |
| Reimbursement | LTCI, Private pay, Veterans |
| Entrance Fee | $1,000 |

## PORTRAIT

Alterra Sterling House of Mansfield is at home on Country Club Drive, near bustling Matlock Street. Whitewood awnings accentuate the building's attractive composition of stone and red brick. Inside, blue carpeting provides a dramatic backdrop to the luxurious sofas, chairs and dark wood tables. The lobby and dining area are adjacent to one another. Residents may reserve a spacious sunroom for banquets and special events. During our visit, residents feasted on chicken fried steak, mashed potatoes and grilled vegetables, as well as more health-conscious items like grilled chicken salad.

ALTERRA STERLING HOUSE OF MANSFIELD (CONTINUED)

Residents' moderately sized rooms each have one window. Natural light, combined with fluorescent lighting and elegant brass lamps and sconces make the interior bright and cheery. The spacious hallways are lined with wooden handrails. An outdoor courtyard is located at the center of the facility. Residents personalize the garden by bringing in their own plants. The parlor is stacked with puzzle boards and games, providing plentiful indoor activities. Scheduled activities such as arts and crafts, baking events, sing-alongs and "Do You Remember When?" discussions among residents all foster a strong community.

The residents we observed were lively; small groups gathered in different corners of the building, filling the halls with chatter and laughter. In spite of a seemingly busy afternoon, management and staff were attentive to residents' needs in addition to being gracious and helpful tour guides.

## ARDEN COURTS OF RICHARDSON A/D

410 Buckingham Road
Richardson, TX 75081

(972) 235-1200
www.hcr-manorcare.com

---

**GILBERT GUIDE OBSERVATIONS**

| | | | |
|---|---|---|---|
| Administration & Staff | g g g g | Dietary & Food Selection | g g g g |
| Facility Aesthetics | g g g g g | Activities | g g g g g |
| Facility Condition & Safety | g g g g g | Alzheimer's & Dementia Capabilities | g g g g g |
| Residents | g g g g g | | |

### DETAILS

Year Built: 1999
Year Remodeled: Ongoing
Current Mgmt. Since: 2001
No. of Floors: 1
Resident Capacity: 60

### SPECIAL

Alzheimer's/Dementia Only Facility
Diets Accommodated: Diabetic, Low-fat, Low-salt
Proximity to Emergency Svcs.: Under 8 miles
Nearby shopping and entertainment
No pets allowed

### STAFF

Nurse/LVN/LPN: 84 hours/week, On-call 24/7
Caregiver Training: Dementia, Ethics, Family communication, Grief, Patient transfers, Stress management, Transition issues, Validation therapy
Criminal Background Check: Yes
Principal Staff Language(s): English
Other Staff Language(s): Spanish

### FACILITY FEATURES

Activities/Recreation
Beauty/Barber Shop ($)
Chapel Services
Facility Parking
Guest Meals ($)
Outside Patio/Gardens
Private Dining Room
24-hour Security

### ROOM FEATURES

Furnished
Grab Bars
Shared & Private Bathrooms
Temperature Controls

### COSTS

PRICES MAY INCREASE. PLEASE CALL FOR MOST CURRENT INFORMATION.

| | |
|---|---|
| Alzheimer's Unit | $3,700/month for private room |
| Respite Stays | $125/day for private room |
| Costs of Care | Included in monthly rate |
| Rate Increase | Every 1½ years |
| Reimbursement | LTCI, Private pay |

### PORTRAIT

Arden Courts is located in an upscale urban neighborhood. The building sits on a large gated lot, allowing residents and their guests to stroll and socialize outdoors. The homelike décor is simple and inviting. Each wing of the building has a kitchen and living room. Residents' rooms are cozy and neat. Each room has a window and shelves for residents to display personal items.

The dining area is set up like an eat-in kitchen, a nice alternative to the standard formal dining room. The kitchen staff offers a menu of hearty lunches and light dinners. For example, country fried steak with mashed potatoes and green beans was served at lunch when we visited. For dinner, residents chose from a menu of assorted soups and sandwiches. The wide hallways are equipped with handrails. Extra seating areas in the halls are perfect for residents to catch up on their reading or bird watch.

The outdoor area is a lovely refuge. Residents enjoy a putting green among the trimmed, open landscape and use their green thumbs in the gardening area. The staff organizes daily activities such as "coffee talk," board games, memory stimulation and fitness instruction. We witnessed a group of residents engaged in a game of dominoes. The activities run by the staff give one the impression that they are well-prepared to accommodate the special needs of these Alzheimer's residents.

## ATRIA GRAPEVINE A/D

3975 William D. Tate Avenue
Grapevine, TX 76051

(817) 416-8907, (817) 913-6415
www.atriaseniorliving.com

| GILBERT GUIDE OBSERVATIONS | | | |
|---|---|---|---|
| Administration & Staff | g g g g | Dietary & Food Selection | g g g g g |
| Facility Aesthetics | g g g g | Activities | g g g g g |
| Facility Condition & Safety | g g g g | Alzheimer's & Dementia Capabilities | g g g g g |
| Residents | g g g g g | | |

### DETAILS

Year Built: 1999
Current Mgmt. Since: 2001
No. of Floors: 3
Resident Capacity: 70

### SPECIAL

Diets Accommodated: Diabetic, Low-fat, Low-salt
Proximity to Emergency Svcs.: Under 8 miles
Nearby shopping and entertainment
Pets allowed

### STAFF

Nurse/LVN/LPN: Onsite 24/7
Caregiver Training: Dementia, Ethics, Family communication, Grief, Patient transfers, Stress management, Transition issues, Validation therapy
Criminal Background Check: Yes
Principal Staff Language(s): English
Other Staff Language(s): Spanish

### FACILITY FEATURES

Activities/Recreation
Beauty/Barber Shop ($)
Chapel Services
Computer/Internet Access
Facility Parking
Fitness Room/Gym
Guest Meals ($)
Outside Patio/Gardens
Pharmaceutical Service
Private Dining Room
Room Service ($)
Separate Therapy Room
Transportation to MD Appointments, Scheduled Outings
24-hour Security

### ROOM FEATURES

Cable TV Ready ($)
Emergency Call System
Private Bathrooms
Telephone Ready ($)
Temperature Controls

## COSTS

PRICES MAY INCREASE. PLEASE CALL FOR MOST CURRENT INFORMATION.

| | |
|---|---|
| Studio Apt. | $2,900/month |
| One Bedroom Apt. | $3,450/month<br>Double occupancy add $995/month |
| Two Bedroom Apt. | $3,775/month<br>Double occupancy add $995/month |
| Alzheimer's Unit | Starting at $3,850/month for shared room<br>$3,850–$5,350/month for private room |
| Respite Stays | $125/day for private room |
| Costs of Care | $325–$1,600/month based on individual need |
| Rate Increase | Annually; usually 5–6% |
| Reimbursement | LTCI, Private pay, SSI, Veterans |
| Entrance Fee | $1,500 |
| Pet Deposit | $750 |

## PORTRAIT

Atria Grapevine is easily accessible to several highways, shopping malls and community centers. Green lawns and oak trees surround the stately building. The large porch area, furnished with tables and rocking chairs, is a relaxing spot where residents and guests visit with one another. Past the secured entrance, the interior is painted in cool blues and pastels.

Residents' rooms are bright and spacious. Residents often gather around the fish tank in the plush common area. The dining room is a lovely setting of mahogany tables draped in white linen. Residents of the Alzheimer's unit dine with the assisted living residents. Assigned seating in the dining room provides added stability for residents with dementia. Residents were enjoying Santa Fe fish with vegetables and fruit cobbler during our visit. The staff accommodates residents with sugar-free diets as well. The secured back patio is a popular retreat for bird watching. Plenty of windows bathe the facility in natural light; lamps and sconces add a warm and homey feel. Broad hallways equipped with handrails are decorated with black-and-white photos of cityscapes.

The staff organizes a full day of activities including Bible study, happy hour, tai chi, piano lessons and card games. On Veteran's Day, residents invited their families for picture taking. We observed residents and staff engaged in many activities together. The residents were entertaining and appeared to be very involved within their community.

## ATRIA RICHARDSON A/D

1493 Richardson Drive
Richardson, TX 75080

(972) 231-3313
(214) 926-4433
www.atriaseniorliving.com

---

### GILBERT GUIDE OBSERVATIONS

| | | | |
|---|---|---|---|
| Administration & Staff | g g g | Dietary & Food Selection | g g g |
| Facility Aesthetics | g g g | Activities | g g g |
| Facility Condition & Safety | g g g g | Alzheimer's & Dementia Capabilities | g g g |
| Residents | g g g g | | |

### DETAILS

Year Built: 1998
Current Mgmt. Since: 1998
No. of Floors: 1
Resident Capacity: 91

### SPECIAL

Diets Accommodated: Diabetic, Low-fat, Low-salt, Renal
Proximity to Emergency Svcs.: Under 8 miles
Nearby shopping and entertainment
Some pets allowed

### STAFF

Nurse/LVN/LPN: 40 hours/week, On-call 24/7
Caregiver Training: Dementia, Ethics, Family communication, Grief, Patient transfers, Stress management, Transition issues, Validation therapy
Criminal Background Check: Yes
Principal Staff Language(s): English
Other Staff Language(s): Spanish

### FACILITY FEATURES

Activities/Recreation
Beauty/Barber Shop ($)
Facility Parking
Guest Meals
Outside Patio/Gardens
Pharmaceutical Service
Private Dining Room
Room Service
Transportation
24-hour Security

### ROOM FEATURES

Cable TV Ready ($)
Emergency Call System
Grab Bars
Kitchenette
Private Bathrooms
Telephone Ready ($)
Temperature Controls

### COSTS

PRICES MAY INCREASE. PLEASE CALL FOR MOST CURRENT INFORMATION.

| | |
|---|---|
| Studio Apt. | $2,895/month |
| One Bedroom Apt. | $3,495/month<br>Double occupancy add $900/month |
| Two Bedroom Apt. | $4,995/month<br>Double occupancy add $900/month |
| Alzheimer's Unit | $4,950–$5,450/month for private room |

| | |
|---|---|
| Respite Stays | $120/day (AL), $200/day (ALZ) for private room |
| Costs of Care | $325–$1,600/month based on individual need |
| Rate Increase | Annually |
| Reimbursement | LTCI, Private pay |
| Entrance Fee | $1,500 |
| Pet Deposit | $900 |

**PORTRAIT**

Visitors can't help but gaze upward to the roof inlaid with beautiful stained glass when entering Atria Richardson. Below, white wooden guardrails stretch around a furnished porch laced with potted greenery. The elegant décor continues inside. Textured wallpaper is a muted backdrop for the prettily upholstered furniture and dark wood pieces that sit atop richly colored rugs. Brass light fixtures and glass globes shed soft light, adding to the homey feel. A grand wood and glass birdcage near the entrance runs the length of the room and houses several finches. We observed a group of residents visiting with one another as the birds twittered in the background.

Residents' rooms run from small to large; each is spacious enough to accommodate personal furnishings. Residents with Alzheimer's enjoy the comfort of private rooms. Natural light cascades over the dining area, making it bright and cheery. A waitstaff serves residents three meals per day; snacks are available around the clock. The enticing dessert menu featured "Florida" lime pie and Irish bread pudding with caramel-whiskey sauce on the day of our visit.

The outdoor area is quite popular among residents. Atria Richardson is adjacent to a private park (also owned by the facility) that features flower-laden paths surrounded by thick wooded areas. Even during winter, the walking club gathers every morning to stroll the meandering walkways that abound. Residents seem to socialize constantly; one group chatted excitedly as they prepared for a scheduled outing. The daughter of one resident paused a moment to share with us how happy she and her mother were with the care at Atria Richardson.

## AUTUMN LEAVES OF GRAPEVINE A/D

2501 Heritage Avenue
Grapevine, TX 76051

(817) 329-8500
(817) 726-2828

**GILBERT GUIDE OBSERVATIONS**

| | | | |
|---|---|---|---|
| Administration & Staff | g g g g | Dietary & Food Selection | g g g g |
| Facility Aesthetics | g g g g g | Activities | g g g g |
| Facility Condition & Safety | g g g g g | Alzheimer's & Dementia Capabilities | g g g g |
| Residents | g g g g g | | |

AUTUMN LEAVES OF GRAPEVINE (CONTINUED)

**DETAILS**

Year Built: 2004
Current Mgmt. Since: 2004
No. of Floors: 1
Resident Capacity: 42

**SPECIAL**

Alzheimer's/Dementia Only Facility
Diets Accommodated: Diabetic, Low-salt
Proximity to Emergency Svcs.: Under 8 miles
Nearby shopping and entertainment
No pets allowed

**STAFF**

Nurse/LVN/LPN: 40 hours/week, On-call 24/7
Caregiver Training: Dementia, Ethics, Family communication, Grief, Patient transfers, Stress management, Transition issues, Validation therapy
Criminal Background Check: Yes
Principal Staff Language(s): English
Other Staff Language(s): Spanish

**FACILITY FEATURES**

Activities/Recreation
Beauty/Barber Shop ($)
Guest Meals ($)
Outside Patio/Gardens
Pharmaceutical Service
Transportation to MD Appointments, Scheduled Outings
24-hour Security

**ROOM FEATURES**

Emergency Call System
Furnished
Telephone Ready ($)
Temperature Controls

**COSTS**

PRICES MAY INCREASE. PLEASE CALL FOR MOST CURRENT INFORMATION.

| | |
|---|---|
| Alzheimer's Unit | $3,350–$4,200/month for private room |
| Costs of Care | Included in monthly rate |
| Rate Increase | Annually; usually 3% |
| Reimbursement | LTCI, Private pay, SSI, Veterans |

**PORTRAIT**

A bubbling fountain greets visitors to Autumn Leaves, a building of stone, crimson brick and red tile. Native Texan shrubs border the walkway to the facility. Multiple windows line the foyer, which features a vaulted ceiling and a fireplace. Lamps brighten the sitting areas and sconces light the wide hallways, which are lined with handrails. Themed "neighborhoods" divide the building. The carpet and wallpaper echo the themes, as do knickknacks in each neighborhood's atrium. Beds and nightstands furnish residents' rooms.

The staff throws a big party every month to celebrate residents' birthdays. Residents also enjoy visiting pet day and therapeutic music hours. The scent of vanilla filled the home during our tour, as several residents baked cookies while others relaxed in front of the TV. A group of residents barbecued in the center courtyard in celebration of Day of the Dead. Two large patios flank the house.

Healthful offerings such as apples and oranges comprise the snacks. The chefs prepare simple meals such as turkey, mashed potatoes and sugar-free cherry pie. Some staff members serve meals; others provide feeding assistance. We noted staff closely monitoring residents who tend to wander. Despite their busy schedules, they engaged in cheerful conversations with residents. Even the owner took the time to say hello and chat with us!

## Autumn Leaves Personal Care Unit

1010 Emerald Isle Drive
Dallas, TX 75218
(214) 328-4161

---

**GILBERT GUIDE OBSERVATIONS**

| | | | |
|---|---|---|---|
| Administration & Staff | g g g g | Residents | g g g g |
| Facility Aesthetics | g g g | Dietary & Food Selection | g g g |
| Facility Condition & Safety | g g g | Activities | g g g |

### DETAILS

Year Built: 1972
Year Remodeled: Ongoing
Current Mgmt. Since: 1972
No. of Floors: 3
Resident Capacity: 58

### SPECIAL

Mild dementia care provided
Diets Accommodated: Diabetic, Low-salt
Proximity to Emergency Svcs.: Under 8 miles
Nearby shopping and entertainment
Pet visits allowed

### STAFF

Nurse/LVN/LPN: Onsite 24/7
Caregiver Training: Ethics, Family communication, Grief, Transition issues, Validation therapy
Criminal Background Check: Yes
Principal Staff Language(s): English
Other Staff Language(s): Spanish

### FACILITY FEATURES

Activities/Recreation
Beauty/Barber Shop ($)
Chapel Services
Computer/Internet Access
Facility Parking
Guest Meals ($)
Outside Patio/Gardens
Pharmaceutical Service ($)
Private Dining Room
Room Service ($)
Transportation
24-hour Security

### ROOM FEATURES

Cable TV Ready ($)
Emergency Call System
Grab Bars
Kitchenette
Private Bathrooms
Telephone Ready ($)
Temperature Controls

AUTUMN LEAVES PERSONAL CARE UNIT (CONTINUED)

## COSTS

PRICES MAY INCREASE. PLEASE CALL FOR MOST CURRENT INFORMATION.

| | |
|---|---|
| Studio Apt. | $2,545/month |
| One Bedroom Apt. | $2,995/month<br>Double occupancy add $545–$630/month |
| Costs of Care | Included in monthly rate |
| Rate Increase | Annually; usually 1–5% |
| Reimbursement | LTCI, Private pay |
| Security Deposit | $500 |

## PORTRAIT

Residents of Autumn Leaves enjoy spectacular views, thanks to the facility's hilltop location overlooking White Rock Lake. The stucco building sits on fancifully named Emerald Isle Drive, in a picturesque Dallas neighborhood that features several historic homes. The leafy canopy above the oak trees that surround the building is a playground for squirrels. Active walking club residents frequent an extensive trail that encircles the nearby lake. Residents are encouraged to suggest new activities to supplement their favorites, which include bingo, happy hour, board games, holiday celebrations and religious services.

Our guide greeted residents by name as we toured the home, prompting them to stop and chat; jokes and outbursts of laughter punctuated the conversations. Several residents offered strong recommendations of the facility. Residents socialized animatedly among the common areas—we spotted one gentleman doing an impromptu jig! The home's interior was under renovation but we were informed that the new décor would include cherry-wood crown moldings, green fabric wallpaper and gold and blue carpet. Sunshine supplements the brass and frosted glass sconces that light the rooms and wide hallways. Light brown carpet extends from wall to wall in residents' large rooms, each of which boasts a balcony or private patio. Bathtubs with low sides in residents' rooms helps ease bathing difficulties.

An expansive glass wall showcases lovely views in the spacious dining hall. Bleached oak floors and comfortable wheeled chairs add practical touches to the elegant room. Hearty offerings include breaded chicken, mashed potatoes and baby carrots followed by buttermilk pie. A salad bar displaying brightly colored vegetables tempts health-minded residents.

## AVALON—ALLENCREST A/D

4330 Allencrest
Dallas, TX 75244

(214) 752-7050
(800) 696-6536
www.avalon-care.com

### GILBERT GUIDE OBSERVATIONS

| Category | Rating | Category | Rating |
|---|---|---|---|
| Administration & Staff | g g g g | Dietary & Food Selection | g g g |
| Facility Aesthetics | g g g g | Activities | g g g |
| Facility Condition & Safety | g g g | Alzheimer's & Dementia Capabilities | g g g |
| Residents | g g g | | |

### DETAILS

Year Built: 1997
Year Remodeled: 2004
Current Mgmt. Since: 2001
No. of Floors: 1
Resident Capacity: 10

### SPECIAL

Alzheimer's/Dementia Only Facility
Diets Accommodated: Diabetic, Low-fat, Low-salt
Proximity to Emergency Svcs.: Under 8 miles
Nearby shopping and entertainment
No pets allowed

### STAFF

Nurse/LVN/LPN: On-call 24/7
Caregiver Training: Dementia, Ethics, Family communication, Grief, Patient transfers, Stress management, Transition issues, Validation therapy
Criminal Background Check: Yes
Principal Staff Language(s): English

### FACILITY FEATURES

Activities/Recreation
Beauty/Barber Shop
Chapel Services
Facility Parking
Guest Meals
Outside Patio/Gardens
24-hour Security

### ROOM FEATURES

Cable TV Ready ($)
Emergency Call System
Furnished
Private Bathrooms
Telephone Ready ($)
Temperature Controls

### COSTS

PRICES MAY INCREASE. PLEASE CALL FOR MOST CURRENT INFORMATION.

| | |
|---|---|
| Alzheimer's Unit | $3,875–$4,275/month for private room |
| Costs of Care | $200/month for incontinence |
| Rate Increase | Every 2–3 years; usually 3–5% |
| Reimbursement | Private pay |
| Security Deposit | $500 |

AVALON—ALLENCREST (CONTINUED)

### PORTRAIT

Avalon Allencrest is a country-style home that offers a refreshingly noninstitutional alternative to traditional Alzheimer's care. Located in a pleasant neighborhood at the end of a cul-de-sac, the home is shaded by tall trees. Dark wood furniture offset by pale walls and tasteful window treatments creates a quaint and rustic atmosphere. Homemade meals are served in the expansive dining room. The dining area is adjacent to the TV room, which also features a library. The open design of the home eliminates hallways. Residents' rooms are sunny, spacious and comfortable. During our visit we were impressed by the state of cleanliness—even the air smelled fresh!

The backyard has well-kept hedges, trees, flowerbeds and a tidy lawn. We witnessed several residents socializing on the patio. Residents commented on some of the activities they enjoyed most—namely, hand and foot massages, cookie socials and trips to nearby shopping malls. The staff was warm and welcoming and we were delighted to see a caregiver dancing excitedly with a resident.

## AVALON—CANNONGATE A/D

7212 CanonGate
Dallas, TX 75252

(214) 752-7050
(800) 696-6536
www.avalon-care.com

---

**GILBERT GUIDE OBSERVATIONS**

| | | | |
|---|---|---|---|
| Administration & Staff | g g g g g | Dietary & Food Selection | g g g |
| Facility Aesthetics | g g g g | Activities | g g g |
| Facility Condition & Safety | g g g g g | Alzheimer's & Dementia Capabilities | g g g g |
| Residents | g g g g g | | |

### DETAILS

Year Built: 1980
Year Remodeled: 2004
Current Mgmt. Since: 2001
No. of Floors: 1
Resident Capacity: 16

### SPECIAL

Alzheimer's/Dementia Only Facility
Diets Accommodated: Diabetic, Low-fat, Low-salt
Proximity to Emergency Svcs.: Under 8 miles
Nearby shopping and entertainment
No pets allowed

### STAFF

Nurse/LVN/LPN: On-call 24/7
Caregiver Training: Dementia, Ethics, Family communication, Grief, Patient transfers, Stress management, Transition issues, Validation therapy
Criminal Background Check: Yes
Principal Staff Language(s): English

### FACILITY FEATURES

Activities/Recreation
Beauty/Barber Shop
Chapel Services
Facility Parking
Guest Meals
Outside Patio/Gardens
Pharmaceutical Service
Private Dining Room
Separate Therapy Room
Transportation
24-hour Security

### ROOM FEATURES

Cable TV Ready ($)
Furnished
Private Bathrooms
Telephone Ready ($)

### COSTS

PRICES MAY INCREASE. PLEASE CALL FOR MOST CURRENT INFORMATION.

| | |
|---|---|
| Alzheimer's Unit | $3,875–$4,275/month for private room |
| Costs of Care | Included in monthly rate |
| Rate Increase | Every 2 years; usually 2.5% |
| Reimbursement | Private pay |
| Security Deposit | $500 |

### PORTRAIT

Squirrels played and birds chirped as we approached Avalon Canongate in North Dallas. A large patio in the rear invites residents to relax in the shade of trees or stroll along the meandering walkway. The attractive common areas inside the facility are furnished with leather sofas and chairs as well as oak occasional tables. Shades of brown and white compose the color scheme. Overhead fixtures and plentiful windows create an abundance of warm lighting throughout the facility. Hallways are wide enough to accommodate wheelchair users. Residents' rooms are furnished with oak nightstands and armoires. The formal dining room serves a dual purpose; it is used for both meals and social gatherings. The table is elegantly dressed in linen and attractive tableware is used in place of plastic dishes, which are typical of most Alzheimer's facilities. The menu of country-style cuisine boasts favorites including meatloaf, baked chicken, and stew.

Daily activities include neighborhood strolls, listening to music, and reminiscence exercises. Field trips are offered weekly. A wide selection of movies is available to residents, who enjoy watching the big-screen TV. The staff was very friendly with us and attentive to residents. This no doubt is a great indicator of quality care; the residents were happy and were noticeably sociable throughout our visit.

## AVALON—CRESTMERE A/D

6217 Crestmere
Dallas, TX 75240

(214) 752-7050
(800) 696-6536
www.avalon-care.com

---

**GILBERT GUIDE OBSERVATIONS**

| | | | |
|---|---|---|---|
| Administration & Staff | g g g g | Dietary & Food Selection | g g g g |
| Facility Aesthetics | g g g g | Activities | g g |
| Facility Condition & Safety | g g g g | Alzheimer's & Dementia Capabilities | g g g |
| Residents | g g g | | |

### DETAILS

Year Built: 1982
Year Remodeled: 2003
Current Mgmt. Since: 2000
No. of Floors: 1
Resident Capacity: 16

### SPECIAL

Alzheimer's/Dementia Only Facility
Diets Accommodated: Diabetic, Low-fat, Low-salt
Proximity to Emergency Svcs.: Under 8 miles
Nearby shopping and entertainment
No pets allowed

### STAFF

Nurse/LVN/LPN: On-call 24/7
Caregiver Training: Dementia, Ethics, Family communication, Grief, Patient transfers, Stress management, Transition issues, Validation therapy
Criminal Background Check: Yes
Principal Staff Language(s): English

### FACILITY FEATURES

Activities/Recreation
Beauty/Barber Shop
Chapel Services
Facility Parking
Outside Patio/Gardens
Pharmaceutical Service
Private Dining Room
Separate Therapy Room
Transportation
24-hour Security

### ROOM FEATURES

Cable TV Ready ($)
Furnished
Private Bathrooms
Telephone Ready ($)

### COSTS

PRICES MAY INCREASE. PLEASE CALL FOR MOST CURRENT INFORMATION.

| | |
|---|---|
| Alzheimer's Unit | $3,875–$4,275/month for private room |
| Costs of Care | $200/month for incontinence |
| Rate Increase | Every 2–3 years; usually 3–5% |
| Reimbursement | Private pay |
| Security Deposit | $500 |

### PORTRAIT

Avalon Crestmere provides a homelike atmosphere for its Alzheimer's residents. The ranch house has a circular driveway flanked by trees. Mirrors and a neutral color scheme give the living room an airy feel. Artwork hangs on the walls of the entryway. Overhead fixtures and lamps brighten the home's interior. The hallways are on the narrow side but can accommodate wheelchair users. The dining room features soft chandelier lighting, a large table and separate bar area. A small window lights the moderately sized residents' rooms, each of which are furnished with a TV. Residents may add personal decorations if they wish.

A fence secures the outdoor area and protects residents' privacy. Large trees shade the patio seating area. There is a well-lit path that provides an excellent spot to walk in agreeable weather. Entrées such as baked chicken and meatloaf are made daily; residents often help in the preparation. Regular activities include exercise, cookie socials and field trips to the zoo. During our visit the staff focused on the residents who, for the most part, were quiet and reserved.

## AVALON—GLENDORA A/D

7315 Glendora
Dallas, TX 75230

(214) 752-7050
(800) 696-6536
www.avalon-care.com

---

| GILBERT GUIDE OBSERVATIONS | | | |
|---|---|---|---|
| Administration & Staff | g g g g g | Dietary & Food Selection | g g g g |
| Facility Aesthetics | g g g | Activities | g g g |
| Facility Condition & Safety | g g g | Alzheimer's & Dementia Capabilities | g g g g |
| Residents | g g g g | | |

### DETAILS

Year Built: 1977
Year Remodeled: 2003
Current Mgmt. Since: 2000
No. of Floors: 2
Resident Capacity: 16

### SPECIAL

Alzheimer's/Dementia Only Facility
Diets Accommodated: Diabetic, Low-fat, Low-salt
Proximity to Emergency Svcs.: Under 8 miles
Nearby shopping and entertainment
No pets allowed

### STAFF

Nurse/LVN/LPN: On-call 24/7
Caregiver Training: Dementia, Ethics, Family communication, Grief, Patient transfers, Stress management, Transition issues, Validation therapy
Criminal Background Check: Yes
Principal Staff Language(s): English

AVALON—GLENDORA (CONTINUED)

## FACILITY FEATURES

Activities/Recreation
Beauty/Barber Shop
Chapel Services
Facility Parking
Guest Meals
Outside Patio/Gardens
Pharmaceutical Service
Private Dining Room
Transportation
24-hour Security

## ROOM FEATURES

Cable TV Ready ($)
Furnished
Private Bathrooms
Telephone Ready ($)
Temperature Controls

## COSTS

PRICES MAY INCREASE. PLEASE CALL FOR MOST CURRENT INFORMATION.

| | |
|---|---|
| Alzheimer's Unit | $3,875–$4,275/month for private room |
| Costs of Care | $200/month for incontinence |
| Rate Increase | Every 3 years; usually 2% |
| Reimbursement | Private pay |
| Security Deposit | $500 |

## PORTRAIT

The philosophy at Avalon Glendora is that institutional settings are inappropriate for people with Alzheimer's. Therefore, the staff strives to provide a genuine feeling of home, working hard to promote residents' self-esteem and dignity. Several of the animated residents thoughtfully asked how we were doing during our visit.

The urban home is close to shopping and entertainment, yet the neighborhood retains a certain country charm. A circular driveway and manicured hedges greet visitors to the ranch home. The retro décor brings to mind a living room, kitchen and den straight from the 1960s. While modern sofas and loveseats provide comfortable seating, dated fixtures shine mellow lighting throughout the home. In contrast to the smallish common area, the adjacent dining room, kitchen and breakfast nook have a spacious feel. The long hallway is wide enough to accommodate wheelchair users. Handmade blankets and artwork created by the residents add coziness to their small bedrooms. Several lamps supplement the limited natural lighting within each room. An oasis of tropical plants and trees near the outdoor swimming pool shades the seating area favored by residents. A wrought iron fence surrounds the pool. Several residents mentioned how they love to spend evenings strolling on the lighted walkway near the pool. Field trips to shopping malls are another favorite pastime.

The menu boasts hearty favorites such as chili, meatloaf and turkey. Cookies and milk and other comforting snacks are served daily.

## AVALON—HUGHES CIRCLE A/D

13215 Hughes Circle
Dallas, TX 75240

214-752-7050
800-696-6536
www.avalon-care.com

---

### GILBERT GUIDE OBSERVATIONS

| | |
|---|---|
| Administration & Staff | g g g g g |
| Facility Aesthetics | g g g g g |
| Facility Condition & Safety | g g g g |
| Residents | g g g g |
| Dietary & Food Selection | g g g |
| Activities | g g g |
| Alzheimer's & Dementia Capabilities | g g g g |

### DETAILS

Year Built: 1997
Year Remodeled: 2002
Current Mgmt. Since: 2001
No. of Floors: 1
Resident Capacity: 16

### SPECIAL

Alzheimer's/Dementia Only Facility
Diets Accommodated: Diabetic, Low-fat, Low-salt
Proximity to Emergency Svcs.: 16+ Miles
Nearby shopping and entertainment
No pets allowed

### STAFF

Nurse/LVN/LPN: On-call 24/7
Caregiver Training: Dementia, Ethics, Family communication, Grief, Patient transfers, Stress management, Transition issues, Validation therapy
Criminal Background Check: Yes
Principal Staff Language(s): English

### FACILITY FEATURES

Activities/Recreation
Beauty/Barber Shop
Chapel Services
Guest Meals
Outside Patio/Gardens
Separate Therapy Room
Transportation
24-hour Security

### ROOM FEATURES

Cable TV Ready ($)
Furnished
Private Bathrooms
Telephone Ready

### COSTS

PRICES MAY INCREASE. PLEASE CALL FOR MOST CURRENT INFORMATION.

| | |
|---|---|
| Alzheimer's Unit | $3,875–$4,275/month for private room |
| Costs of Care | $200/month for incontinence |
| Rate Increase | Annually; usually 2–3% |
| Reimbursement | Private pay |
| Security Deposit | $500 |

AVALON—HUGHES CIRCLE (CONTINUED)

### PORTRAIT

Avalon Hughes Circle provides a safe and loving environment for Alzheimer's residents. The ranch home is tucked away in a serene and elegant neighborhood. The front yard is dotted with groomed bushes and mature trees. An off-white color scheme, tasteful décor, live plants and spotless upkeep are among the physical hallmarks of the home. Light-colored oak furniture and a large sectional furnish the common area where residents and guests gather to watch the big-screen TV. Overhead fixtures and floor lamps provide bright yet soothing light. There are no hallways due to the open design of the home. The residents' rooms are large and furnished with tables, chairs and armoires. Residents' personal belongings add elements of comfort to the rooms. The spacious dining room has two tables, which are also used for activities such as card games. During our visit, several residents were enjoying an afternoon snack at one of the tables. The simple menu features homemade meals made from fresh ingredients; the entrées are high in protein, usually incorporating chicken, turkey or beef.

A shady walkway in the backyard encourages residents to stroll while a sitting area provides a comfortable resting spot. Daily activities include field trips, morning exercise and cookie socials. The highly attentive staff knows each resident by name. During our visit, we noticed one caregiver helping a resident tie her shoe; both suddenly burst out laughing as the resident accidentally stepped on her.

## AVALON—QUARTERWAY A/D

6908 Quarterway
Dallas, TX 75248

(214) 752-7050
(800) 696-6536
www.avalon-care.com

---

**GILBERT GUIDE OBSERVATIONS**

| | | | |
|---|---|---|---|
| Administration & Staff | g g g g g | Dietary & Food Selection | g g g g |
| Facility Aesthetics | g g g g | Activities | g g g g |
| Facility Condition & Safety | g g g g g | Alzheimer's & Dementia Capabilities | g g g g |
| Residents | g g g g | | |

### DETAILS

Year Built: 1980
Year Remodeled: 2003
Current Mgmt. Since: 2001
No. of Floors: 1
Resident Capacity: 16

### SPECIAL

Alzheimer's/Dementia Only Facility
Diets Accommodated: Diabetic, Low-fat, Low-salt
Proximity to Emergency Svcs.: Under 8 miles
Nearby shopping and entertainment
No pets allowed

### STAFF

Nurse/LVN/LPN: On-call 24/7

Caregiver Training: Dementia, Ethics, Family communication, Grief, Patient transfers, Stress management, Transition issues, Validation therapy
Criminal Background Check: Yes
Principal Staff Language(s): English

## FACILITY FEATURES

Activities/Recreation
Beauty/Barber Shop
Chapel Services
Facility Parking
Guest Meals
Outside Patio/Gardens
Private Dining Room
Separate Therapy Room
Transportation
24-hour Security

## ROOM FEATURES

Cable TV Ready ($)
Furnished
Grab Bars
Private Bathrooms
Telephone Ready ($)

## COSTS

PRICES MAY INCREASE. PLEASE CALL FOR MOST CURRENT INFORMATION.

| | |
|---|---|
| Alzheimer's Unit | $3,875–$4,275/month for private room |
| Costs of Care | $200/month for incontinence |
| Rate Increase | Annually; usually 2–3% |
| Reimbursement | Private pay |
| Security Deposit | $500 |

## PORTRAIT

Avalon Quarterway is one of several Alzheimer's facilities owned by Avalon Residential Care Homes, a nonprofit agency that offers care within homelike settings. Tall cottonwood trees shade the charming home, which is set in a peaceful area.

During our visit, the rosebushes in the landscaped yard were in full bloom. Residents were enjoying an afternoon iced tea social on the patio. Residents often spend time watching TV in the den. Weekly field trips include neighborhood strolls and picnics. We were impressed by the vivacious nature of the residents. Several friendly residents related stories of their past to us. The staff members are attentive and caring. Avalon Quarterway possesses a definite air of family.

The attractively decorated interior imparts a sense of home. Silk flower arrangements brighten the common room, bathed in warm earth tones and furnished with well-maintained sofas and chairs. The lighting in the den is a bit dim. The single hallway is short and wide enough for wheelchair users. Although residents' rooms are small, they are flooded with sunlight, which creates a more spacious feeling. Oak bedside tables and hanging art are in every room. The cozy formal dining area features a beautiful crystal chandelier, linen tablecloths and freshly picked flowers from the garden. The variety of homemade options at breakfast, which include oatmeal, eggs, pancakes and the "omelet station" on Fridays, has made it a favorite mealtime.

## Avalon—Royal Circle A/D

7355 Royal Circle
Dallas, TX 75230

(214) 752-7050
(800) 696-6536

---

### GILBERT GUIDE OBSERVATIONS

| | | | |
|---|---|---|---|
| Administration & Staff | g g g g | Dietary & Food Selection | g g g |
| Facility Aesthetics | g g g | Activities | g g g |
| Facility Condition & Safety | g g g g | Alzheimer's & Dementia Capabilities | g g g g |
| Residents | g g g g | | |

### DETAILS

Year Built: 1966
Year Remodeled: 2004
Current Mgmt. Since: 2000
No. of Floors: 1
Resident Capacity: 16

### SPECIAL

Alzheimer's/Dementia Only Facility
Diets Accommodated: Diabetic, Low-fat, Low-salt
Proximity to Emergency Svcs.: Under 8 miles
Nearby shopping and entertainment
No pets allowed

### STAFF

Nurse/LVN/LPN: On-call 24/7
Caregiver Training: Dementia, Ethics, Family communication, Grief, Patient transfers, Stress management, Transition issues, Validation therapy
Criminal Background Check: Yes
Principal Staff Language(s): English

### FACILITY FEATURES

Activities/Recreation
Beauty/Barber Shop
Chapel Services
Facility Parking
Guest Meals
Outside Patio/Gardens
Pharmaceutical Service
Private Dining Room
Transportation
24-hour Security

### ROOM FEATURES

Furnished
Private Bathrooms

### COSTS

PRICES MAY INCREASE. PLEASE CALL FOR MOST CURRENT INFORMATION.

| | |
|---|---|
| Alzheimer's Unit | $3,875–$4,275/month for private room |
| Costs of Care | $200/month for incontinence |
| Rate Increase | Every 3 years; usually 2.5% |
| Reimbursement | Private pay |
| Security Deposit | $500 |

## PORTRAIT

When the owners of Avalon could not find a homey care facility for their grandparents, they founded Avalon Royal Circle. The comfortable house in upscale North Dallas is complete with hedges and rosebushes. It was designed to be as homelike as possible. Residents are encouraged to furnish their rooms to evoke familiarity and comfort. Each of the rooms is spacious and has a large window.

Balanced meals, homemade with fresh ingredients, are served in an airy dining room. During our visit, a resident helped the kitchen staff prepare an appetizing beef stew. Fruit, cookies, crackers and other snacks are available daily. The dining area and the breakfast nook are both popular spots for residents and staff to visit with each other. Photos of the residents decorate the walls of the sunny den. We observed residents walking about and chatting together in this space. Comfortable new recliners and a sofa invite residents to watch movies on the big-screen TV. The staff seemed to enjoy their work and interacted warmly with the residents.

The secured backyard contains trees and a small patio with a seating area. An umbrella provides afternoon shade. In the early morning, residents often gather to watch hummingbirds at the bird feeder.

# Bentley Assisted Living at Christian Care Center

1000 Wiggins Parkway
Mesquite, TX 75150

(972) 686-3789
www.christiancarecenters.org

---

## GILBERT GUIDE OBSERVATIONS

| | | | |
|---|---|---|---|
| Administration & Staff | g g g g g | Residents | g g g g g |
| Facility Aesthetics | g g g | Dietary & Food Selection | g g g g g |
| Facility Condition & Safety | g g g g | Activities | g g g g g |

## DETAILS

Year Built: 1988
Year Remodeled: Ongoing
Current Mgmt. Since: 1988
No. of Floors: 4
Resident Capacity: 69

## SPECIAL

Mild dementia care provided
Diets Accommodated: Diabetic, Low-fat, Low-salt
Proximity to Emergency Svcs.: Under 8 miles
Nearby shopping and entertainment
No pets allowed

## STAFF

Nurse/LVN/LPN: 32 hours/week, On-call 24/7
Caregiver Training: Dementia, Ethics, Grief, Stress management
Criminal Background Check: Yes

BENTLEY ASSISTED LIVING AT CHRISTIAN CARE CENTER (CONTINUED)

Principal Staff Language(s): English
Other Staff Language(s): Spanish

**FACILITY FEATURES**

Activities/Recreation
Beauty/Barber Shop ($)
Chapel Services
Facility Parking
Guest Meals ($)
Outside Patio/Gardens
Private Dining Room
Room Service
Separate Therapy Room
Transportation to MD Appointments, Scheduled Outings
24-hour Security

**ROOM FEATURES**

Cable TV Ready
Emergency Call System
Grab Bars
Kitchenette
Private Bathrooms
Telephone Ready
Temperature Controls

**COSTS**

PRICES MAY INCREASE. PLEASE CALL FOR MOST CURRENT INFORMATION.

| | |
|---|---|
| Studio Apt. | $2,029–$2,312/month |
| One Bedroom Apt. | $2,941/month<br>Double occupancy add $650/month |
| Costs of Care | Starting at $125/month based on individual need |
| Rate Increase | Annually; usually 3–4% |
| Reimbursement | Private pay |
| Application Fee | $100 |
| Security Deposit | $500 |

**PORTRAIT**

Bentley Assisted Living is situated on the expansive Christian Care campus, next to Mesquite Golf Course. Two of the entrances are along glass-walled hallways that showcase beautiful views of the grounds. Covered walkways lead to a few of the decorative gazebos. The interior design maximizes window space and natural light. There are five floor plans, which range from studios to one-bedrooms. Crown moldings and two-tone paint make the rooms quaint and homey. Residents on one side are treated to views of the golf course; rooms on the other side look out onto the courtyard. The halls feature seating areas and are wide enough to accommodate walker and wheelchair use.

A few staff members have been at Christian Care since its opening; others have worked there for more than twenty years. Strong teamwork makes a large staff unnecessary. The staff nurse conducts monthly medication counseling with residents who administer their own medications.

Regular activities include a Red Hat Society, men's club, tai chi, and mental stimulation games. Outings are common: the rodeo and professional sporting events are among recent offerings. Bentley's activity director developed "bingo bucks," to reward residents for wearing their nametags and participating in activities. An auctioneer holds a monthly auction where residents make purchases with their bingo bucks. We were delighted to meet Bill Cannon, a resident and author of several books about Texas. Mr. Cannon is also the long-time host of a radio talk show.

The staff contacts residents who do not attend meals. A variety of sugar-free desserts are always available. Although the dining area has one glass wall, it is not particularly sunny; however, there are plans to remodel in order to maximize natural light.

## Broadway Plaza at Pecan Park A/D

915 North Fielder Road
Arlington, TX 76012

(817) 265-6900, (877) 219-5437
www.arclp.com

---

### GILBERT GUIDE OBSERVATIONS

| | | | |
|---|---|---|---|
| Administration & Staff | g g g | Dietary & Food Selection | g g g |
| Facility Aesthetics | g g g | Activities | g g g |
| Facility Condition & Safety | g g g g | Alzheimer's & Dementia Capabilities | g g g |
| Residents | g g g | | |

### DETAILS

Year Built: 2000
Current Mgmt. Since: 2002
No. of Floors: 2
Resident Capacity: 40 (AL), 40 (ALZ)

### SPECIAL

Diets Accommodated: Diabetic, Low-salt
Proximity to Emergency Svcs.: Under 8 miles
Nearby shopping and entertainment
Some pets allowed

### STAFF

Nurse/LVN/LPN: 48 hours/week, On-call 24/7
Caregiver Training: Dementia, Ethics, Family communication, Grief, Patient transfers, Stress management, Transition issues, Validation therapy
Criminal Background Check: Yes
Principal Staff Language(s): English
Other Staff Language(s): Spanish

### FACILITY FEATURES

Activities/Recreation
Beauty/Barber Shop ($)
Facility Parking
Guest Meals ($)
Outside Patio/Gardens
Pharmaceutical Service
Private Dining Room
Separate Therapy Room

### ROOM FEATURES

Cable TV Ready ($)
Emergency Call System
Kitchenette
Private Bathrooms
Telephone Ready ($)
Temperature Controls

BROADWAY PLAZA AT PECAN PARK (CONTINUED)

**FACILITY FEATURES (CONTINUED)**

Transportation
24-hour Security

## COSTS

PRICES MAY INCREASE. PLEASE CALL FOR MOST CURRENT INFORMATION.

| | |
|---|---|
| Studio Apt. | $2,395/month |
| One Bedroom Apt. | $2,892/month |
| Costs of Care | $200–$1,000/month based on individual need |
| Rate Increase | Annually; usually 3% |
| Reimbursement | LTCI, Private pay, Veterans |
| Entrance Fee | $2,000 |
| Security Deposit | $500 |
| Pet Deposit | $500 |

## PORTRAIT

Broadway Plaza at Pecan Park is an opulent property at the corner of North Fielder Road and Wright Street. A wrought iron fence surrounds the park-like setting of towering trees and colored shrubbery. Inside the main building, lavish seating areas with rich blue, maroon and green upholstered chairs beckon residents to gather. The walls are hung with elegant paintings of landscapes and floral arrangements. Although residents with Alzheimer's share the same staff and activity calendar with assisted living residents, their rooms are located in a separate building on the same campus.

Residents furnish and decorate their moderately sized rooms to suit their tastes. The grand staircase in the lobby leads to the upstairs dining area and common room. The dining area, an attractive arrangement of upholstered chairs and oak tables, has a "resident kitchen," which is used for cooking and baking activities. The kitchen staff prepares menus that include various Mexican and American entrées. The main common area on the first floor accommodates large group activities, while the upstairs area is a quieter refuge with a TV and lounge furniture. We observed residents engaged in activities throughout the facility; some were enjoying potato salad and shrimp entrées in the dining area; others gathered in front of the television; and one group was spotted lounging on patio furniture enjoying the unusually warm winter day.

The hallways are bright and airy. Soft artificial lighting and natural light are prevalent throughout the building. Memory-enhancing games, which include "Resident Stories" and word games, stimulate cognitive faculties while fostering familiarity with one another. Trips to Wal-Mart, Nordstrom and Babe's Chicken are resident favorites. We observed many active residents at Broadway Plaza gathering in the hallways and chatting while they walked together. The staff seemed very attentive, greeting each passing resident by name.

## Cambridge Court & Memory Care Community A/D

711 Matador Lane
Mesquite, TX 75149

(972) 285-9800
www.cambridgecourtalf.com

### GILBERT GUIDE OBSERVATIONS

| | | | |
|---|---|---|---|
| Administration & Staff | g g g | Dietary & Food Selection | g g |
| Facility Aesthetics | g g g g | Activities | g |
| Facility Condition & Safety | g g g g g | Alzheimer's & Dementia Capabilities | g g |
| Residents | g g | | |

### DETAILS

Year Built: 2002
Current Mgmt. Since: 2003
No. of Floors: 2
Resident Capacity: 75

### SPECIAL

Diets Accommodated: Diabetic, Low-fat, Low-salt
Proximity to Emergency Svcs.: Under 8 miles
Nearby shopping and entertainment
Pets allowed

### STAFF

Nurse/LVN/LPN: 40 hours/week, On-call 24/7
Caregiver Training: Dementia, Ethics, Family communication, Patient transfers, Stress management
Criminal Background Check: Yes
Principal Staff Language(s): English
Other Staff Language(s): Spanish

### FACILITY FEATURES

Activities/Recreation
Beauty/Barber Shop ($)
Chapel Services
Facility Parking
Guest Meals ($)
Outside Patio/Gardens
Overnight Guest Room ($)
Pharmaceutical Service
Private Dining Room
Room Service
Transportation
24-hour Security

### ROOM FEATURES

Cable TV Ready
Emergency Call System
Grab Bars
Kitchenette
Private Bathrooms
Telephone Ready
Temperature Controls

### COSTS

PRICES MAY INCREASE. PLEASE CALL FOR MOST CURRENT INFORMATION.

| | |
|---|---|
| Studio Apt. | $2,145–$3,425/month |
| One Bedroom Apt. | $2,675–$2,875/month<br>Double occupancy add $500/month |
| Alzheimer's Unit | $3,125/month for shared room |
| Respite Stays | Call for shared room rates |
| Costs of Care | Included in monthly rate |

CAMBRIDGE COURT & MEMORY CARE COMMUNITY (CONTINUED)

| | |
|---|---|
| Rate Increase | Annually |
| Reimbursement | LTCI, Private pay |
| Security Deposit | $100 (refundable) |

### PORTRAIT

Cambridge Court is located south of Highway 80 and east of Interstate 635, nestled in a quiet residential area, minutes from shopping and other local businesses. The grand portico at the entrance is surrounded by trimmed lawns and manicured flowerbeds.

All residents' rooms have windows. Residents furnish and decorate the rooms to suit their tastes. The dining room doubles as an activity space, comfortably furnished with tables and chairs. The menu on the day of our visit featured fried entrées with few alternatives. The building is illuminated with soft artificial lighting. Hallways are spacious and well-kept; handrails are more decorative than functional.

The well-groomed outdoor area provides lovely walkways for residents to stroll. We observed residents lounging on patio furniture and enjoying the warm weather. Another group was participating in a scheduled art activity. The event calendar listed fitness instruction, church services, baking and arts and crafts. Residents and staff greeted each other pleasantly throughout the day. The staff seemed very attentive to residents' needs. Although the administrator and marketing representative were both fairly new to management, they interacted warmly with residents. The marketing representative shared her excitement about the arrival of a new resident who might help initiate participation from the rest of the Memory Care unit.

## CARRIAGE HOUSE ASSISTED LIVING

1357 Bernard Street
Denton, TX 76201

(940) 484-1066
www.carriagehouseofdenton.com

### GILBERT GUIDE OBSERVATIONS

| | | | |
|---|---|---|---|
| Administration & Staff | g g | Residents | g g g |
| Facility Aesthetics | g g g | Dietary & Food Selection | g g g |
| Facility Condition & Safety | g g g | Activities | g g g g |

### DETAILS

Year Built: 1990
Current Mgmt. Since: Unknown
No. of Floors: 1
Resident Capacity: 80

### SPECIAL

Mild dementia care provided
Diets Accommodated: Diabetic, Low-fat, Low-salt, Renal
Proximity to Emergency Svcs.: Under 8 miles
Nearby shopping and entertainment
Pets allowed

## STAFF

Nurse/LVN/LPN: 40 hours/week, On-call 24/7
Caregiver Training: Stress management
Criminal Background Check: Yes
Principal Staff Language(s): English

## FACILITY FEATURES

Activities/Recreation
Beauty/Barber Shop ($)
Outside Patio/Gardens
Private Dining Room
Transportation
24-hour Security

## ROOM FEATURES

Cable TV Ready
Emergency Call System
Grab Bars
Kitchenette
Private Bathrooms
Telephone Ready ($)
Temperature Controls

## COSTS

PRICES MAY INCREASE. PLEASE CALL FOR MOST CURRENT INFORMATION.

| | |
|---|---|
| Studio Apt. | $2,075–$2,275/month |
| One Bedroom Apt. | $2,600/month<br>Double occupancy add $750/month |
| Costs of Care | $450–$1,300/month based on individual need |
| Rate Increase | Annually; usually 1% |
| Reimbursement | LTCI, Private pay |
| Security Deposit | $800 |

## PORTRAIT

Carriage House is just minutes away from Interstate 35, the University of North Texas, and downtown Denton. A groomed lawn surrounds the exterior of the facility. Wingback chairs and coffee tables in the spacious entry make for an atmosphere not unlike a library. The facility's cozy restaurant-style dining area is furnished with sturdy chairs, and tables topped with pretty flower arrangements. A combination of sunlight and fluorescent lighting illuminate the facility.

Residents decorate their rooms with personal belongings to create a homey feeling. Some of the rooms feature bay windows and skylights. The bathrooms have walk-in showers, skid-resistant tiles and handy grab bars. Watching movies in the TV room and reading daily newspapers are among residents' favorite activities. Daily activities, such as games and arts and crafts, give residents an opportunity to socialize. Listening to music is another resident favorite.

One unique aspect of Carriage House is that it provides annual health assessments and temporary illness care for its residents.

## Caruth Haven Court

5585 Caruth Haven Lane
Dallas, TX 75225

(214) 368-8545
www.caruthhavencourt.com

### GILBERT GUIDE OBSERVATIONS

| | | | |
|---|---|---|---|
| Administration & Staff | g g g | Residents | g g g g |
| Facility Aesthetics | g g g g g | Dietary & Food Selection | g g g g g |
| Facility Condition & Safety | g g g g g | Activities | g g g |

### DETAILS

Year Built: 1999
Current Mgmt. Since: 1999
No. of Floors: 3
Resident Capacity: 91

### SPECIAL

Mild dementia care provided
Diets Accommodated: Diabetic, Low-fat, Low-salt, Renal
Proximity to Emergency Svcs.: Under 8 miles
Nearby shopping and entertainment
Pets allowed

### STAFF

Nurse/LVN/LPN: 56 hours/week, On-call 24/7
Caregiver Training: Dementia, Ethics, Family communication, Grief, Patient transfers, Transition issues
Criminal Background Check: Yes
Principal Staff Language(s): English
Other Staff Language(s): Spanish

### FACILITY FEATURES

Activities/Recreation
Beauty/Barber Shop ($)
Chapel Services
Facility Parking
Guest Meals ($)
Outside Patio/Gardens
Pharmaceutical Service
Room Service ($)
Transportation
24-hour Security

### ROOM FEATURES

Cable TV Ready
Emergency Call System
Grab Bars
Kitchenette
Private Bathrooms
Telephone Ready
Temperature Controls

### COSTS

PRICES MAY INCREASE. PLEASE CALL FOR MOST CURRENT INFORMATION.

| | |
|---|---|
| Studio Apt. | $3,500–$3,700/month |
| One Bedroom Apt. | $4,502–$5,600/month<br>Double occupancy add $600/month |
| Two Bedroom Apt. | $7,500–$8,000/month<br>Double occupancy add $600/month |
| Respite Stays | $150/day for private room |
| Costs of Care | $200–$1,000/month based on individual need |
| Rate Increase | Annually; usually 4% |

| | |
|---|---|
| Reimbursement | LTCI, Private pay |
| Application Fee | $1,000 |
| Security Deposit | $1,000 (refundable) |
| Pet Deposit | $500 (refundable) |

**PORTRAIT**

Caruth Haven Court is located in an upscale neighborhood off of Central Expressway just minutes from banking, restaurants and the famed NorthPark Mall. The property's colorful shrubbery and shapely hedges are beautifully trimmed. The two front porches, furnished with rattan rocking chairs, overlook a beautiful fountain and a nearby birdfeeder. The lobby is a comfortably furnished seating area where residents may browse the bookshelves, compose letters at the writing desk, or brew a fresh pot of coffee for morning gatherings. The concierge, administrative offices, living and dining rooms and residents' mailboxes are all on the first floor. The facility is brightened by a combination of natural and artificial lighting.

An elegant stairwell leads upstairs to the residents' rooms. High ceilings impart a spacious feel to the rooms, which are carpeted in green. Each has windows that let in natural light, large closets with mirrored doors and a lighted vanity. Meals are served restaurant-style in the dining room, which features a lovely view of the garden and the gazebo. Residents who require special assistance dine on the third floor to reduce their walking distance. The tinkling sounds of the grand piano in the comfortable living room can often be heard throughout the facility. The screened porch is an excellent spot for outdoor lounging. Residents stroll along trimmed walkways or gather in the charming gazebo in the garden. The spacious hallways are equipped with handrails. Cozy furnished areas throughout the halls invite residents to socialize. Caruth's event calendar is brimming with activities. The activity director schedules movie nights, gardening and field trips to neighboring suburbs, retail shops and bookstores. During the recent Thanksgiving feast, management arranged for a musician to entertain the residents with a piano performance.

## C.C. Young & The Cove A/D

4829 Lawther Lane
Dallas, TX 75214

(214) 827-8080
www.ccyoung.org

**GILBERT GUIDE OBSERVATIONS**

| | | | |
|---|---|---|---|
| Administration & Staff | g g g | Dietary & Food Selection | g g g g |
| Facility Aesthetics | g g g | Activities | g g g |
| Facility Condition & Safety | g g g | Alzheimer's & Dementia Capabilities | g g g |
| Residents | g g g | | |

C.C. YOUNG & THE COVE (CONTINUED)

### DETAILS
Year Built: 1922
Year Remodeled: 1999
Current Mgmt. Since: 1917
No. of Floors: 4
Resident Capacity: 65 (AL), 54 (ALZ)

### SPECIAL
Diets Accommodated: Diabetic
Proximity to Emergency Svcs.: Under 8 miles
Nearby shopping and entertainment
Pets allowed

### STAFF
Nurse/LVN/LPN: Onsite 24/7
Caregiver Training: Dementia, Ethics, Family communication, Patient transfers, Stress management
Criminal Background Check: Yes
Principal Staff Language(s): English
Other Staff Language(s): Spanish

### FACILITY FEATURES
Activities/Recreation
Beauty/Barber Shop
Chapel Services
Facility Parking
Guest Meals
Outside Patio/Gardens
Pharmaceutical Service
Transportation
24-hour Security

### ROOM FEATURES
Cable TV Ready
Emergency Call System
Furnished
Grab Bars
Kitchenette
Shared & Private Bathrooms
Telephone Ready
Temperature Controls

### COSTS
PRICES MAY INCREASE. PLEASE CALL FOR MOST CURRENT INFORMATION.

| | |
|---|---|
| Studio Apt. | $2,603/month |
| One Bedroom Apt. | $3,043/month<br>Double occupancy add $559/month |
| Alzheimer's Unit | $122/day for shared room<br>$157/day for private room |
| Costs of Care | Included in monthly and daily rates |
| Rate Increase | Annually; usually 1–5% |
| Reimbursement | LTCI, Private pay |
| Application Fee | $250 |
| Security Deposit | $3,000 (refundable) |

### PORTRAIT
C.C. Young's retirement community is spread out over twenty acres of manicured landscaping. The property, which overlooks White Rock Lake, is close to entertainment and medical facilities. We observed a group of residents waiting for the bus, alert and eager for their ride around town. The entrance to the Alzheimer's unit is secured.

Residents' snug living quarters are intended to encourage them to devote more time in the common areas socializing with one another. The look is somewhat institutional, but residents decorate to suit their tastes. The main activity room, adjacent to the dining room, is a spacious and bright atmosphere. Residents enjoy 1920s music while lounging on the plush furniture. A decorative quilt hangs next to a lovely wall calendar. Soft lighting from hanging lamps is a nice accent to the sunlight that already brightens the facility. Residents often play the piano, watch television or entertain themselves in the puzzle room. Appetizing selections such as chicken fried steak, grilled vegetables, mashed potatoes and assorted fruit pies are regular menu options. An alternate menu of lighter entrées is also available. Activities are routinely scheduled after dinner.

Beautifully groomed outdoor areas offer quiet refuge. One area sports a fountain and a raised planter for residents to plant seasonal blossoms. Another features comfortable patio chairs. The long halls are equipped with handrails. Residents with dementia might find the expansive layout somewhat disconcerting at first, but from their station, nurses have a clear vantage point of the residents' rooms, which helps them to quickly identify and alleviate any confusion.

## Chambrel at Club Hill

1321 Colonel Drive
Garland, TX 75043

(972) 278-8500
www.brookdaleliving.com

---

**GILBERT GUIDE OBSERVATIONS**

| | | | |
|---|---|---|---|
| Administration & Staff | g g g g g | Residents | g g g g |
| Facility Aesthetics | g g g g g | Dietary & Food Selection | g g g |
| Facility Condition & Safety | g g g g g | Activities | g g g g |

### DETAILS

Year Built: 1987
Year Remodeled: Ongoing
Current Mgmt. Since: 2002
No. of Floors: 3
Resident Capacity: 134

### SPECIAL

Mild dementia care provided
Diets Accommodated: Diabetic, Low-fat, Low-salt
Proximity to Emergency Svcs.: Under 8 miles
Nearby shopping and entertainment
Pets allowed

### STAFF

Nurse/LVN/LPN: Onsite 24/7
Caregiver Training: Dementia, Ethics, Family communication, Grief, Patient transfers, Stress management, Transition issues
Criminal Background Check: Yes
Principal Staff Language(s): English
Other Staff Language(s): Russian, Spanish

CHAMBREL AT CLUB HILL (CONTINUED)

**FACILITY FEATURES**

Activities/Recreation
Beauty/Barber Shop ($)
Chapel Services
Computer/Internet Access
Facility Parking
Fitness Room/Gym
Guest Meals ($)
Outside Patio/Gardens
Overnight Guest Room ($)
Pharmaceutical Service
Private Dining Room
Room Service
24-hour Security

**ROOM FEATURES**

Cable TV Ready
Emergency Call System
Grab Bars
Kitchenette
Private Bathrooms
Telephone Ready
Temperature Controls

**COSTS**

PRICES MAY INCREASE. PLEASE CALL FOR MOST CURRENT INFORMATION.

| | |
|---|---|
| Studio Apt. | $1,900–$2,210/month |
| One Bedroom Apt. | $2,310–$2,710/month<br>Double occupancy add $350/month |
| Two Bedroom Apt. | $2,935–$3,155/month<br>Double occupancy add $450/month |
| Costs of Care | $50–$700/month based on individual need |
| Rate Increase | Annually; usually 3% |
| Reimbursement | Private pay |
| Application Fee | $200 |
| Security Deposit | One month's rent (refundable) |
| Pet Deposit | $500 |

**PORTRAIT**

Chambrel offers a country club atmosphere in an upscale facility. The attractively landscaped campus sits on a tranquil street where green belt of lawn separates the cluster of buildings from a shopping area. The bridge spanning a fish pond and a bubbling fountain provides access to Chambrel from the main building. The concierge welcomes visitors to the main building, which houses the dining area and gym. All outer doors are locked to prevent intruders; residents and their families have card keys.

The lobby features a large aquarium with colorful fish. Options abound with seven different floor plans. Some of the rooms boast outdoor patios. The recessed cabinets in the bathrooms are wheelchair-accessible and the walk-in showers have seats and handheld showerheads. Each room comes with additional storage space.

Chambrel is licensed as ambulatory, which means that all residents must be able to evacuate the building without assistance. Skylights and arched windows flood the hallways with sunlight. The tables in the formal dining area are set with linen tablecloths and napkins. Assigned seating enables staff to quickly recognize any absences.

Residents engaged in animated conversation as they waited for dinner and chatted with staff at the nurses' desk. The staff seemed well acquainted with the residents, even greeting family members by name. Many of the staff members, including aides, CNAs and administration, have been at Chambrel for several years. The roster of activities includes Red Hat Society meetings, a men's club, daily current events discussions and a low-vision support group. A popular family night celebration occurs every other month. This facility is typically at capacity, with a waiting list.

## Courtyard at Christian Care A/D

950 Wiggins Parkway
Mesquite, TX 75150

(972) 698-2626, (972) 698-2628
www.christiancarecenters.org

---

**GILBERT GUIDE OBSERVATIONS**

| | | | |
|---|---|---|---|
| Administration & Staff | g g g | Dietary & Food Selection | g g g |
| Facility Aesthetics | g g g | Activities | g g |
| Facility Condition & Safety | g g g | Alzheimer's & Dementia Capabilities | g g g |
| Residents | g g | | |

### DETAILS

Year Built: 2002
Current Mgmt. Since: 2002
No. of Floors: 2
Resident Capacity: 44

### SPECIAL

Alzheimer's/Dementia Only Facility
Diets Accommodated: Diabetic, Low-fat, Low-salt
Proximity to Emergency Svcs.: Under 8 miles
Nearby shopping and entertainment
Pet visits allowed

### STAFF

Nurse/LVN/LPN: On-call 24/7
Caregiver Training: Dementia, Ethics, Family communication, Grief, Stress management, Transition issues
Criminal Background Check: Yes
Principal Staff Language(s): English
Other Staff Language(s): Spanish

### FACILITY FEATURES

Activities/Recreation
Beauty/Barber Shop ($)
Chapel Services
Facility Parking
Guest Meals ($)
Outside Patio/Gardens

### ROOM FEATURES

Cable TV Ready
Emergency Call System
Grab Bars
Private Bathrooms
Telephone Ready
Temperature Controls

COURTYARD AT CHRISTIAN CARE (CONTINUED)

**FACILITY FEATURES (CONTINUED)**

Private Dining Room
24-hour Security

## COSTS

PRICES MAY INCREASE. PLEASE CALL FOR MOST CURRENT INFORMATION.

| | |
|---|---|
| Alzheimer's Unit | $3,780–$4,732/month for private room |
| Costs of Care | Included in monthly rate |
| Rate Increase | Annually; usually 3–4% |
| Reimbursement | Private pay |
| Application Fee | $40 |
| Security Deposit | $500 |

## PORTRAIT

Courtyard sits on the large Christian Care campus. Sliding glass doors open onto the somewhat dim lobby. The secured area for Alzheimer's residents is much brighter, however, and features a plethora of windows and recessed lighting. There is a seating area at the end of the hall. Artwork, and bulletin boards covered with photographs of the residents, hang on the walls. The nurses' office features a library stocked with books and information on dementia; family members and caregivers have found these resources invaluable.

Residents often dine on the outdoor patio in pleasant weather, where there are picnic tables and umbrellas. A secure walking path is available for residents' use. Both dining rooms, one on each floor, are used for activities. Bright wallpaper adds cheer. The facility uses practical furnishings, such as chairs with sturdy arms, that make it easy for residents to sit and rise on their own. The aides in the dining area seem particularly well-acquainted with residents. Snacks are offered during most of the activities. The carpeted living room, which features an electric fireplace and large TV, doubles as the main activity room. An additional room upstairs is used for private dining, doctors' visits and a few activities.

The staff makes a point of actively encouraging residents to participate in activities. The activities director has been in place since the facility opened. There is an activity planned every evening, but few are scheduled on the weekends, when family members tend to visit. We noted an impressive number of volunteers in various roles.

## Covenant Place of Waxahachie

401 Solon Road
Waxahachie, TX 75165

(972) 923-9911
www.thecovenantgroup.com

### GILBERT GUIDE OBSERVATIONS

| | | | |
|---|---|---|---|
| Administration & Staff | g g g g g | Residents | g g g g |
| Facility Aesthetics | g g g g | Dietary & Food Selection | g g g |
| Facility Condition & Safety | g g g g g | Activities | g g g g g |

### DETAILS

Year Built: 1999
Current Mgmt. Since: 1999
No. of Floors: 1
Resident Capacity: 62

### SPECIAL

Mild dementia care provided
Diets Accommodated: Diabetic, Low-fat, Low-salt, Renal
Proximity to Emergency Svcs.: Under 8 miles
Nearby shopping and entertainment
Pets allowed

### STAFF

Nurse/LVN/LPN: 40 hours/week, On-call 24/7
Caregiver Training: Dementia, Ethics, Family communication, Patient transfers, Stress management
Criminal Background Check: Yes
Principal Staff Language(s): English
Other Staff Language(s): Spanish

### FACILITY FEATURES

Activities/Recreation
Beauty/Barber Shop ($)
Chapel Services
Facility Parking
Guest Meals ($)
Outside Patio/Gardens
Pharmaceutical Service
Private Dining Room
Separate Therapy Room
Transportation

### ROOM FEATURES

Cable TV Ready ($)
Emergency Call System
Grab Bars
Kitchenette
Private Bathrooms
Telephone Ready ($)
Temperature Controls

### COSTS

PRICES MAY INCREASE. PLEASE CALL FOR MOST CURRENT INFORMATION.

| | |
|---|---|
| Studio Apt. | $2,470–$3,370/month |
| One Bedroom Apt. | $2,570–$3,470/month |
| | Double occupancy add $400–$1,300/month |
| Costs of Care | Included in monthly rate |
| Rate Increase | Annually; usually 2–4% |
| Reimbursement | LTCI, Private pay, SSI, Veterans |
| Security Deposit | $500 (refundable) |

COVENANT PLACE OF WAXAHACHIE (CONTINUED)

## PORTRAIT

Covenant Place of Waxahachie may seem an unlikely place to find love but that is just what Mary, seventy-eight, and Harold, seventy-four, found with each other. Mary lived at the facility for three years before Harold moved in and caught her eye. In addition to the occasional romance, some of the more usual activities include bingo, exercise, worship, sing-alongs and trivia games. We observed staff members leading residents in a baking activity as well as a stretching class. Residents tend a large garden in the courtyard, which also features a walkway and a number of benches. A sunroom overlooks the landscaped grounds. The library holds a vast array of books, which ranges from history to fantasy. The activity room is furnished with tables, a refrigerator, a stove and a popcorn maker.

The U.S. flag snaps in the breeze in front of the red brick building. A tall gray fireplace dominates the foyer, where artificial trees highlight green accents in the maroon carpet. Mahogany chairs upholstered in pink and white encircle a wrought iron table. Oil paintings adorn the walls. A combination of artificial and natural light brightens the facility. Handrails edge the broad hallways. Beige carpet extends from wall to wall in residents' moderately sized rooms. Each of the rooms is clearly labeled with the occupant's name. All feature spacious showers.

American food is a staple here, but once a week Mexican meals such as chili con carne, cheese enchiladas and Spanish rice are featured. Tomato soup and grilled cheese sandwiches were offered on the day of our visit. Fixtures accented in gold shed light on the oil paintings that decorate the dining area, where floral-patterned upholstered chairs surround the dining tables. A floor-to-ceiling mirror also trimmed in gold, a china cabinet and an oak table furnish the luxurious private dining room.

## GRACE PRESBYTERIAN & GRACE PRESBYTERIAN VILLAGE A/D

550 East Ann Arbor
Dallas, TX 75216

(214) 376-1701
www.gracepresbyterianvillage.org

---

**GILBERT GUIDE OBSERVATIONS**

| | | | |
|---|---|---|---|
| Administration & Staff | g g g | Dietary & Food Selection | g g g g g |
| Facility Aesthetics | g g g g | Activities | g g g |
| Facility Condition & Safety | g g g g g | Alzheimer's & Dementia Capabilities | g g g g |
| Residents | g g g | | |

**DETAILS**

Year Built: 1962
Year Remodeled: 2001
Current Mgmt. Since: 1999

**SPECIAL**

Diets Accommodated: Diabetic, Low-fat, Low-salt, Renal
Proximity to Emergency Svcs.: Under 8 miles

DETAILS (CONTINUED)
No. of Floors: 2
Resident Capacity: 160 (AL), 60 (ALZ)

SPECIAL (CONTINUED)
Nearby shopping and entertainment
Pets allowed

## STAFF

Nurse/LVN/LPN: 24 hours/week, On-call 24/7
Caregiver Training: Dementia, Family communication, Grief, Stress management
Criminal Background Check: Yes
Principal Staff Language(s): English
Other Staff Language(s): Spanish

## FACILITY FEATURES

Activities/Recreation
Beauty/Barber Shop ($)
Chapel Services
Computer/Internet Access
Facility Parking
Fitness Room/Gym
Guest Meals
Outside Patio/Gardens
Overnight Guest Room ($)
Pharmaceutical Service
Private Dining Room
Separate Therapy Room
Transportation to MD Appointments, Personal Outings, Scheduled Outings
24-hour Security

## ROOM FEATURES

Cable TV Ready ($)
Emergency Call System
Furnished
Grab Bars
Kitchenette
Private Bathrooms
Telephone Ready ($)
Temperature Controls

## COSTS

PRICES MAY INCREASE. PLEASE CALL FOR MOST CURRENT INFORMATION.

| | |
|---|---|
| Studio Apt. | $1,398–$1,868/month |
| One Bedroom Apt. | $2,855–$2,990/month |
| Respite Stays | $119–$133/day for shared room, $165–$252/day for private room |
| Costs of Care | Included in monthly rate |
| Rate Increase | Annually |
| Reimbursement | LTCI, Private pay, SSI, Veterans |
| Application Fee | $500 (portion applied to rent/security deposit) |
| Security Deposit | $500 |
| Pet Deposit | $250 (refundable) |

## PORTRAIT

Grace Presbyterian and its sister Alzheimer's facility share a lovely wooded campus. Trails and walkways meander throughout the twenty-seven acres, punctuated by mature shade trees, flowers and creeks. A striking glass walkway links the skilled nursing and assisted living areas.

Shadow boxes outside of residents' rooms contain photographs and personal items to aid residents with recall. The bathroom entrances in residents' small rooms are highly visible, to assist those who have difficulty seeing at night. The lighting is soft and colors are muted in

GRACE PRESBYTERIAN & GRACE PRESBYTERIAN VILLAGE (CONTINUED)

the Alzheimer's facility, which is illuminated by overhead fixtures and lamps. The hallways are wide and equipped with handrails.

There was an array of appetizing entrées when we visited, including baked chicken and meatloaf. Snacks are available all day. The large dining area in the Alzheimer's unit has a 1950s diner motif. In contrast, the common areas feature modern TVs, couches and chairs. All areas are comfortable and well maintained. The dining room boasts views of the front courtyard and garden and provides a good vantage point for residents and staff to enjoy viewing the many species of birds that are native to the area. The landscaped outdoor areas are all comfortably furnished. A family of rabbits living in one of the patio areas provides entertainment for the residents.

The staff is very attentive to the residents and we noted a friendly connection between them. Because many of the residents are hard of hearing, the staff takes care to speak loudly and clearly. The activities calendar lists bingo, ceramics, movie night and religious services, among others. One resident told us that she enjoys relaxing in the jacuzzi.

## Hearthstone of Garland

1246 Colonel Drive
Garland, TX 75043

(972) 278-4004
www.hearthstoneassisted.com

**GILBERT GUIDE OBSERVATIONS**

| | | | |
|---|---|---|---|
| Administration & Staff | g g g | Residents | g g g g |
| Facility Aesthetics | g g g g | Dietary & Food Selection | g g g g g |
| Facility Condition & Safety | g g g g g | Activities | g g g g |

**DETAILS**

Year Built: 1999
Year Remodeled: Ongoing
Current Mgmt. Since: 1999
No. of Floors: 1
Resident Capacity: 118

**SPECIAL**

Mild dementia care provided
Diets Accommodated: Diabetic, Low-salt
Proximity to Emergency Svcs.: Under 8 miles
Nearby shopping and entertainment
Some pets allowed

**STAFF**

Nurse/LVN/LPN: 40 hours/week, On-call 24/7
Caregiver Training: Dementia, Ethics, Family communication, Grief, Patient transfers, Stress management, Transition issues, Validation therapy
Criminal Background Check: Yes
Principal Staff Language(s): English
Other Staff Language(s): Spanish

### FACILITY FEATURES

Activities/Recreation
Beauty/Barber Shop ($)
Chapel Services
Facility Parking
Guest Meals ($)
Outside Patio/Gardens
Pharmaceutical Service ($)
Private Dining Room
Room Service
Transportation
24-hour Security

### ROOM FEATURES

Cable TV Ready
Emergency Call System
Grab Bars
Kitchenette
Private Bathrooms
Telephone Ready
Temperature Controls

### COSTS

PRICES MAY INCREASE. PLEASE CALL FOR MOST CURRENT INFORMATION.

| | |
|---|---|
| Studio Apt. | $1,995/month |
| Two Bedroom Apt. | $2,995–$3,345/month |
| Costs of Care | $175–$1,025/month based on individual need |
| Rate Increase | Annually; usually 3% |
| Reimbursement | Private pay |
| Application Fee | $1,750 |
| Pet Deposit | $250 (refundable) |

### PORTRAIT

Near the busy intersection of Broadway and Centerville, Hearthstone Garland is nevertheless a quiet and private refuge. The shady front porch with wicker rockers is our first glimpse of this slice of Southern comfort.

The spacious hallways are a decorated tribute to residents and staff. Hearthstone staff considers getting to know each other vital to the community environment they foster. Residents display personal items outside their rooms, giving passersby a clue to their identity. A bulletin board designated for photos of residents and staff promotes further familiarity with one another. Staff members "adopt" new residents during their first month to help ease the transition. The facility surrounds a screened porch that opens onto a beautifully groomed, enclosed courtyard. During the winter, the screens are covered with plexiglass so that residents can relax outside in warmth. Benches line curved sidewalks, manicured flowerbeds and various shrubs. The dining room is appealing with its skylights, vaulted ceiling and dark green carpeting. The menu changes regularly. Aside from basic meal plans, residents enjoy room service with snacks like sandwiches and milk, as well as a 24-hour beverage bar with coffee, tea and juice.

Residents use an area adjacent to the dining room for "messy" activities like cooking.
Other regular activities include dominoes, card games and bingo—all take place in the activity parlor. Residents also have the option of attending weekly mass. During our visit, the director proudly informed us that over half of the residents attend musical events regularly, and 100% of the residents participated in family night that month.

## Hearthstone of Irving

2425 Texas Drive
Irving, TX 75062

(972) 659-6800
(801) 830-9060
www.hearthstoneassisted.com

---

**GILBERT GUIDE OBSERVATIONS**

| | | | |
|---|---|---|---|
| Administration & Staff | g g g g g | Residents | g g g g g |
| Facility Aesthetics | g g g g g | Dietary & Food Selection | g g g g g |
| Facility Condition & Safety | g g g g g | Activities | g g g g g |

### DETAILS

Year Built: 1999
Current Mgmt. Since: 1999
No. of Floors: 1
Resident Capacity: 90

### SPECIAL

Mild dementia care provided
Diets Accommodated: Low-fat, Low-salt
Proximity to Emergency Svcs.: Under 8 miles
Nearby shopping and entertainment
Pets allowed

### STAFF

Nurse/LVN/LPN: 20 hours/week, On-call 24/7
Caregiver Training: Dementia, Ethics, Family communication, Grief, Patient transfers, Stress management, Transition issues, Validation therapy
Criminal Background Check: Yes
Principal Staff Language(s): English
Other Staff Language(s): Spanish

### FACILITY FEATURES

Activities/Recreation
Beauty/Barber Shop ($)
Chapel Services
Facility Parking
Guest Meals ($)
Outside Patio/Gardens
Private Dining Room ($)
Room Service
Separate Therapy Room
Transportation
24-hour Security

### ROOM FEATURES

Cable TV Ready ($)
Emergency Call System
Grab Bars
Kitchenette
Private Bathrooms
Telephone Ready ($)
Temperature Controls

### COSTS

PRICES MAY INCREASE. PLEASE CALL FOR MOST CURRENT INFORMATION.

| | |
|---|---|
| Studio Apt. | $2,895–$2,945/month |
| One Bedroom Apt. | $3,295/month<br>Double occupancy add $1,995/month |
| Two Bedroom Apt. | $4,790/month |
| Costs of Care | $175–$425/month based on individual need |
| Rate Increase | Annually; usually 2–3% |
| Reimbursement | Private pay |

| | |
|---|---|
| Entrance Fee | $1,500 |
| Pet Deposit | $250 |

**PORTRAIT**

Hearthstone is located in a quiet neighborhood off of Highway 183. The circular driveway that leads to the attractive brick building showcases its manicured landscape of boxwood shrubs, crepe myrtles, pansies and freshly cut lawns. As we entered the building, residents greeted us in the foyer—a spacious seating area with rich green carpeting, maroon couches and chairs, dark wooden tables and a fireplace. 1930 Chevy model trucks decorate the mantle. The artificial lighting in the building is complemented by an abundance of natural light. Broad hallways are equipped with handrails; there are furnished rest areas throughout.

Residents' rooms are moderately sized. Each has a large window and is furnished according to preference. The rooms vary in pastel colors and furnishings, some of which are antique, others contemporary. Common areas are located in the four corners of the building and offer different types of entertainment. Depending on their mood, residents can listen to their favorite radio show, socialize or work on puzzles. The dining room is an elegant setting of chandeliers and tables draped with white linen. The kitchen staff prepares appetizing selections such as beef burgundy, rice pilaf, baby carrots and key lime pie. The staff uses color-coded plates to identify the specific dietary needs of each resident.

The center courtyard is equipped with patio furniture as well as a barbeque. Lush landscapes of palm fronds, elephant's ears, seasonal flowers and shrubs surround a decorative fountain. Residents are encouraged to use their green thumbs in this area. Organized activities include bingo, dominoes and field trips to local stores and the library. Hearthstone's Red Hat Society hosts meetings, social events and luncheons. One staff member informed us that an open-door policy allows residents, families and staff to communicate with management at any time.

## JACKSON LIVING CENTER

1250 Abrams Road
Dallas, TX 75214

(214) 827-0813
www.fowlerhomes.org

**GILBERT GUIDE OBSERVATIONS**

| | | | |
|---|---|---|---|
| Administration & Staff | g g g g g | Residents | g g g |
| Facility Aesthetics | g g g g g | Dietary & Food Selection | g g g g g |
| Facility Condition & Safety | g g g g g | Activities | g g g g g |

JACKSON LIVING CENTER (CONTINUED)

### DETAILS

Year Built: 2001
Current Mgmt. Since: 2001
No. of Floors: 2
Resident Capacity: 32

### SPECIAL

Mild dementia care provided
Diets Accommodated: Diabetic, Low-fat, Low-salt, Renal
Proximity to Emergency Svcs.: Under 8 miles
Nearby shopping and entertainment
Some pets allowed

### STAFF

Nurse/LVN/LPN: Onsite 24/7
Caregiver Training: Dementia, Family communication, Grief, Patient transfers, Stress management
Criminal Background Check: Yes
Principal Staff Language(s): English
Other Staff Language(s): Spanish

### FACILITY FEATURES

Activities/Recreation
Beauty/Barber Shop ($)
Chapel Services
Facility Parking
Fitness Room/Gym
Guest Meals ($)
Outside Patio/Gardens
Pharmaceutical Service
Private Dining Room
Separate Therapy Room
Transportation to MD Appointments ($), Personal Outings ($), Scheduled Outings
24-hour Security

### ROOM FEATURES

Cable TV Ready
Emergency Call System
Grab Bars
Kitchenette
Private Bathrooms
Telephone Ready
Temperature Controls

### COSTS

PRICES MAY INCREASE. PLEASE CALL FOR MOST CURRENT INFORMATION.

| | |
|---|---|
| Studio Apt. | $2,375–$2,455/month |
| One Bedroom Apt. | $2,765/month |
| Costs of Care | $200–$800/month based on individual need |
| Rate Increase | Annually; usually 2% |
| Reimbursement | LTCI, Private pay, SSI, Veterans |
| Application Fee | $250 |
| Security Deposit | $750 |
| Pet Deposit | $350 (refundable) |

### PORTRAIT

Jackson Living Center sits on a sixteen-acre campus, which is also the home of Pearl Nordan Care Center and Fowler Christian Apartments, an independent living complex for seniors. The campus is mere minutes from parks, shopping centers and downtown Dallas. A cherry-wood reception desk, nearly fifteen feet long, dominates the atrium. The facility's dark green carpeting is interspersed with floral patterns. Spiral staircases rise to the second floor. Handrails and botanical paintings line the walls of the extra-wide hallways. Natural lighting brightens the facility. Textured walls and crown moldings add luxurious elements to the sunny residents' rooms.

Pink, red, and white tablecloths dress the dining room tables. Staff members kindly invited us to share the midday snack of cookies and hot chocolate. The chefs prepared tomato soup and turkey sandwiches for lunch that day. The staff at Jackson Living Center interacted with residents as if they were old friends.

Popular activities include dancing, playing ping pong and swimming. Residents also enjoy attending chapel services, weekly outings and tea with Marla, a local musician. We saw residents walking the hallways and playing chess in the library. Several other were picnicking outside, beneath towering maple and cedar trees. Pathways meander through the grass and past sundials in the garden.

## Kingsley Place at Stonebridge Ranch

1650 South Stonebridge Drive
McKinney, TX 75070
(972) 529-1420
www.emeritus.com

---

### GILBERT GUIDE OBSERVATIONS

| | | | |
|---|---|---|---|
| Administration & Staff | g g g g g | Residents | g g g g g |
| Facility Aesthetics | g g g g g | Dietary & Food Selection | g g g g g |
| Facility Condition & Safety | g g g g g | Activities | g g g g g |

### DETAILS

Year Built: 1998
Year Remodeled: Ongoing
Current Mgmt. Since: Unknown
No. of Floors: 1
Resident Capacity: 80

### SPECIAL

Mild dementia care provided
Diets Accommodated: Diabetic, Low-fat, Low-salt
Proximity to Emergency Svcs.: Under 8 miles
Nearby shopping and entertainment
Pets allowed

### STAFF

Nurse/LVN/LPN: 40 hours/week
Caregiver Training: Dementia, Ethics, Family communication, Stress management
Criminal Background Check: Yes
Principal Staff Language(s): English

KINGSLEY PLACE AT STONEBRIDGE RANCH (CONTINUED)

**FACILITY FEATURES**

Activities/Recreation
Beauty/Barber Shop ($)
Chapel Services
Facility Parking
Guest Meals
Outside Patio/Gardens
Pharmaceutical Service ($)
Room Service
Separate Therapy Room
Transportation to MD Appointments, Scheduled Outings

**ROOM FEATURES**

Cable TV Ready
Emergency Call System
Grab Bars
Kitchenette
Private Bathrooms
Telephone Ready ($)
Temperature Controls

**COSTS**

PRICES MAY INCREASE. PLEASE CALL FOR MOST CURRENT INFORMATION.

| | |
|---|---|
| Shared Room | $1,800/month |
| Studio Apt. | $2,435/month |
| One Bedroom Apt. | $2,540–$2,905/month |
| Costs of Care | $325–$950/month based on individual need |
| Rate Increase | Every 18–24 months |
| Reimbursement | Private pay, Veterans |
| Entrance Fee | $1,000 |
| Pet Deposit | $250 |

**PORTRAIT**

Kingsley Place is a lovely addition to the affluent McKinney area. The building is designed like a grand home with lush landscaping gracing the entrance. The interior is a lavish scene of gold and brass chandeliers, sconces filled with fresh flower arrangements and decorative rugs. Skylights and windows provide plenty of natural light throughout the building. Soft artificial lighting brightens the broad hallways.

Residents' rooms are moderately sized. Many come with French doors that open onto the courtyard. The dining room is furnished with antique pieces. Residents select an entrée, dessert and drink from the menu card prepared by the kitchen staff. The antique bar in the common room hosts happy hours. The furniture in the common areas is upholstered in pretty floral patterns.

The secured courtyard in the center of the building is well-maintained. During our visit, the staff cleared foliage to prepare for fall. Residents at Kingsley Place enjoy theater outings, movies, shopping, arts and crafts, and watching local college activities. We observed approximately forty residents participating in the home's daily exercise program. Kingsley residents enjoy the comfort of an elegant home and the attention of a caring and accommodating staff.

## Loyalton of Lake Highlands A/D

9715 Plano Road
Dallas, TX 75238

(214) 343-7445
www.emeritus.com

### GILBERT GUIDE OBSERVATIONS

| | |
|---|---|
| Administration & Staff | g g g |
| Facility Aesthetics | g g g |
| Facility Condition & Safety | g g g g |
| Residents | g g g |
| Dietary & Food Selection | g g |
| Activities | g g |
| Alzheimer's & Dementia Capabilities | g g g |

### DETAILS

Year Built: 1996
Year Remodeled: 2004
Current Mgmt. Since: 2001
No. of Floors: 1
Resident Capacity: 18

### SPECIAL

Diets Accommodated: Diabetic, Low-fat, Low-salt
Proximity to Emergency Svcs.: Under 8 miles
Nearby shopping and entertainment
No pets allowed

### STAFF

Nurse/LVN/LPN: On-call 24/7
Caregiver Training: Dementia, Ethics, Family communication, Grief, Patient transfers, Stress management, Transition issues, Validation therapy
Criminal Background Check: Yes
Principal Staff Language(s): English
Other Staff Language(s): Spanish

### FACILITY FEATURES

Activities/Recreation
Beauty/Barber Shop ($)
Chapel Services
Facility Parking
Fitness Room/Gym
Guest Meals
Outside Patio/Gardens
Pharmaceutical Service ($)
Private Dining Room
Transportation
24-hour Security

### ROOM FEATURES

Cable TV Ready
Emergency Call System
Grab Bars
Shared & Private Bathrooms
Telephone Ready
Temperature Controls

### COSTS

PRICES MAY INCREASE. PLEASE CALL FOR MOST CURRENT INFORMATION.

| | |
|---|---|
| Shared Room | $1,600/month |
| Private Room | $2,250/month |
| Studio Apt. | $2,450/month |
| One Bedroom Apt. | $2,750/month |
| Alzheimer's Unit | $3,250–$3,450/month for shared room |
| Costs of Care | $300–$1,000/month based on individual need |
| Rate Increase | Annually |

LOYALTON OF LAKE HIGHLANDS (CONTINUED)

| | |
|---|---|
| Reimbursement | LTCI, Private pay |
| Security Deposit | $1,000 |

**PORTRAIT**

Loyalton of Lake Highlands resides on Plano Road, across from a beautiful park. Abundant parking and an emerald lawn dotted with manicured shrubs lay before the red brick facility. The secured Alzheimer's unit is located at the rear of the square building. Soft lighting abounds throughout the interior. Pretty lace curtains dress the expansive windows that line the dining room, which is furnished with dark wood tables and chairs upholstered in blue. The staff members are familiar with each resident's eating preferences, so they ensure that the menu offers those options. The wide hallways are decorated with "life stations" that stimulate residents' memories; one example includes a bassinet and baby clothes, which reminds residents of raising their children. Shadow boxes that feature photographs and mementos hang outside the doors of residents' rooms—these, too, jog residents' memories. Mirrored closet doors, white walls and large windows create a spacious atmosphere in residents' rooms.

The staff informed us that plans to install a fountain in the outdoor patio of the Alzheimer's unit are underway. Residents enjoy growing plants and eating at the picnic tables in this area. A fence separates the patio from the facility's main courtyard. The homey activity room opens to the secured patio. Here, we observed a few residents sitting on couches and watching the fish swim in an aquarium. Others were napping, as our visit took place directly after lunch.

## Medallion Assisted Living & Memory Care Community A/D

12400 Preston Road
Dallas, TX 75230

(972) 661-3111
(214) 500-9705
www.medallionalf.com

**GILBERT GUIDE OBSERVATIONS**

| | | | |
|---|---|---|---|
| Administration & Staff | g g g g | Dietary & Food Selection | g g g |
| Facility Aesthetics | g g g | Activities | g g g |
| Facility Condition & Safety | g g g | Alzheimer's & Dementia Capabilities | g g g g |
| Residents | g g g g | | |

## DETAILS

Year Built: 1997
Year Remodeled: Ongoing
Current Mgmt. Since: 1997
No. of Floors: 2
Resident Capacity: 107

## SPECIAL

Diets Accommodated: Diabetic, Low-salt
Proximity to Emergency Svcs.: Under 8 miles
Nearby shopping and entertainment
No pets allowed

## STAFF

Nurse/LVN/LPN: 40 hours/week, On-call 24/7
Caregiver Training: Dementia, Ethics, Family communication, Grief, Patient transfers, Stress management, Transition issues
Criminal Background Check: Yes
Principal Staff Language(s): English
Other Staff Language(s): Spanish

## FACILITY FEATURES

Activities/Recreation
Beauty/Barber Shop ($)
Facility Parking
Guest Meals ($)
Outside Patio/Gardens
Pharmaceutical Service ($)
Private Dining Room
Separate Therapy Room
Transportation
24-hour Security

## ROOM FEATURES

Cable TV Ready
Emergency Call System
Grab Bars
Private Bathrooms
Telephone Ready ($)
Temperature Controls

## COSTS

PRICES MAY INCREASE. PLEASE CALL FOR MOST CURRENT INFORMATION.

| | |
|---|---|
| Studio Apt. | $2,095–$3,100/month |
| Alzheimer's Unit | $2,095–$3,100/month for private room |
| Respite Stays | $25/day for private room |
| Costs of Care | Included in monthly rate |
| Rate Increase | Annually; usually 1–5% |
| Reimbursement | LTCI, Private pay |

## PORTRAIT

Medallion Assisted Living and Memory Care Community boasts two local advantages: upscale residential surroundings and proximity to Galleria shopping and restaurants on Preston Road. Splendid oak trees border the red brick building. Visitors and residents travel through a long covered walkway, away from the clamor of the street to enter the facility. The interior décor is somewhat dated; the furniture appears well-worn but comfortable. At the time of our visit, the freshly painted walls indicated management's ongoing remodeling project. The secured Alzheimer's unit is located in the main building.

Residents' rooms are small, but each has a view of the street or garden. Residents are encouraged to decorate their rooms to suit their tastes. The dining room, which doubles as the primary common area, is bathed in natural light. The freshly stocked salad bar supplements tasty entrées such as baked chicken and grilled vegetables.

The interior courtyard features lush greenery and soaring oak trees. Residents often relax on comfortable patio furniture or tend to their plants in the "potting station." A varied event calendar that includes morning worship, Shabbat services, fitness instruction, social hour, "movie and popcorn night," sing-alongs and bingo games promotes familiarity. The staff coordinates memory-stimulating tasks, including "life" activities such as table setting, laundry folding and flower arranging for residents with Alzheimer's. We observed a group of residents engaged in pleasant banter on the patio. The friendly staff and residents made our visit an enjoyable one.

## Merrill Gardens (Sterling House on the Parkway)

2525 Lillian Miller Parkway (940) 320-1926
Denton, TX 76210

---

**GILBERT GUIDE OBSERVATIONS**

| | | | |
|---|---|---|---|
| Administration & Staff | g g g g g | Residents | g g g g |
| Facility Aesthetics | g g g g g | Dietary & Food Selection | g g g g g |
| Facility Condition & Safety | g g g g g | Activities | g g g g g |

### DETAILS

Year Built: 1996
Year Remodeled: Ongoing
Current Mgmt. Since: 2006
No. of Floors: 1
Resident Capacity: 44

### SPECIAL

Mild dementia care provided
Diets Accommodated: Diabetic, Low-fat, Low-salt, Renal
Proximity to Emergency Svcs.: Under 8 miles
Nearby shopping and entertainment
Pets allowed

### STAFF

Nurse/LVN/LPN: 40 hours/week, On-call 24/7
Caregiver Training: Dementia, Ethics, Family communication, Grief, Stress management, Transition issues
Criminal Background Check: Yes
Principal Staff Language(s): English

### FACILITY FEATURES

Activities/Recreation
Beauty/Barber Shop ($)
Chapel Services
Facility Parking
Fitness Room/Gym

### ROOM FEATURES

Cable TV Ready ($)
Emergency Call System
Grab Bars
Kitchenette
Private Bathrooms

FACILITY FEATURES (CONTINUED)

Guest Meals
Outside Patio/Gardens
Pharmaceutical Service ($)
Private Dining Room
Transportation to MD Appointments, Personal Outings ($)
24-hour Security

ROOM FEATURES (CONTINUED)

Telephone Ready ($)
Temperature Controls

## COSTS

PRICES MAY INCREASE. PLEASE CALL FOR MOST CURRENT INFORMATION.

| | |
|---|---|
| Studio Apt. | $2,125/month |
| Two Bedroom Apt. | $2,960–$3,375/month |
| Costs of Care | $500–$850/month based on individual need |
| Rate Increase | Annually; usually 2% |
| Reimbursement | Private pay |
| Entrance Fee | $600 |
| Pet Deposit | $400 |

## PORTRAIT

Sterling House on the Parkway, formerly Merrill Gardens of Denton, rests on winding Lillian Miller Parkway. Centrally located in Denton, it offers the conveniences of nearby medical facilities as well as shopping centers. A cordial staff greeted us upon entering the facility, which is bright with artificial lighting. Plentiful seating areas create a comfortable atmosphere. Residents warm themselves by the fireplaces on cold winter evenings and enjoy the sunlight streaming in from the windows. A mixture of artificial and live plants throughout the building adda touches of greenery.

Residents' suites are bright and roomy. Outside each room, residents organize individual displays to introduce others to their personal histories. Hallways are wide and neat. The dining room is spacious enough to easily accommodate wheelchair users. The dinner menu is posted outside the dining hall. An alternative selection is always offered. The lounges and libraries all feature ample seating. On movie nights, residents gather in the fully equipped house theater. Residents seem to love the theater furniture and the authenticity of the popcorn and Coke bar. It is definitely a house favorite!

Walking paths set among the gardens are a peaceful escape. Pretty flowerbeds, blossoming trees and shaped hedges pepper the outdoor landscape. The activity director has arranged a special music therapy program with students from the University of Texas, an activity enjoyed by all. Many residents have become computer savvy through "Touch Town", a senior email program. The staff and residents of Sterling House seemed very comfortable with one another. The staff is familiar not only with the residents but with their families as well; we observed the staff greeting many of the visitors by name.

## Monticello West A/D

5114 McKinney Avenue
Dallas, TX 75205

(214) 528-0660

---

### GILBERT GUIDE OBSERVATIONS

| | | | |
|---|---|---|---|
| Administration & Staff | g g g g | Dietary & Food Selection | g g g |
| Facility Aesthetics | g g g g | Activities | g g g g g |
| Facility Condition & Safety | g g g g | Alzheimer's & Dementia Capabilities | g g g |
| Residents | g g g | | |

### DETAILS

Year Built: 1980
Year Remodeled: 2004
Current Mgmt. Since: 1980
No. of Floors: 4
Resident Capacity: 159

### SPECIAL

Diets Accommodated: Diabetic, Low-fat, Low-salt, Renal
Proximity to Emergency Svcs.: Under 8 miles
Nearby shopping and entertainment
Some pets allowed

### STAFF

Nurse/LVN/LPN: Onsite 24/7
Caregiver Training: Dementia, Family communication, Grief, Transition issues
Criminal Background Check: Yes
Principal Staff Language(s): English
Other Staff Language(s): Spanish

### FACILITY FEATURES

Activities/Recreation
Beauty/Barber Shop ($)
Chapel Services
Computer/Internet Access
Facility Parking
Fitness Room/Gym
Outside Patio/Gardens
Pharmaceutical Service
Private Dining Room
Room Service
Separate Therapy Room
Transportation to MD Appointments, Personal Outings, Scheduled Outings
24-hour Security

### ROOM FEATURES

Cable TV Ready ($)
Emergency Call System
Grab Bars
Kitchenette
Private Bathrooms
Telephone Ready ($)
Temperature Controls

### COSTS

PRICES MAY INCREASE. PLEASE CALL FOR MOST CURRENT INFORMATION.

| | |
|---|---|
| Studio Apt. | $2,650–$3,300/month |
| One Bedroom Apt. | $4,100–$5,300/month<br>Double occupancy add $750–$1,000/month |
| Alzheimer's Unit | $3,300–$3,400/month for shared room<br>$4,000–$5,400/month for private room |

| | |
|---|---|
| Costs of Care | $300–$350/month based on individual need |
| Rate Increase | Annually; usually 3% |
| Reimbursement | LTCI, Private pay |
| Security Deposit | One month's rent (refundable) |

**PORTRAIT**

A stucco exterior punctuated by green awnings gives Monticello West the appearance of an apartment building. Mature oak trees border the parking lot in front of the portico. Despite its bustling location between McKinney Avenue and North Central Expressway, the nearby traffic does not mar the facility's serene atmosphere. The upscale interior features beautiful earth-toned carpeting. Silk floral arrangements grace the lovely dark wood bookcases, hutches and tables. The white domed ceiling seems to float overhead. The elegance extends to the computer room (which has internet access) and other common areas. Tasteful glass and metal fixtures shed soft light throughout the facility. Handrails trace the broad hallways. Residents furnish their rooms, where pretty off-white curtains frame the windows.

During our visit, mouthwatering aromas from the kitchen announced a meal of sesame chicken, sweet and sour pork, steamed rice and sautéed squash. Active residents enjoy buffet-style dining in the main dining room, which also hosts sing-alongs and guest musicians. Residents are served by a waitstaff in the other dining areas. The helpful staff knows each resident by name. Genuine affection marks the interaction between the two groups. Bingo, movies, bowling, exercise and various games are among the many scheduled activities. Two extensively landscaped courtyards entice residents to walk among the shade trees and vine-covered trellises.

The Alzheimer's unit at Monticello West occupies its own floor. The unit is divided between residents in the early stages of Alzheimer's and those in advanced stages. During the tour, our guide soothed a distressed resident who was lost. She was relieved to be escorted back to her room, which she believed to be the home that she had lived in with her family. Our guide validated her belief and the resident was visibly comforted.

## Presbyterian Village North—Joyce Hall

8600 Skyline Drive
Dallas, TX 75243

(214) 355-9018
www.presbyterianvillagenorth.org

### GILBERT GUIDE OBSERVATIONS

| | | | |
|---|---|---|---|
| Administration & Staff | g g g g | Residents | g g g |
| Facility Aesthetics | g g g g | Dietary & Food Selection | g g g |
| Facility Condition & Safety | g g g | Activities | g |

### DETAILS

Year Built: 1989
Year Remodeled: Ongoing
Current Mgmt. Since: 1989
No. of Floors: 3
Resident Capacity: 87

### SPECIAL

Mild dementia care provided
Diets Accommodated: Diabetic, Low-salt
Proximity to Emergency Svcs.: Under 8 miles
Nearby shopping and entertainment
No pets allowed

### STAFF

Nurse/LVN/LPN: 40 hours/week, On-call 24/7
Caregiver Training: Dementia, Ethics, Family communication, Stress management, Transition issues
Criminal Background Check: Yes
Principal Staff Language(s): English
Other Staff Language(s): Spanish

### FACILITY FEATURES

Activities/Recreation
Beauty/Barber Shop ($)
Facility Parking
Guest Meals ($)
Outside Patio/Gardens
Pharmaceutical Service
Transportation
24-hour Security

### ROOM FEATURES

Cable TV Ready
Emergency Call System
Grab Bars
Kitchenette
Private Bathrooms
Telephone Ready
Temperature Controls

### COSTS

PRICES MAY INCREASE. PLEASE CALL FOR MOST CURRENT INFORMATION.

| | |
|---|---|
| Studio Apt. | $2,800–$3,005/month |
| One Bedroom Apt. | $3,790–$4,215/month<br>Double occupancy add $650/month |
| Two Bedroom Apt. | $4,265/month<br>Double occupancy add $750/month |
| Costs of Care | Included in monthly rate |
| Rate Increase | Annually; usually 4% |
| Reimbursement | Private pay |
| Entrance Fee | $1,000 |

### PORTRAIT

Joyce Hall, Presbyterian Village North's assisted living facility, sits on a sixty-three acre campus. A creek runs beneath trees and through open spaces on the property. The three-story atrium creates a stunning entrance to the building. The lobby area, at the confluence of the main resident halls, houses the concierge desk. A grandfather clock ticks nearby in a cozy living room that features a fireplace and bookshelves. The lighting was somewhat dim in areas; this was particularly the case in the long hallways, which terminate in arched windows.

The friendly nurse manager conducted our tour. Residents enjoy luxurious apartments; all have spacious bathrooms featuring mirrored closets, heat lamps and a long vanity. Curtains dress the expansive windows. A small closet near the bathroom adds extra storage space. Some of the apartments boast balconies and vaulted ceilings.

The upscale dining room is used exclusively for meals. The facility has multiple common areas; one has a sewing machine, a second is set up for games, and sofas furnish yet another with a balcony and a full-service kitchen. Due to the limited activities offered by the facility, which include exercise, outings, and performances by local entertainers, most residents create their own activities. This seems to work well, as many residents know each other from living in other areas of the campus.

## Preston Hollow Assisted Living & Memory Care A/D

4205 West Northwest Highway
Dallas, TX 75220

(214) 357-7900
www.prestonhollowalf.com

### GILBERT GUIDE OBSERVATIONS

| | | | |
|---|---|---|---|
| Administration & Staff | g g g g | Dietary & Food Selection | g g g |
| Facility Aesthetics | g g g g g | Activities | g g g |
| Facility Condition & Safety | g g g g | Alzheimer's & Dementia Capabilities | g g g |
| Residents | g g g | | |

### DETAILS

Year Built: 1997
Current Mgmt. Since: 2004
No. of Floors: 2
Resident Capacity: 64

### SPECIAL

Diets Accommodated: Diabetic, Low-fat, Low-salt
Proximity to Emergency Svcs.: Under 8 miles
Nearby shopping and entertainment
Pets allowed

PRESTON HOLLOW ASSISTED LIVING & MEMORY CARE (CONTINUED)

## STAFF

Nurse/LVN/LPN: 40–45 hours/week, On-call 24/7
Caregiver Training: Dementia, Ethics, Family communication, Grief, Patient transfers, Stress management, Transition issues
Criminal Background Check: Yes
Principal Staff Language(s): English
Other Staff Language(s): Spanish

## FACILITY FEATURES

Activities/Recreation
Beauty/Barber Shop ($)
Chapel Services
Facility Parking
Guest Meals ($)
Outside Patio/Gardens
Pharmaceutical Service
Private Dining Room
Room Service
Transportation to MD Appointments, Scheduled Outings
24-hour Security

## ROOM FEATURES

Cable TV Ready ($)
Emergency Call System
Furnished
Grab Bars
Kitchenette
Private Bathrooms
Telephone Ready ($)
Temperature Controls

## COSTS

PRICES MAY INCREASE. PLEASE CALL FOR MOST CURRENT INFORMATION.

| | |
|---|---|
| Studio Apt. | $2,380–$2,800/month |
| One Bedroom Apt. | $3,160/month<br>Double occupancy add $850/month |
| Respite Stays | $100/day for private room |
| Costs of Care | Included in monthly rate |
| Rate Increase | Annually; usually 3% |
| Reimbursement | LTCI, Private pay, Veterans |
| Entrance Fee | $500 |
| Security Deposit | $100 (refundable) |
| Pet Deposit | $500 |

## PORTRAIT

Preston Hollow is part of an affluent Dallas neighborhood that features multi-million dollar homes. The Alzheimer's unit is a well-blended addition to its sister assisted living facility. The building enjoys proximity to NorthPark Center and the city's vibrant downtown area. The stately home with white columns that houses the facility fits right in with its residential neighbors.

A winding wooden staircase is the stunning focal point in the foyer. The floral carpet coordinates nicely with the rich maroon and forest green furniture and drapes. Oak columns and moldings add lovely elements throughout the home. The Alzheimer's unit was clearly designed with the residents' special needs in mind; the décor reflects only the simplest patterns. Alarms and security pads control access to the home. The hallways are clear of obstructions and are equipped with handrails. Residents' rooms have expansive windows that let in plentiful sunlight. Nametags and room numbers label the doors of the private rooms.

Tables dressed in linen and leather-like rolling chairs furnish the dining area. Large windows offer a pleasant view of the small courtyard, where oak trees shade the seating area. A typical menu includes oven fried chicken, roasted new potatoes with gravy, seasoned broccoli and raspberry parfait squares. During our visit, many residents enjoyed a post-lunch nap. Activities include exercise, gardening, ceramics, baking, watching movies and listening to guest musical performances. Residents also attend scheduled outings to church services, shopping areas and tourist attractions. The Life Engagement program at Preston Hollow is based on each resident's interests, abilities, history and routine. The engagements promote cognitive, physical, sensory, and creative skills, allowing residents to maintain a comfortable level of independence, while they are fully supported by staff members.

Staff members and residents interacted warmly with one another. A nod to charming Southern roots, the staff politely address residents by title and first name—for example, "Ms. Betty" or "Mr. Daniel." Perhaps the most noteworthy aspect among Preston Hollow's special offerings includes a five-day respite stay—at no charge—for potential residents to "test drive" the facility.

## St. Josephs Residence

330 West Pembrook Avenue
Dallas, TX 75208

(214) 948-3597
www.stjr.org

---

**GILBERT GUIDE OBSERVATIONS**

| | | | |
|---|---|---|---|
| Administration & Staff | g g g g g | Residents | g g g g g |
| Facility Aesthetics | g g g g | Dietary & Food Selection | g g g |
| Facility Condition & Safety | g g g g g | Activities | g g g g |

### DETAILS

Year Built: 1955
Year Remodeled: 2004
Current Mgmt. Since: 1955
No. of Floors: 1
Resident Capacity: 65

### SPECIAL

Mild dementia care provided
Diets Accommodated: Diabetic, Low-fat, Low-salt
Proximity to Emergency Svcs.: Under 8 miles
Nearby shopping and entertainment
Pet visits allowed

### STAFF

Nurse/LVN/LPN: Onsite 24/7
Caregiver Training: Dementia, Ethics, Family communication

ST. JOSEPHS RESIDENCE (CONTINUED)

Criminal Background Check: Yes
Principal Staff Language(s): English
Other Staff Language(s): Spanish

**FACILITY FEATURES**

Activities/Recreation
Beauty/Barber Shop
Chapel Services
Facility Parking
Fitness Room/Gym
Outside Patio/Gardens
Pharmaceutical Service
Private Dining Room
Separate Therapy Room
24-hour Security

**ROOM FEATURES**

Cable TV Ready ($)
Emergency Call System
Furnished
Grab Bars
Shared & Private Bathrooms
Telephone Ready ($)
Temperature Controls

**COSTS**

PRICES MAY INCREASE. PLEASE CALL FOR MOST CURRENT INFORMATION.

| | |
|---|---|
| One Bedroom Apt. | $1,200–$1,500/month<br>Double occupancy add $750/month |
| Costs of Care | $200–$600/month based on individual need |
| Rate Increase | Annually; usually 10% |
| Reimbursement | LTCI, Private pay |
| Application Fee | $100 |
| Security Deposit | $1,000 (refundable) |

**PORTRAIT**

Located in a quiet neighborhood off Pembrook Avenue, St. Joseph's is a staple in the community. The well-maintained red brick frame and classic wrought iron fence surrounding the front yard belie its age of fifty years. Park-like landscapes of mature trees and pretty flowerbeds add elegance to the exterior.

A hodgepodge of old and modern décor, including ceramic tile floors, freshly painted walls adorned with artwork, antique furniture and oak bookcases creates a homey atmosphere. Residents' rooms are spacious enough for personal furnishings and are equipped with hospital beds. Each has a garden view. Soft lamps and overhead fixtures complement the abundance of natural lighting throughout the facility. Residents gather in the comfortably furnished, roomy common areas. We observed residents on walkers and wheelchairs move about these rooms with ease. The living room features a big-screen TV and the hallways are equipped with handrails.

During our visit, the smell of home-cooked meals and fragrant spices filled the air. Residents bring in personal snacks or choose from a wide selection offered by the staff. Visiting near the outdoor hummingbird feeder is among residents' favorite pastimes. Three seating areas with patio furniture beckon residents to relax and enjoy the surrounding nature. St. Joseph's hosts daily religious activities at the onsite church, as well as weekly performances by visiting singing groups. Toward the end of our tour, one gentleman (a resident) offered to finish the tour so that our guide could rest her feet. He mentioned how he "loves everyone and everything" about St. Joseph's and feels "very much at home" there.

## Stone Bridge Alzheimer's Special Care Center A/D

9271 White Rock Trail
Dallas, TX 75238

(214) 691-7400
www.jeaseniorliving.com

---

**GILBERT GUIDE OBSERVATIONS**

| Category | Rating | Category | Rating |
|---|---|---|---|
| Administration & Staff | g g g g | Dietary & Food Selection | g g g |
| Facility Aesthetics | g g g g g | Activities | g g g g |
| Facility Condition & Safety | g g g g | Alzheimer's & Dementia Capabilities | g g g g |
| Residents | g g g | | |

### DETAILS

Year Built: 1999
Current Mgmt. Since: 1999
No. of Floors: 1
Resident Capacity: 56

### SPECIAL

Alzheimer's/Dementia Only Facility
Diets Accommodated: Diabetic, Low-fat, Low-salt
Proximity to Emergency Svcs.: Under 8 miles
Nearby shopping and entertainment
No pets allowed

### STAFF

Nurse/LVN/LPN: Onsite 24/7
Caregiver Training: Dementia, Ethics, Family communication, Grief, Patient transfers, Stress management, Transition issues, Validation therapy
Criminal Background Check: Yes
Principal Staff Language(s): English
Other Staff Language(s): Spanish

### FACILITY FEATURES

Activities/Recreation
Beauty/Barber Shop ($)
Chapel Services
Facility Parking
Guest Meals ($)
Outside Patio/Gardens
Pharmaceutical Service
Private Dining Room
Separate Therapy Room
Transportation to MD Appointments, Scheduled Outings
24-hour Security

### ROOM FEATURES

Cable TV Ready ($)
Emergency Call System
Furnished
Shared & Private Bathrooms
Telephone Ready ($)
Temperature Controls

STONE BRIDGE ALZHEIMER'S SPECIAL CARE CENTER (CONTINUED)

## COSTS

PRICES MAY INCREASE. PLEASE CALL FOR MOST CURRENT INFORMATION.

| | |
|---|---|
| Alzheimer's Unit | $1,760–$3,400/month for shared room<br>Up to $3,400/month for private room |
| Respite Stays | $125/day for shared room |
| Costs of Care | $200–$1,000/month based on individual need |
| Rate Increase | Annually; usually 3% |
| Reimbursement | LTCI, Private pay, Veterans |

## PORTRAIT

Stone Bridge is located just off Walnut Hill Lane, adjacent to White Rock Lake Park. The exterior stucco walls are washed in pale yellow and accented by a stone base trim. Flowerbeds, shrubs and trees grace the circular driveway. Victorian furniture surrounds a cherrywood coffee table in the elegant lobby. The facility is decorated with silk flowers and hanging prints of equally stunning floral arrangements.

Residents' rooms are moderately sized. Each has two windows with matching curtains and berber carpeting. Both dining rooms are furnished with dark wood tables and chairs. Placemats and fragrant flowers give the rooms a homey feel. Activity rooms are adjacent to the courtyard. During our visit, the kitchen staff prepared an appetizing lemon pepper chicken with fresh vegetables and sweet cinnamon apples. The staff offers a variety of snacks that includes fresh fruit, cookies, crackers and breads. Residents gathered in the kitchen to make peanut butter and jelly sandwiches as part of the weekly cooking calendar.

The building surrounds the outdoor courtyard. Residents enjoy the shady patio, with its comfy lawn furniture. Garden paths wind between colorful flowerbeds and shrubs. The three-tier stone fountain is a lovely centerpiece. The building is bathed in natural light; fluorescent lighting adds to the warm glow. The hallways are spacious and neat.

The residents of Stone Bridge are a lively group. They enjoy weekly activities including movie matinees, manicures, fitness instruction, gardening and weekly devotional services. The atmosphere buzzed with energy on our visit, while staff and residents mingled comfortably in every corner of the building.

## Summer Ridge

3020 Ridge Road
Rockwall, TX 75032

(972) 771-2800
www.scc-texas.com

### GILBERT GUIDE OBSERVATIONS

| | | | |
|---|---|---|---|
| Administration & Staff | g g g g | Residents | g g g g g |
| Facility Aesthetics | g g g g g | Dietary & Food Selection | g g g g g |
| Facility Condition & Safety | g g g g g | Activities | g g g g g |

### DETAILS

Year Built: 1999
Current Mgmt. Since: 1999
No. of Floors: 1
Resident Capacity: 77

### SPECIAL

Diets Accommodated: Low-fat
Proximity to Emergency Svcs.: 9–15 Miles
Nearby shopping and entertainment
Pets allowed

### STAFF

Nurse/LVN/LPN: On-call 24/7
Caregiver Training: Ethics, Family communication, Grief, Patient transfers, Stress management, Transition issues, Validation therapy
Criminal Background Check: Yes
Principal Staff Language(s): English

### FACILITY FEATURES

Activities/Recreation
Beauty/Barber Shop
Chapel Services
Facility Parking
Fitness Room/Gym
Guest Meals
Outside Patio/Gardens
Private Dining Room
Room Service
Transportation to MD Appointments ($), Personal Outings ($), Scheduled Outings
24-hour Security

### ROOM FEATURES

Cable TV Ready
Emergency Call System
Grab Bars
Kitchenette
Private Bathrooms
Telephone Ready
Temperature Controls

### COSTS

PRICES MAY INCREASE. PLEASE CALL FOR MOST CURRENT INFORMATION.

| | |
|---|---|
| Studio Apt. | $2,195–$2,495/month |
| One Bedroom Apt. | $2,395–$3,295/month<br>Double occupancy add $800–$1,100/month |
| Two Bedroom Apt. | $3,295–$3,995/month<br>Double occupancy add $800–$1,100/month |
| Costs of Care | Call for rates |
| Rate Increase | Annually; usually 2–3% |
| Reimbursement | Private pay |

SUMMER RIDGE (CONTINUED)

| | |
|---|---|
| Entrance Fee | $350 |
| Pet Deposit | $200 (refundable) |

**PORTRAIT**

Ridge Road curves gently past the grassy knolls and colorful flowerbeds of Summer Ridge's lovely entrance. Although located in a quiet residential area, it neighbors a major shopping center with retail shopping, a grocery store, nail salon and theater. The foyer is a striking display of cherrywood tables, contemporary green and maroon couches, hanging chandeliers, a handmade tapestry and a grandfather clock. The hallways are decorated with fresh floral arrangements in oriental vases and hanging impressionist lithographs.

Residents' rooms are especially bright and airy. Each has large windows and extra storage space. Residents furnish to suit their tastes. The dining area is equipped with tables for four, strategically spaced to accommodate residents using wheelchairs. The soothing mauve and green color scheme creates a serene dining atmosphere. The kitchen staff prepares a healthy and appetizing menu featuring selections such as beef burgundy, butternut squash, steak fingers with gravy, and lemon cake. The soup, sandwich and pizza menu provides lighter alternatives.

Residents gather in the common area for social hour and various activities. Plush couches and chairs are arranged in a U-shape in front of the big-screen TV—perfect for popcorn and movie nights! Residents stay busy with bingo, arts and crafts, fitness programs, painting classes, board games and holiday activities. The secured patio and courtyard features lush greenery and birdlife. Residents enjoy outdoor barbeques and lounging on comfy patio furniture. A lovely walkway curves through bright gardens of rainbow-colored flowers. The residents were quite neighborly with each other and seemed very comfortable around the staff, with whom they were quick to strike up conversations. The cheerful energy at Summer Ridge is absolutely infectious.

## Summerville at Lakeland Hills

3305 Dilido
Dallas, TX 75228

(214) 321-7300
www.seniorstar.com

**GILBERT GUIDE OBSERVATIONS**

| | | | |
|---|---|---|---|
| Administration & Staff | g g g g g | Residents | g g g g g |
| Facility Aesthetics | g g g g g | Dietary & Food Selection | g g g |
| Facility Condition & Safety | g g g g g | Activities | g g g g g |

**DETAILS**

Year Built: 1997
Year Remodeled: 2003

**SPECIAL**

Mild dementia care provided
Diets Accommodated: Diabetic, Low-fat, Low-salt

DETAILS (CONTINUED)
Current Mgmt. Since: November 2005
No. of Floors: 1
Resident Capacity: 45

SPECIAL (CONTINUED)
Proximity to Emergency Svcs.: Under 8 miles
Nearby shopping and entertainment
Some pets allowed

## STAFF

Nurse/LVN/LPN: None on staff
Caregiver Training: Dementia, Ethics, Family communication, Grief, Patient transfers, Transition issues
Criminal Background Check: Yes
Principal Staff Language(s): English
Other Staff Language(s): Spanish

## FACILITY FEATURES

Activities/Recreation
Beauty/Barber Shop
Chapel Services
Computer/Internet Access
Facility Parking
Fitness Room/Gym
Guest Meals
Outside Patio/Gardens
Overnight Guest Room ($)
Pharmaceutical Service
Room Service
Separate Therapy Room
Transportation
24-hour Security

## ROOM FEATURES

Cable TV Ready ($)
Emergency Call System
Grab Bars
Kitchenette
Private Bathrooms
Telephone Ready ($)
Temperature Controls

## COSTS

PRICES MAY INCREASE. PLEASE CALL FOR MOST CURRENT INFORMATION.

| | |
|---|---|
| Studio Apt. | $2,395/month |
| Costs of Care | $400–$800/month based on individual need |
| Rate Increase | Annually; usually 5% |
| Reimbursement | Private pay |
| Entrance Fee | $1,000 |
| Pet Deposit | $200 |

## PORTRAIT

Summerville at Lakeland Hills was among the first accredited assisted living programs in Texas. Its location near a major intersection provides easy access to the surrounding urban area while also retaining a tranquil, homey feel. The Victorian décor features classic paintings, beautiful lamps and antique occasional tables.

Activities include sing-alongs, religious services, birthday parties, performances by outside entertainers and field trips to casinos and shopping malls. There are three common areas where residents relax among the overstuffed sofas and ottomans to visit or watch televi-

SUMMERVILLE AT LAKELAND HILLS (CONTINUED)

sion. During our visit, the kitchen was filled with the delicious smell of baked chicken. Popcorn and ice cream are among residents' favorite snacks.

One resident introduced us to the two parakeets that live at the facility, explaining that she loves to visit them as they remind her of her children. As she put it, "they never shut up!" Two other residents were enjoying themselves in the beauty salon. Residents' spacious rooms are freshly painted and adorned with personal touches such as antique nightstands and hanging art. The hallways are wide and have unique seating options including a daybed-style bench.

## VERANDA PRESTON HOLLOW A/D

11409 North Central
Dallas, TX 75243

(214) 363-5100
www.verandaprestonhollow.com

### GILBERT GUIDE OBSERVATIONS

| | | | |
|---|---|---|---|
| Administration & Staff | g g g | Dietary & Food Selection | g g g |
| Facility Aesthetics | g g g g | Activities | g g g g |
| Facility Condition & Safety | g g g g | Alzheimer's & Dementia Capabilities | g g g g |
| Residents | g g g | | |

### DETAILS

Year Built: 2001
Current Mgmt. Since: 2003
No. of Floors: 2
Resident Capacity: 41

### SPECIAL

Diets Accommodated: Diabetic, Low-fat, Low-salt
Proximity to Emergency Svcs.: Under 8 miles
Nearby shopping and entertainment
Pets allowed

### STAFF

Nurse/LVN/LPN: Onsite 24/7
Caregiver Training: Dementia, Family communication, Grief, Patient transfers, Stress management
Criminal Background Check: Yes
Principal Staff Language(s): English
Other Staff Language(s): Spanish

### FACILITY FEATURES

Activities/Recreation
Beauty/Barber Shop ($)
Chapel Services
Facility Parking
Fitness Room/Gym
Guest Meals ($)
Outside Patio/Gardens

### ROOM FEATURES

Cable TV Ready
Emergency Call System
Grab Bars
Kitchenette
Shared & Private Bathrooms
Telephone Ready
Temperature Controls

FACILITY FEATURES (CONTINUED)

Pharmaceutical Service ($)
Private Dining Room
Room Service
Separate Therapy Room
Transportation
24-hour Security

## COSTS

PRICES MAY INCREASE. PLEASE CALL FOR MOST CURRENT INFORMATION.

| | |
|---|---|
| Studio Apt. | $2,900/month |
| One Bedroom Apt. | $3,900–$5,600/month<br>Double occupancy add $600/month |
| Alzheimer's Unit | $2,380–$3,160/month for private room |
| Respite Stays | $100/day for private room |
| Costs of Care | Based on individual need |
| Rate Increase | Annually; usually 4% |
| Reimbursement | LTCI, Private pay |
| Security Deposit | $1,000 (refundable) |

## PORTRAIT

Veranda Preston Hollow sits on a shady road just off of Central Expressway in an upscale Dallas neighborhood. Residents are treated to a plush lobby equipped with a small library, a grand piano, an aquarium (with eels!) and a cappuccino station. The conference room in the entry doubles as the private dining room. Large windows usher in plentiful sunlight and offer lovely garden views. Veranda Preston Hollow offers assisted living services as well as Alzheimer's and dementia care. The dementia unit is secured. There is a front desk attendant on duty all night, and video monitoring provides additional security.

Residents' rooms vary in size from small to medium. The dining room is an elegant setting of dark wood chairs upholstered in pretty fabric, soft lighting from decorative sconces, fine china and fresh flowers atop white linen tablecloths. A waitstaff serves three meals a day. One furnished common area features a big-screen TV and a popcorn machine; the other serves as a game room. Each floor has a beverage bar that offers coffee, and assorted teas and juices. The outdoor patio on the second floor is an inviting spot for residents to relax on comfortable rocking chairs while enjoying the quiet outdoors. The hallways are broad and clean. Recessed lighting throughout the building complements the flood of natural light from numerous windows.

Residents participate in various organized activities. Trivia and word play are an important part of cognitive stimulation, and fitness instruction provides regular physical activity. Residents also attend field trips to botanical gardens and state fairs. Residents have access to physical and occupational therapy equipment on the fourth floor, which also houses Veranda Preston Hollow's skilled nursing facility. Prospective residents are encouraged to take advantage of Veranda's free five-day respite trial period.

## The Vintage Retirement Community Assisted Living

205 North Bonnie Brae
Denton, TX 76201

(940) 384-1500
www.scc-texas.com

---

**GILBERT GUIDE OBSERVATIONS**

| | | | |
|---|---|---|---|
| Administration & Staff | g g g | Residents | g g g |
| Facility Aesthetics | g g g | Dietary & Food Selection | g g g |
| Facility Condition & Safety | g g g | Activities | g g g g g |

### DETAILS

Year Built: 1985
Year Remodeled: Ongoing
Current Mgmt. Since: Unknown
No. of Floors: 2
Resident Capacity: 105
Transportation

### SPECIAL

Mild dementia care provided
Diets Accommodated: Diabetic, Low-fat, Low-salt
Proximity to Emergency Svcs.: Under 8 miles
Nearby shopping and entertainment
Pets allowed

### STAFF

Nurse/LVN/LPN: On-call 24/7
Caregiver Training: Ethics, Grief, Stress management
Criminal Background Check: Yes
Principal Staff Language(s): English
Other Staff Language(s): Spanish

### FACILITY FEATURES

Activities/Recreation
Beauty/Barber Shop
Chapel Services
Facility Parking
Private Dining Room
Transportation

### ROOM FEATURES

Cable TV Ready ($)
Emergency Call System
Grab Bars
Kitchenette
Private Bathrooms
Telephone Ready ($)
Temperature Controls

### COSTS

PRICES MAY INCREASE. PLEASE CALL FOR MOST CURRENT INFORMATION.

| | |
|---|---|
| Studio Apt. | $2,160–$2,460/month |
| One Bedroom Apt. | $2,300–$2,600/month<br>Double occupancy add $800/month |
| Two Bedroom Apt. | $3,050–$3,350/month<br>Double occupancy add $800–$1,100/month |
| Costs of Care | $300/month |
| Rate Increase | Annually; usually 3% |
| Reimbursement | LTCI, Private pay |
| Security Deposit | $500 (refundable) |

### PORTRAIT

Our first impression of The Vintage was of a historic upscale hotel. Located in an older neighborhood, it is right next to Presbyterian Hospital of Denton. The exterior is freshly painted and the manicured lawn is dotted with large shade trees. Brass fixtures in the décor add to the hotel-like ambiance. Maroon, green and floral patterns give The Vintage a stately feel.

Residents' apartments are modestly sized. The showers, cabinets and carpet all appear to be recently updated. The large two-bedroom apartments easily accommodate personal furnishings. Residents in rooms that feature balconies often use the space to grow plants. Residents frequently use the many common areas that the facility boasts, including a game room with a big-screen TV, a bridge parlor, and a private library and reading room. The facility also features a piano and an organ. The wide hallways are kept free of obstructions. Landscaping is minimal in the outdoor area, which has horseshoe pits and personal gardening spaces.

At the time of our visit, the staff was occupied with various tasks; therefore our interaction was minimal. Activities satisfy a mix of interests—from walking groups, theater and sightseeing trips, to arts and crafts, worship services, discussion groups, musical performances and the "Out to Lunch Bunch".

## WALNUT PLACE A/D

5515 Glen Lakes
Dallas, TX 75231

(214) 361-8923
www.walnutplacedallas.com

---

### GILBERT GUIDE OBSERVATIONS

| | | | |
|---|---|---|---|
| Administration & Staff | g g g g g | Dietary & Food Selection | g g g g g |
| Facility Aesthetics | g g g | Activities | g g g g g |
| Facility Condition & Safety | g g g g g | Alzheimer's & Dementia Capabilities | g g g g g |
| Residents | g g g g g | | |

### DETAILS

Year Built: 1985
Year Remodeled: 2002
Current Mgmt. Since: 1980
No. of Floors: 6
Resident Capacity: 85 (AL), 32 (ALZ)

### SPECIAL

Diets Accommodated: Diabetic, Low-fat, Low-salt
Proximity to Emergency Svcs.: Under 8 miles
Nearby shopping and entertainment
Some pets allowed

### STAFF

Nurse/LVN/LPN: Onsite 24/7
Caregiver Training: Dementia, Ethics, Family communication, Grief, Patient transfers, Stress management, Transition issues, Validation therapy

WALNUT PLACE (CONTINUED)

Criminal Background Check: Yes
Principal Staff Language(s): English
Other Staff Language(s): Spanish

### FACILITY FEATURES

Activities/Recreation
Beauty/Barber Shop ($)
Chapel Services
Facility Parking
Guest Meals
Pharmaceutical Service
Private Dining Room
Room Service
Separate Therapy Room
Transportation
24-hour Security

### ROOM FEATURES

Cable TV Ready
Emergency Call System
Grab Bars
Kitchenette
Private Bathrooms
Telephone Ready
Temperature Controls

### COSTS

PRICES MAY INCREASE. PLEASE CALL FOR MOST CURRENT INFORMATION.

| | |
|---|---|
| Studio Apt. | $2,600–$2,800/month |
| One Bedroom Apt. | $3,300–$3,600/month |
| Two Bedroom Apt. | $3,800/month |
| Alzheimer's Unit | $3,600–$4,000/month for shared room<br>$4,500/month for private room |
| Costs of Care | Included in monthly rate |
| Rate Increase | Annually; usually 4% |
| Reimbursement | Private pay |
| Security Deposit | $500 (refundable) |

### PORTRAIT

The unassuming exterior of Walnut Place conceals a treasure trove. The facility boasts a wonderful reputation built on twenty-five years of service. The administrator has been with the facility since its opening; other staff members have worked there nearly as long. The staff maintains an open-door policy, but are rarely in their offices, due to constant resident interaction. The seasoned gerontologist who manages the Alzheimer's unit frequently calls residents' families to keep them abreast of recent developments. The staff dietician knows most of the residents personally and can discuss most cases without referencing their charts.

The activities director coordinates activities geared toward residents' interests and abilities. Nearly all residents attend Friday Happy Hour to enjoy the snacks and live entertainment. Field trips include a weekly ice cream run. Residents thoroughly enjoyed a recent trip to Six Flags Theme Park. One resident organized a men's club and another shares his collection of movies with other residents by playing them in a fourth floor common area.

The formal dining area is used for meetings and support groups as well as private dining. It is furnished with a big-screen TV and a piano. The dining area looks out onto the open atrium, where birds can be seen flying in and out. Pet birds in decorative cages and a pond with colorful koi add charm to the area. The halls have handrails and are wide enough to accommodate three wheelchair users abreast. They feature seating at both ends, which often serve as informal meeting areas. Natural light supplements the overhead lighting. The dark carpeting has a slight pattern, which may be problematic for some dementia residents.

Residents' rooms have large windows with views of the grounds or the atrium. Crown moldings and double closets with mirrored doors make the rooms feel luxurious. When residents require nursing care, they simply move to another floor, where familiar staff members provide care. One resident developed a fear of bathing, as a result of Alzheimer's. In response, an aide provided dry shampoos and baths. The resident later suffered a severe stroke and it was plain that she would not live much longer. Instead of moving her to the nursing unit, she was provided with hospice care in her room, allowing her to maintain contact with familiar aides and favorite neighbors for the remainder of her life.

## Windsor Court Assisted Living

2535 West Pleasant Run Road (972) 228-8059
Lancaster, TX 75146

### GILBERT GUIDE OBSERVATIONS

| | | | |
|---|---|---|---|
| Administration & Staff | g g g | Residents | g g g |
| Facility Aesthetics | g g g g | Dietary & Food Selection | g g g g g |
| Facility Condition & Safety | g g g | Activities | g g g |

### DETAILS

Year Built: 1999
Current Mgmt. Since: 2001
No. of Floors: 1
Resident Capacity: 32

### SPECIAL

Mild dementia care provided
Diets Accommodated: Diabetic, Low-fat, Low-salt
Proximity to Emergency Svcs.: Under 8 miles
Pet visits allowed

### STAFF

Nurse/LVN/LPN: On-call 24/7
Caregiver Training: Dementia, Ethics, Family communication, Grief, Patient transfers, Stress management, Transition issues, Validation therapy
Criminal Background Check: Yes
Principal Staff Language(s): English
Other Staff Language(s): Spanish

WINDSOR COURT ASSISTED LIVING (CONTINUED)

## FACILITY FEATURES

Activities/Recreation
Beauty/Barber Shop
Chapel Services
Computer/Internet Access
Facility Parking
Fitness Room/Gym
Guest Meals
Outside Patio/Gardens
Pharmaceutical Service
Private Dining Room
Transportation
24-hour Security

## ROOM FEATURES

Cable TV Ready ($)
Emergency Call System
Furnished
Grab Bars
Private Bathrooms
Telephone Ready ($)
Temperature Controls

## COSTS

PRICES MAY INCREASE. PLEASE CALL FOR MOST CURRENT INFORMATION.

| | |
|---|---|
| Studio Apt. | $2,100/month |
| One Bedroom Apt. | $2,600/month |
| Costs of Care | Based on individual need |
| Rate Increase | Annually; usually 2% |
| Reimbursement | Private pay |
| Application Fee | $500 |

## PORTRAIT

Windsor Court is located in a posh suburb on West Pleasant Road, minutes from Highway 35. White columns mark the entrance of the red brick building. Hanging artwork adorns the soft green and white walls inside. Contemporary furniture complements the charming modern décor.

Partially furnished with a TV, armoire and table, residents' rooms are spacious and get plenty of natural light. Residents add knickknacks and other belongings to personalize their space. A combination of overhead fixtures and lamps bathe the facility in soft light. Elegant wooden handrails in the wide hallways add a decorative—and practical—touch. The oak tables and chairs in the main dining room provide the comfort and familiarity of home. Distinguished by a grand cherrywood table, the fine dining room is reserved for special gatherings; the "resident of the week" is rewarded the use of this space as well. The kitchen staff, who specialize in homestyle meals, served appetizing meatloaf with roasted potatoes during our visit. Residents enjoy weekend ice cream socials. The outdoor patios provide refuge among a manicured landscape of trees and flowers. Residents and staff use an old fountain in the courtyard to grow seasonal plants and flowers.

A wide variety of activities is offered—daily morning exercise (a house favorite), game hour and weekly manicures, to name a few. Residents waved and smiled as we toured the facility. The staff is familiar with all facets of resident care, because management emphasizes promoting from within; for example, the director of marketing began in housekeeping. She was serving meals when we arrived. Lots of smiling residents contributed to a cheerful environment and made our visit a pleasant one.

## SKILLED NURSING FACILITIES

### Ashley Court at Turtle Creek

3611 Dickason Avenue (214) 559-0140
Dallas, TX 75219

**TOTAL GOVERNMENT DEFICIENCIES: 2** Reviewed on: October 28, 2004

| Administration | Resident Assessment |
|---|---|
| 1 | 1 |

* IMPORTANT: REVIEW DETAILS OF EACH DEFICIENCY AT WWW.MEDICARE.GOV

**GILBERT GUIDE OBSERVATIONS**

| | | | |
|---|---|---|---|
| Administration & Staff | g g g g | Dietary & Food Selection | g g g |
| Facility Aesthetics | g g g | Activities | g g g |
| Facility Condition & Safety | g g g g | Access to Medical Care | g g g g g |
| Residents | g g g | | |

#### DETAILS

Year Built: 1997
Year Remodeled: 2000
Current Mgmt. Since: 2000
No. of Floors: 1
Resident Capacity: 54
Facility Type: Long-term care

#### SPECIAL

Special diets accommodated
Proximity to Emergency Svcs.: Less than 8 miles

#### STAFF

Caregiver Training: Dementia, Ethics, Family communication, Grief, Pain management, Patient transfers, Stress management, Universal precautions, Wound care
Criminal Background Check: Yes
Principal Staff Language(s): English
Other Staff Language(s): Russian, Spanish

#### FACILITY FEATURES

Activities/Recreation
Beauty/Barber Shop ($)
Chapel Services
Outside Patio/Gardens
Private Dining Room
Separate Therapy Room

#### ROOM FEATURES

Cable TV Ready
Space for personal items
Shared & Private Bathrooms
Telephone Ready ($)

ASHLEY COURT AT TURTLE CREEK (CONTINUED)

### COSTS

PRICES MAY INCREASE. PLEASE CALL FOR MOST CURRENT INFORMATION.

| | |
|---|---|
| Shared Room | $149/day |
| Private Room | $169/day |
| Rate Increase | Periodically |
| Reimbursement | Medicare, Medicaid, LTCI, Private pay |

### PORTRAIT

Ashley Court is tucked away in Turtle Creek, a wealthy residential neighborhood in Dallas. Residents are just minutes from the vibrant downtown area, which offers endless entertainment options, ranging from movie theaters to art galleries. The facility is located in a small, cheerful yellow house with green shutters, which blends seamlessly with the surrounding condos and town homes. Large plants decorate the front porch. Tall trees and a manicured lawn surround the property.

The tidy facility is furnished in a practical manner. The hallways are free of obstacles. Residents' moderately sized rooms have limited windows. The common room features TVs, couches and separate seating areas. Tasteful floral arrangements are placed throughout the facility. Plentiful natural light supplements the soft artificial lighting. During our visit, the facility was bustling with staff, residents and visitors, which contributed to an energetic atmosphere—somewhat unusual for a SNF. The staff appeared to be quite attentive to residents' needs. The manager is an RN who is involved in every aspect of residents' care.

## AUTUMN LEAVES PERSONAL CARE UNIT

1010 Emerald Isle Drive (214) 328-4161
Dallas, TX 75218

---

**TOTAL GOVERNMENT DEFICIENCIES: 8** Reviewed on: June 17, 2005

| Environmental | Nutrition and Dietary | Pharmacy Service |
|---|---|---|
| 2 | 2 | 1 |
| **Quality Care** | **Resident Rights** | |
| 2 | 1 | |

* IMPORTANT: REVIEW DETAILS OF EACH DEFICIENCY AT WWW.MEDICARE.GOV

**GILBERT GUIDE OBSERVATIONS**

| | | | |
|---|---|---|---|
| Administration & Staff | g g g g | Dietary & Food Selection | g g g |
| Facility Aesthetics | g g g | Activities | g g g |
| Facility Condition & Safety | g g g | Access to Medical Care | g g g |
| Residents | g g g | | |

### DETAILS

Year Built: 1972
Year Remodeled: Ongoing
Current Mgmt. Since: 1972
No. of Floors: 3
Resident Capacity: 98
Facility Type: Long-term care

### SPECIAL

Special diets accommodated
Proximity to Emergency Svcs.: 9–15 Miles

### STAFF

Caregiver Training: Dementia, Ethics, Family communication, Grief, Pain management, Patient transfers, Stress management, Transition issues, Universal precautions, Validation therapy, Wound care
Criminal Background Check: Yes
Principal Staff Language(s): English
Other Staff Language(s): Spanish

### FACILITY FEATURES

Activities/Recreation
Beauty/Barber Shop ($)
Chapel Services
Guest Meals ($)
Outside Patio/Gardens
Private Dining Room
Separate Therapy Room
24-hour Security
Wanderguard

### ROOM FEATURES

Cable TV Ready ($)
Space for personal items
Shared & Private Bathrooms
Telephone Ready ($)

### COSTS

PRICES MAY INCREASE. PLEASE CALL FOR MOST CURRENT INFORMATION.

| | |
|---|---|
| Shared Room | $126/day |
| Private Room | $170/day |
| Rate Increase | Annually; usually 1–5% |
| Reimbursement | Medicare, LTCI, Private pay, Veterans |

### PORTRAIT

A number of residents have been able to extend their stay at Autumn Leaves for several years thanks to its wide spectrum of care, which includes independent living, assisted living and skilled nursing. The owners are two doctors who take a hands-on approach to ensure the facility's smooth operation. They spend one day each month working at the home. Their philosophy, that no job is too small, is refreshing. They perform tasks that range from cleaning and attending to resident care and administrative work.

As we toured the skilled nursing unit, our guide greeted the handful of animated residents in the common areas by name. Cherrywood crown molding, light green wallpaper and earth-toned carpet accented with blue and gold comprise the luxurious décor in the common rooms and broad hallways. Brass and frosted glass sconces, recessed fluorescent fixtures and generously sized windows fill the home with light. Residents' sunny rooms are

AUTUMN LEAVES PERSONAL CARE UNIT (CONTINUED)

moderately sized and feature additional space for personal belongings. Residents usually take meals in their rooms, although they occasionally use the spacious dining area. A glass wall in the dining room displays attractive views of White Rock Lake, which the stucco building overlooks from atop a hill. Residents enjoy watching squirrels scamper among the oak trees surrounding their home.

## Castle Manor

1922 Castle Drive
Garland, TX 75040

(972) 494-1471
www.nexion-health.com

**TOTAL GOVERNMENT DEFICIENCIES: 17** — Reviewed on: August 19, 2005

| Administration | Environmental | Nutrition and Dietary | Pharmacy Service |
|---|---|---|---|
| 2 | 6 | 1 | 2 |
| Quality Care | Resident Rights | | |
| 3 | 3 | | |

* IMPORTANT: REVIEW DETAILS OF EACH DEFICIENCY AT WWW.MEDICARE.GOV

**GILBERT GUIDE OBSERVATIONS**

| | | | |
|---|---|---|---|
| Administration & Staff | g g g | Dietary & Food Selection | g g g |
| Facility Aesthetics | g g g | Activities | g g g |
| Facility Condition & Safety | g g g | Access to Medical Care | g g g g |
| Residents | g g g g | | |

### DETAILS

Year Built: 1960
Year Remodeled: 2003
Current Mgmt. Since: 1960
No. of Floors: 1
Resident Capacity: 84
Facility Type: Long-term care, Short-term rehab

### SPECIAL

Special diets accommodated
Proximity to Emergency Svcs.: Less than 8 miles

### STAFF

Caregiver Training: Dementia, Ethics, Family communication, Grief, Pain management, Patient transfers, Stress management, Transition issues, Universal precautions, Validation therapy, Wound care
Criminal Background Check: Yes
Principal Staff Language(s): English
Other Staff Language(s): Spanish

### FACILITY FEATURES

Activities/Recreation
Beauty/Barber Shop
Chapel Services
Guest Meals ($)
Outside Patio/Gardens
24-hour Security

### ROOM FEATURES

Cable TV Ready ($)
Space for personal items
Shared Bathrooms
Telephone Ready

### COSTS

PRICES MAY INCREASE. PLEASE CALL FOR MOST CURRENT INFORMATION.

| | |
|---|---|
| Shared Room | $106/day |
| Private Room | $165/day |
| Rate Increase | Every 1½ years; usually 1% |
| Reimbursement | Medicare, Medicaid, Private pay |

### PORTRAIT

Castle Manor is in a residential area that has a rural feel to it. A large pasture sprinkled with blue, yellow and purple flowers surrounds the white brick building. The stone birdbath in the shape of a flower adds an additional pastoral element to the entrance. The foyer doubles as the main common area, wallpapered in hues of green and complemented by polished hardwood floors. Comfortable couches and chairs arranged in front of the big-screen TV are strategically spaced for residents and guests who use wheelchairs or walkers.

Residents' rooms are cozy and inviting. Each has a large window and is furnished with a nightstand, bed and TV table. The cherrywood furniture with brass accents is somewhat worn, but elegant nevertheless. Residents decorate the rooms to suit their personal tastes.

The dining room is bright and airy. The furniture is generously spaced, allowing for easy maneuvering in wheelchairs. Clean, broad hallways are equipped with handrails for added support. Castle Manor boasts a front and back patio. Residents enjoy comforting rocking chairs out front and lively card games on the back patio (a favorite activity in warm weather).

Residents and staff mingled comfortably during lunch hour. Staff members delivered meals while engaging residents in friendly banter. During our visit, we observed the administrator visiting residents throughout the day.

## CHRISTIAN CARE CENTER A/D

1000 Wiggins Parkway
Mesquite, TX 75150

(972) 686-3014
www.christiancarecenters.org

**TOTAL GOVERNMENT DEFICIENCIES: 8** — Reviewed on: June 10, 2005

| Environmental | Nutrition and Dietary | Resident Rights |
|---|---|---|
| 2 | 4 | 2 |

* IMPORTANT: REVIEW DETAILS OF EACH DEFICIENCY AT WWW.MEDICARE.GOV

**GILBERT GUIDE OBSERVATIONS**

| | | | |
|---|---|---|---|
| Administration & Staff | g g g g g | Dietary & Food Selection | g g |
| Facility Aesthetics | g g g | Activities | g g |
| Facility Condition & Safety | g g g | Alzheimer's & Dementia Capabilities | g g g g g |
| Residents | g g g | Access to Medical Care | g g g g |

### DETAILS

Year Built: 1973
Year Remodeled: 1985
Current Mgmt. Since: 1973
No. of Floors: 1
Resident Capacity: 180
Facility Type: Long-term care, Short-term rehab, Alzheimer's unit

### SPECIAL

Special diets accommodated
Proximity to Emergency Svcs.: Less than 8 miles

### STAFF

Caregiver Training: Dementia, Ethics, Family communication, Grief, Pain management, Patient transfers, Stress management, Transition issues, Universal precautions, Wound care
Criminal Background Check: Yes
Principal Staff Language(s): English
Other Staff Language(s): Spanish

### FACILITY FEATURES

Activities/Recreation
Beauty/Barber Shop
Chapel Services
Guest Meals ($)
Outside Patio/Gardens
Private Dining Room
Private Visiting Room
Separate Therapy Room
24-hour Security
Wanderguard
Whirlpool Baths

### ROOM FEATURES

Cable TV Ready
Space for personal items
Shared & Private Bathrooms
Telephone Ready

## COSTS

PRICES MAY INCREASE. PLEASE CALL FOR MOST CURRENT INFORMATION.

| | |
|---|---|
| Shared Room | $136–$144/day |
| Private Room | $156–$168/day |
| Respite Stays | $136–$144/day for shared room<br>$156–$168/day for private room |
| Rate Increase | Annually; usually 3–4% |
| Reimbursement | Medicare, Medicaid, LTCI, Private pay, Veterans |

## PORTRAIT

Christian Care Center sits on an expansive twenty-five acre campus. The administrator and numerous staff members have worked for Christian Care for more than a decade. The facility boasts three full-time activity directors. The activities staff prioritizes resident participation, and it shows: as many as ninety residents participate in some of the activities!

The covered entrance is convenient when entering and exiting the building in bad weather. The wide hallways are filled with artwork. Christian Care is well-maintained and has undergone several major renovations. Residents' rooms are housed in two sections; each wing has sixty beds. The rooms in the older section are certified by Medicaid. Most of these beds are filled by residents who have spent down their resources. There are rarely openings for seniors from outside of the facility. The new wing, built in 1985, has larger rooms with faux wood flooring, which is easier to maintain than carpeting. There are plans to add a dividing wall to the semi-private accommodations. All of the rooms have lovely views of the landscaped grounds.

The main dining room has linoleum floors and doubles as an activities room. The tables are on rollers so they can easily be moved out of the way for activities or cleaning. Management plans to divide the dining room into smaller areas to make it more homelike. The common area has floor-to-ceiling windows that look out onto the gardens.

## Doctors Healthcare Center

9009 Whiterock Trail
Dallas, TX 75238

(214) 348-8100
(214) 355-3304

**TOTAL GOVERNMENT DEFICIENCIES: 23** — Reviewed on: October 28, 2005

| Administration | Environmental | Pharmacy Service | Nutrition and Dietary |
|---|---|---|---|
| 2 | 7 | 2 | 3 |
| **Quality Care** | **Resident Rights** | **Mistreatment** | |
| 4 | 3 | 2 | |

* IMPORTANT: REVIEW DETAILS OF EACH DEFICIENCY AT WWW.MEDICARE.GOV

**GILBERT GUIDE OBSERVATIONS**

| | | | |
|---|---|---|---|
| Administration & Staff | g g g | Dietary & Food Selection | g g g |
| Facility Aesthetics | g g g | Activities | g g g |
| Facility Condition & Safety | g g g | Access to Medical Care | g g g |
| Residents | g g g | | |

### DETAILS

Year Built: 1967
Year Remodeled: 2005
Current Mgmt. Since: 2004
No. of Floors: 1
Resident Capacity: 230
Facility Type: Long-term care, Short-term rehab

### SPECIAL

Special diets accommodated
Proximity to Emergency Svcs.: Less than 8 miles

### STAFF

Caregiver Training: Dementia, Ethics, Family communication, Grief, Pain management, Patient transfers, Stress management, Transition issues, Universal precautions, Validation therapy, Wound care
Criminal Background Check: Yes
Principal Staff Language(s): English
Other Staff Language(s): Spanish

### FACILITY FEATURES

Activities/Recreation
Beauty/Barber Shop ($)
Chapel Services
Guest Meals ($)
Private Visiting Room
Separate Therapy Room
24-hour Security
Wanderguard
Whirlpool Baths

### ROOM FEATURES

Cable TV Ready
Space for personal items
Shared & Private Bathrooms
Telephone Ready

## COSTS

PRICES MAY INCREASE. PLEASE CALL FOR MOST CURRENT INFORMATION.

| | |
|---|---|
| Shared Room | $116/day; $3,596/month |
| Private Room | $141/day; $4,371/month |
| Rate Increase | Annually; usually 3% |
| Reimbursement | Medicare, Medicaid, LTCI, HMO, Private pay, Veterans |

## PORTRAIT

White Rock Lake Park provides a lovely view from the rear of the brick building that houses Doctors Healthcare Center. A creek runs beneath majestic trees, and colorful flowerbeds and black lampposts line the facility's walkways. Sunlight streams into the entry through floor-to-ceiling windows. A china cabinet and reception desk furnish the foyer, which is carpeted in a soothing light blue.

Staff members dressed in scrubs carried on friendly conversations with residents as they assisted them in various tasks. Staff members informed us that plans to remodel include eliminating the assisted living unit, which will create larger rooms for residents in the skilled nursing area. Burgundy carpet covers the floors of the moderately sized residents' rooms. Crimson comforters and window treatments contrast with the pale cloth-covered walls. The rooms are furnished with TVs, nightstands and mirrored vanity areas with storage.

Natural and fluorescent lights brighten the interior. Wooden handrails trace the wide hallways. White tablecloths dress the small dining tables in the facility's numerous dining areas. Tables and a big-screen TV furnish the spacious activities room. The gift shop sells trinkets and snacks. The facility boasts five aviaries that house different species of birds, including the canaries we heard singing cheerfully during our tour.

## THE FORUM AT PARK LANE

7827 Park Lane
Dallas, TX 75225

(214) 369-9905
www.sunriseseniorliving.com

**TOTAL GOVERNMENT DEFICIENCIES: 7** Reviewed on: October 6, 2005

| Administration | Mistreatment | Pharmacy Service |
|---|---|---|
| 1 | 1 | 3 |
| Quality Care | Resident Assessment | |
| 1 | 1 | |

* IMPORTANT: REVIEW DETAILS OF EACH DEFICIENCY AT WWW.MEDICARE.GOV

**GILBERT GUIDE OBSERVATIONS**

| | | | |
|---|---|---|---|
| Administration & Staff | g g g g | Dietary & Food Selection | g g g |
| Facility Aesthetics | g g | Activities | g g g |
| Facility Condition & Safety | g g g | Access to Medical Care | g g g |
| Residents | g g g | | |

### DETAILS

Year Built: 1990
Year Remodeled: 2006
Current Mgmt. Since: 2003
No. of Floors: 2
Resident Capacity: 90
Facility Type: Long-term care, Short-term rehab

### SPECIAL

Special diets accommodated
Proximity to Emergency Svcs.: Less than 8 miles

### STAFF

Caregiver Training: Dementia, Ethics, Family communication, Grief, Pain management, Patient transfers, Stress management, Universal precautions, Wound care
Criminal Background Check: Yes
Principal Staff Language(s): English
Other Staff Language(s): Spanish

### FACILITY FEATURES

Activities/Recreation
Beauty/Barber Shop ($)
Chapel Services
Facility Parking ($)
Guest Meals ($)
Outside Patio/Gardens
Private Dining Room
Separate Therapy Room
24-hour Security
Whirlpool Baths

### ROOM FEATURES

Cable TV Ready
Space for personal items
Shared Bathrooms
Telephone Ready

## COSTS

PRICES MAY INCREASE. PLEASE CALL FOR MOST CURRENT INFORMATION.

| | |
|---|---|
| Shared Room | $125/day |
| Private Room | $180–$245/day |
| Respite Stays | $125/day for shared room<br>$180–$245/day for private room |
| Rate Increase | Annually; usually 3% |
| Reimbursement | Medicare, LTCI, Private pay |

## PORTRAIT

The Forum at Park Lane possesses curb appeal, thanks to its red brick exterior and beautiful landscaping. It is located in an upscale Metroplex neighborhood near NorthPark Mall. The facility's outdoor area is small due to its urban location, but residents seem to thoroughly enjoy the garden, where abundant plants and flowers thrive. The caring and supportive staff members know each resident by name.

The bottom floor houses assisted living, while the second and third floors feature skilled nursing and independent living. Our tour coincided with a renovation of the two sunny upper floors. Elegant burgundy and gold furnishings create a comfortable sitting area in the spacious foyer. White columns support the visible second floor landing. Crown moldings accent soft yellow walls. Large windows allow plentiful sunlight into the dining room, which doubles as an activities area. The dining area becomes slightly crowded once wheelchair users are at the tables. Other common areas include a sunny lounge and a living room furnished with Queen Anne pieces, including a floral sofa and a cherrywood hutch. Seating areas are conveniently arranged at the ends of the hallways. Residents' rooms range from small to large and are somewhat institutional-looking, although simple efforts have been made to make the spaces homier, such as the attractive curtains that hang from residents' expansive windows.

## GOLDEN ACRES A/D

2525 Centerville Road
Dallas, TX 75225

(214) 327-4503
www.goldenacres.org

**TOTAL GOVERNMENT DEFICIENCIES: 8** Reviewed on: February 11, 2005

| Administration | Mistreatment | Nutrition and Dietary |
|---|---|---|
| 2 | 2 | 1 |
| Pharmacy Service | Quality Care | |
| 1 | 2 | |

* IMPORTANT: REVIEW DETAILS OF EACH DEFICIENCY AT WWW.MEDICARE.GOV

**GILBERT GUIDE OBSERVATIONS**

| | | | |
|---|---|---|---|
| Administration & Staff | g g g g g | Dietary & Food Selection | g g g g g |
| Facility Aesthetics | g g g g | Activities | g g g g g |
| Facility Condition & Safety | g g g g g | Alzheimer's & Dementia Capabilities | g g g g g |
| Residents | g g g g g | Access to Medical Care | g g g |

### DETAILS

Year Built: 1953
Year Remodeled: 2005
Current Mgmt. Since: 1953
No. of Floors: 4
Resident Capacity: 260
Facility Type: Long-term care, Short-term rehab, Alzheimer's unit

### SPECIAL

Special diets accommodated
Proximity to Emergency Svcs.: Less than 8 miles

### STAFF

Caregiver Training: Dementia, Ethics, Family communication, Grief, Pain management, Patient transfers, Stress management, Transition issues, Universal precautions, Validation therapy, Wound care
Criminal Background Check: Yes
Principal Staff Language(s): English
Other Staff Language(s): Hebrew, Spanish

### FACILITY FEATURES

Activities/Recreation
Beauty/Barber Shop
Chapel Services
Guest Meals ($)
Outside Patio/Gardens
Private Dining Room
Private Visiting Room
Separate Therapy Room
24-hour Security
Whirlpool Baths

### ROOM FEATURES

Cable TV Ready
Space for personal items
Shared & Private Bathrooms
Telephone Ready

## COSTS

PRICES MAY INCREASE. PLEASE CALL FOR MOST CURRENT INFORMATION.

| | |
|---|---|
| Shared Room | $142–$153/day |
| Private Room | $171–$223/day |
| Dementia Unit | Call for shared and private room rates |
| Respite Stays | $142–$153/day for shared room<br>$171–$223/day for private room |
| Rate Increase | Annually |
| Reimbursement | Medicare, Medicaid, LTCI, HMO, Private pay |

## PORTRAIT

Fifty-three sprawling acres surround the stately facility, which boasts a beautiful frame crawling with Carolina jasmine! Majestic trees shade the garden paths and outdoor seating areas. Inside, beautiful photos of seniors from around the world adorn the walls of the lobby. The space also hosts plush seating arrangements, where the residents enjoy live piano entertainment. Several residents were visiting with one another in the lovely garden room when we arrived.

Residents' generously sized rooms receive ample natural light. Most feature alcoves, which is a nice departure from the usual square layout. Two Alzheimer's units accommodate thirty residents each; most of these rooms are private. Both secured units are bathed in natural light, as is the rest of the facility. One unit has a birdcage that runs the length of one wall; the other, a grand aquarium!

The main dining area is a spacious setting of circular and square tables, matching chairs and spotless linoleum floors. Oversized windows capture lovely views of the outdoor sculpture garden. The "Country Store," also operated by the kitchen and volunteer staff, serves soups and sandwiches, salads, coffee and assorted beverages. Ample seating throughout the facility provides many opportunities for residents to sit and visit. Each common area features a different type of entertainment: one room has a big-screen TV and sound equipment; others have birdcages with singing starlings and various birdlife. Passing one common area, we saw a resident working on a jigsaw puzzle, as an antique radio played in the background. Across from the library is a spacious beauty parlor, where residents receive complimentary manicures and pedicures from the staff! An unbelievable thirteen staff therapists use the fully equipped therapy space. Flanking the house synagogue, which doubles as a chapel, is an auditorium with a stage and choir loft.

Much of Golden Acres' resident population and management are Jewish, but people of all faiths and backgrounds are welcomed. The management's complete dedication to the residents has spawned numerous ongoing remodeling projects, which have greatly enhanced the facility. Currently, the community is raising funds to add a pediatric wing for children with chronic illnesses.

## Grace Presbyterian Village

550 East Ann Arbor
Dallas, TX 75126

(214) 376-1701
www.gracepresbyterianvillage.org

**TOTAL GOVERNMENT DEFICIENCIES: 1** Reviewed on: September 9, 2005

| Nutrition and Dietary |
|---|
| 1 |

* IMPORTANT: REVIEW DETAILS OF EACH DEFICIENCY AT WWW.MEDICARE.GOV

**GILBERT GUIDE OBSERVATIONS**

| | | | |
|---|---|---|---|
| Administration & Staff | g g g | Dietary & Food Selection | g g g |
| Facility Aesthetics | g g g g | Activities | g g g |
| Facility Condition & Safety | g g g g | Access to Medical Care | g g g |
| Residents | g g g | | |

### DETAILS

Year Built: 1962
Year Remodeled: 2001
Current Mgmt. Since: 1999
No. of Floors: 3
Resident Capacity: 160
Facility Type: Long-term care

### SPECIAL

Special diets accommodated
Proximity to Emergency Svcs.: Less than 8 miles

### STAFF

Caregiver Training: Dementia, Ethics, Family communication, Grief, Pain management, Patient transfers, Stress management, Transition issues, Universal precautions, Validation therapy, Wound care
Criminal Background Check: Yes
Principal Staff Language(s): English
Other Staff Language(s): Spanish

### FACILITY FEATURES

Activities/Recreation
Beauty/Barber Shop ($)
Chapel Services
Facility Parking
Guest Meals
Outside Patio/Gardens
Private Dining Room
Private Visiting Room
Separate Therapy Room
24-hour Security
Whirlpool Baths

### ROOM FEATURES

Cable TV Ready ($)
Space for personal items
Shared & Private Bathrooms
Telephone Ready ($)

## COSTS

PRICES MAY INCREASE. PLEASE CALL FOR MOST CURRENT INFORMATION.

| | |
|---|---|
| Shared Room | $125–$133/day |
| Private Room | $162–$252/day |
| Rate Increase | Periodically |
| Reimbursement | Medicare, Medicaid, LTCI, HMO, Private pay, Veterans |

## PORTRAIT

Grace Presbyterian Village is located on a large campus south of downtown Dallas. The entrance was under construction when we visited, but the rest of the facility was beautifully maintained. An attractive glass walkway connects the skilled nursing and assisted living areas. Many staff members have been with Grace Presbyterian Village for more than thirteen years.

Music played softly in the background as we toured the facility. The interior is homelike, although the lighting is somewhat institutional. Well-kept common areas include TVs, couches and chairs. The hallways are wide and equipped with handrails. The large dining area is spotless and comfortable. Residents' rooms feature elegant and practical furnishings. Windows allow natural light. Special pressure-relieving mattresses help prevent bedsores. The facility is equipped with lifting devices to help transfer residents between beds, walkers and wheelchairs when necessary.

Residents and their families enjoy the lovely twenty-seven acre grounds, which are wooded and hilly. The campus is landscaped with grass, flowers and shade trees. A stream runs across the property. Flocks of native birds call the area home, much to the pleasure of resident bird-watchers.

## Huguley Nursing and Rehabilitation Center

301 Huguley Boulevard
Burleson, TX 76028

(817) 551-5900
www.adventistcare.org

**TOTAL GOVERNMENT DEFICIENCIES: 13** Reviewed on: November 4, 2005

| Quality Care | Resident Assessment | Resident Rights | Nutrition and Dietary |
|---|---|---|---|
| 4 | 1 | 2 | 1 |
| **Pharmacy Service** | **Environmental** | **Administration** | |
| 1 | 3 | 1 | |

* IMPORTANT: REVIEW DETAILS OF EACH DEFICIENCY AT WWW.MEDICARE.GOV

**GILBERT GUIDE OBSERVATIONS**

| | | | |
|---|---|---|---|
| Administration & Staff | g g g | Dietary & Food Selection | g g g |
| Facility Aesthetics | g g g g | Activities | g g g |
| Facility Condition & Safety | g g g | Access to Medical Care | g g g g |
| Residents | g g g | | |

### DETAILS

Year Built: 1977
Year Remodeled: 1991
Current Mgmt. Since: 1999
No. of Floors: 1
Resident Capacity: 178
Facility Type: Long-term care, Short-term rehab

### SPECIAL

Special diets accommodated
Proximity to Emergency Svcs.: Less than 8 miles

### STAFF

Caregiver Training: Ethics, Family communication, Grief, Pain management, Patient transfers, Stress management, Transition issues, Universal precautions, Validation therapy, Wound care
Criminal Background Check: Yes
Principal Staff Language(s): English
Other Staff Language(s): Spanish

### FACILITY FEATURES

Activities/Recreation
Beauty/Barber Shop ($)
Chapel Services
Guest Meals ($)
Outside Patio/Gardens
Separate Therapy Room
Wanderguard
Whirlpool Baths

### ROOM FEATURES

Cable TV Ready
Space for personal items
Private Bathrooms
Telephone Ready

## COSTS

PRICES MAY INCREASE. PLEASE CALL FOR MOST CURRENT INFORMATION.

| | |
|---|---|
| Shared Room | $114/day |
| Rate Increase | Annually |
| Reimbursement | Medicare, Medicaid, LTCI, HMO, Private pay, SSI, Veterans |

## PORTRAIT

Located off of Interstate 35, Huguley Nursing and Rehabilitation is one of several health care facilities on the Huguley Health System campus; also on campus are a medical center, a retirement community, a diabetes management center and a fitness center. The nursing building is surrounded by freshly cut lawns, potted shrubs and towering oak trees. The lobby doubles as a common area—a homey setting with floral lithographs, rich maroon sofas and blue speckled carpeting.

Decorative curtains divide residents' moderately sized rooms in half. Each room has two windows, which let in plenty of natural light. The spacious dining area is also used for activities. Numerous windows make the facility especially bright and cheery. Residents enjoy three furnished outdoor areas replete with shaded garden paths that wind throughout the grassy landscape; the paths are broad enough to accommodate residents who use wheelchairs. The wooden gazebo is the centerpiece of the main courtyard.

The day of our visit seemed especially busy for Huguley's staff. Energetic residents hosted visitors while management and staff tended to business operations.

# LANCASTER NURSING AND REHAB

1515 North Elm Street (972) 227-6066
Lancaster, TX 75134

---

**TOTAL GOVERNMENT DEFICIENCIES: 1** Reviewed on: February 3, 2005

| Environmental |
|---|
| 1 |

* IMPORTANT: REVIEW DETAILS OF EACH DEFICIENCY AT WWW.MEDICARE.GOV

**GILBERT GUIDE OBSERVATIONS**

| | | | |
|---|---|---|---|
| Administration & Staff | g g g | Dietary & Food Selection | g g g |
| Facility Aesthetics | g g g | Activities | g g g |
| Facility Condition & Safety | g g g | Access to Medical Care | g g g |
| Residents | g g g | | |

LANCASTER NURSING AND REHAB (CONTINUED)

### DETAILS

Year Built: 1978
Year Remodeled: 1998
Current Mgmt. Since: 2003
No. of Floors: 1
Resident Capacity: 110
Facility Type: Long-term care, Short-term rehab

### SPECIAL

Special diets accommodated
Proximity to Emergency Svcs.: Less than 8 miles

### STAFF

Caregiver Training: Dementia, Ethics, Family communication, Grief, Patient transfers, Stress management, Universal precautions, Wound care
Criminal Background Check: Yes
Principal Staff Language(s): English
Other Staff Language(s): Spanish

### FACILITY FEATURES

Activities/Recreation
Beauty/Barber Shop ($)
Guest Meals ($)
Outside Patio/Gardens
Separate Therapy Room
Wanderguard

### ROOM FEATURES

Space for personal items
Private Bathrooms
Telephone Ready ($)

### COSTS

PRICES MAY INCREASE. PLEASE CALL FOR MOST CURRENT INFORMATION.

| | |
|---|---|
| Shared Room | $96/day |
| Private Room | $150/day |
| Rate Increase | Annually; usually 3–5% |
| Reimbursement | Medicare, Medicaid, HMO, Private pay, SSI, Veterans |

### PORTRAIT

Lancaster Nursing and Rehab enjoys the best of both worlds: it is close to Interstate 35, a major Dallas thoroughfare, yet it is tucked away from the urban hustle and bustle in a peaceful residential area. The facility is housed in a white brick building decorated with several beautiful plants at the entrance.

Lancaster specializes in physical, occupational and speech therapy programs. It also offers wound care, IV and pain management therapy, which is somewhat unusual for a SNF. Staff members encourage residents to walk about the building and enjoy themselves; we noted several residents doing so on our visit. Staff members and residents dine together in the two newly furnished dining rooms, adding to the homey atmosphere. It was a particularly hot day when we visited, so no one was on the small outdoor patio, although the staff informed us that residents enjoy socializing there in cooler weather.

The facility's state of cleanliness impressed us. The white tile flooring, spartan décor and spotless but outdated furniture are reminiscent of a hospital. The bright fluorescent lighting allows residents to navigate the building without fear of an unseen obstacle. The wide, uncluttered hallways are equipped with handrails. New hospital beds furnish the residents' spacious, sunny rooms. Each room has an area for personal belongings, which many of the residents have decorated with floral arrangements, knickknacks and family photographs.

## The Meadows Nursing & North Dallas Rehab

8383 Meadows Road
Dallas, TX 75231
(214) 238-6000

---

**TOTAL GOVERNMENT DEFICIENCIES: 1** Reviewed on: December 1, 2005

Environmental Deficiencies
1

* IMPORTANT: REVIEW DETAILS OF EACH DEFICIENCY AT WWW.MEDICARE.GOV

**GILBERT GUIDE OBSERVATIONS**

| | | | |
|---|---|---|---|
| Administration & Staff | g g g g | Dietary & Food Selection | g g g g g |
| Facility Aesthetics | g g g | Activities | g g |
| Facility Condition & Safety | g g g | Access to Medical Care | g g g |
| Residents | g g g | | |

### DETAILS

Year Built: 1977
Year Remodeled: 1998
Current Mgmt. Since: 1996
No. of Floors: 2
Resident Capacity: 148
Facility Type: Long-term care, Short-term rehab

### SPECIAL

Special diets accommodated
Proximity to Emergency Svcs.: Less than 8 miles

### STAFF

Caregiver Training: Ethics, Family communication, Grief, Pain management, Patient transfers, Stress management, Universal precautions, Wound care
Criminal Background Check: Yes
Principal Staff Language(s): English
Other Staff Language(s): Spanish

### FACILITY FEATURES

Activities/Recreation
Beauty/Barber Shop ($)
Chapel Services
Guest Meals

### ROOM FEATURES

Cable TV Ready
Space for personal items
Shared & Private Bathrooms
Telephone Ready

THE MEADOWS NURSING & NORTH DALLAS REHAB (CONTINUED)

**FACILITY FEATURES (CONTINUED)**

Outside Patio/Gardens
Private Dining Room
Private Visiting Room
Separate Therapy Room
24-hour Security
Wanderguard
Whirlpool Baths

## COSTS

PRICES MAY INCREASE. PLEASE CALL FOR MOST CURRENT INFORMATION.

| | |
|---|---|
| Shared Room | $122/day |
| Private Room | $166/day |
| Respite Stays | $122/day for shared room<br>$166/day for private room |
| Rate Increase | Every 2 years; usually 3% |
| Reimbursement | Medicare, Medicaid, LTCI, Private pay, SSI, Veterans |

## PORTRAIT

The Meadows is situated on a bustling commercial street. The building is a prototypical "big city" structure, utilizing concrete throughout. The administrator informed us that plans for valet parking are underway and will alleviate the current parking inconveniences.

The interior is well-worn, but homey nevertheless. Residents' rooms are bathed in sunlight. The recently refurbished dining room has vaulted ceilings and skylights, which are complemented by brightly painted walls adorned with art deco pieces. Residents lounge on plush chairs in the common room. The outdoor area is a lovely alternative to the building's concrete facade. Residents enjoy patio seating amidst blossoming plants. The hallways are narrow but well-lit.

Staff "angels" assigned to each hall foster greater familiarity between residents and staff members. Be it an impromptu visit or daily assistance, residents welcome the company. The interaction between residents and staff buzzed with enthusiasm. The Meadows' administrator is spearheading many projects to upgrade the building. The management's philosophy promotes integrating patients back into the community as soon as they are comfortable; the organization prides itself on a high resident discharge ratio. The environment at The Meadows is a familial one. Residents and staff welcomed us as if we were newcomers to their tight-knit community. Everyone was delighted to host us.

## Northgate Plaza

2101 West Northgate Drive
Irving, TX 75062

(982) 255-4460
(214) 783-9746
www.stonegateseniorcare.com

**TOTAL GOVERNMENT DEFICIENCIES: 5** — Reviewed on: February 25, 2005

| Environmental | Mistreatment | Nutrition and Dietary | Quality Care |
|---|---|---|---|
| 1 | 1 | 1 | 2 |

* IMPORTANT: REVIEW DETAILS OF EACH DEFICIENCY AT WWW.MEDICARE.GOV

**GILBERT GUIDE OBSERVATIONS**

| | | | |
|---|---|---|---|
| Administration & Staff | g g g g | Dietary & Food Selection | g g g |
| Facility Aesthetics | g g g | Activities | g g g |
| Facility Condition & Safety | g g g g | Access to Medical Care | g g g g |
| Residents | g g g g | | |

### DETAILS

Year Built: 2003
Current Mgmt. Since: 2003
No. of Floors: 1
Resident Capacity: 110
Facility Type: Long-term care, Short-term rehab

### SPECIAL

Special diets accommodated
Proximity to Emergency Svcs.: Less than 8 miles

### STAFF

Caregiver Training: Dementia, Ethics, Family communication, Grief, Pain management, Patient transfers, Stress management, Transition issues, Universal precautions, Validation therapy, Wound care
Criminal Background Check: Yes
Principal Staff Language(s): English
Other Staff Language(s): Spanish

### FACILITY FEATURES

Activities/Recreation
Beauty/Barber Shop ($)
Chapel Services
Private Dining Room ($)
Separate Therapy Room
24-hour Security
Wanderguard

### ROOM FEATURES

Cable TV Ready ($)
Space for personal items
Shared Bathrooms
Telephone Ready

### COSTS

PRICES MAY INCREASE. PLEASE CALL FOR MOST CURRENT INFORMATION.

| | |
|---|---|
| Shared Room | $114–$150/day |
| Respite Stays | $114–$150/day for shared room |

NORTHGATE PLAZA (CONTINUED)

| | |
|---|---|
| Rate Increase | Every 2–3 years; usually 1–2% |
| Reimbursement | Medicare, Medicaid, LTCI, Private pay, Veterans |

**PORTRAIT**

Northgate Plaza is nestled in a hilly residential area. The expansive grounds are brightened with red photinias, pansies and pink crepe myrtles. The interior of this brick building is accented in shades of maroon, cream and green. The foyer is comfortably furnished with plush couches, cushioned wooden chairs and tables. Prints of Italian villas, Grecian urns and pastoral scenes decorate the walls.

Residents' rooms are spacious and bright. Each has a large window and is furnished with a bed, nightstand, dresser and food tray. Glass chandeliers add elegance to the dinning room. The two common areas that flank the dining room are furnished with modern blue and gray couches. A group of residents were laughing and socializing in front of the big-screen TV during our visit. Wooden benches on the cozy back porch invite residents to enjoy the outdoors.

The hallways are uncluttered and lined with white handrails. The nurses' station is situated in the middle of the star-shaped building; it is an excellent vantage point. The building is brightened by fluorescent lighting. We witnessed plenty of interaction between residents and staff. Whether socializing in the halls or engaged in Bible study, residents seemed vibrant and content. Northgate's nursing staff struck us as attentive, patient and professional.

## PEARL NORDAN CARE CENTER

1234 Abrams Road
Dallas, TX 75214

(214) 827-0813
www.fowlerhomes.org

**TOTAL GOVERNMENT DEFICIENCIES: 11** — Reviewed on: June 23, 2005

| Administration | Environmental | Nutrition and Dietary | Pharmacy Service |
|---|---|---|---|
| 1 | 2 | 1 | 2 |
| **Quality Care** | **Resident Rights** | | |
| 2 | 3 | | |

* IMPORTANT: REVIEW DETAILS OF EACH DEFICIENCY AT WWW.MEDICARE.GOV

**GILBERT GUIDE OBSERVATIONS**

| | | | |
|---|---|---|---|
| Administration & Staff | g g g g g | Dietary & Food Selection | g g g g g |
| Facility Aesthetics | g g g g g | Activities | g g g g g |
| Facility Condition & Safety | g g g g g | Access to Medical Care | g g g g g |
| Residents | g g g | | |

## DETAILS

Year Built: 2001
Current Mgmt. Since: 2001
No. of Floors: 2
Resident Capacity: 61
Facility Type: Long-term care

## SPECIAL

Special diets accommodated
Proximity to Emergency Svcs.: Less than 8 miles

## STAFF

Caregiver Training: Dementia, Family communication, Grief, Patient transfers, Stress management
Criminal Background Check: Yes
Principal Staff Language(s): English
Other Staff Language(s): Spanish

## FACILITY FEATURES

Activities/Recreation
Beauty/Barber Shop ($)
Chapel Services
Guest Meals ($)
Outside Patio/Gardens
Private Dining Room
Private Visiting Room
Separate Therapy Room
24-hour Security

## ROOM FEATURES

Cable TV Ready
Space for personal items
Private Bathrooms
Telephone Ready

## COSTS

PRICES MAY INCREASE. PLEASE CALL FOR MOST CURRENT INFORMATION.

| | |
|---|---|
| Private Room | $2,400–$2,600/month |
| Rate Increase | Annually; usually 2% |
| Reimbursement | Medicare, Medicaid, LTCI, Private pay, SSI, Veterans |

## PORTRAIT

Pearl Nordan is a gorgeous addition to the sixteen-acre campus of Juliette Fowler Homes; also members of the community are independent and assisted living residents from Fowler Christian Apartments and the Jackson Living Center. Green foliage envelops the attractive brick frame. The building is minutes from downtown Dallas and the Lakewood area. Residents and their families enjoy outings to any of several nearby parks. The reception area is an elegant setting of cherrywood furniture with floral upholstery and dark green carpeting. The building is bathed in sunlight that streams in from windows on all sides.

Residents' luxurious rooms are accented with crown moldings and textured walls. Residents socialize and gather in the many common areas, which include a fitness room, club rooms, libraries, a swimming pool and a chapel. In the dining room, a group of residents were sharing a meal of turkey and cheese sandwiches with tomato soup, prepared by the kitchen staff. The expansive outdoor area is well-maintained. Shaded picnic tables in grassy areas, curved pathways and majestic cedar and maple trees are all a part of this picturesque

PEARL NORDAN CARE CENTER (CONTINUED)

refuge. The hallways are spacious and equipped with handrails. Residents' mailboxes also line the halls.

The community at Pearl Nordan is an active one. The combination of independent living and assisted living residents gives the campus a feeling of vitality. We observed residents checking mail, walking with staff through the halls, playing chess in one of the common areas and preparing for outdoor picnics. Staff and residents were very pleasant with one another, adding to the vibrant, homelike environment.

## Senior Care Beltline

106 North Beltline Road
Garland, TX 75040

(972) 495-7700
www.scc-texas.com

**TOTAL GOVERNMENT DEFICIENCIES: 20** — Reviewed on: October 7, 2005

| Administration | Environmental | Nutrition and Dietary | Pharmacy Service |
|---|---|---|---|
| 1 | 7 | 4 | 5 |
| **Quality Care** | **Resident Rights** | | |
| 2 | 1 | | |

* IMPORTANT: REVIEW DETAILS OF EACH DEFICIENCY AT WWW.MEDICARE.GOV

**GILBERT GUIDE OBSERVATIONS**

| | | | |
|---|---|---|---|
| Administration & Staff | g g g g | Dietary & Food Selection | g g g |
| Facility Aesthetics | g g | Activities | g |
| Facility Condition & Safety | g g g | Access to Medical Care | g g g g |
| Residents | g g g | | |

### DETAILS

Year Built: 1976
Year Remodeled: 2001
Current Mgmt. Since: 2000
No. of Floors: 1
Resident Capacity: 118
Facility Type: Long-term care, Short-term rehab

### SPECIAL

Special diets accommodated
Proximity to Emergency Svcs.: Less than 8 miles

### STAFF

Caregiver Training: Dementia, Ethics, Family communication, Grief, Pain management, Patient transfers, Stress management, Transition issues, Universal precautions, Validation therapy, Wound care
Criminal Background Check: Yes

Principal Staff Language(s): English
Other Staff Language(s): Spanish

## FACILITY FEATURES

Activities/Recreation
Beauty/Barber Shop ($)
Guest Meals ($)
Outside Patio/Gardens
Separate Therapy Room
24-hour Security
Wanderguard

## ROOM FEATURES

Cable TV Ready
Space for personal items
Shared Bathrooms
Telephone Ready

## COSTS

PRICES MAY INCREASE. PLEASE CALL FOR MOST CURRENT INFORMATION.

| | |
|---|---|
| Shared Room | $107/day |
| Private Room | $214/day |
| Respite Stays | $107/day for shared room<br>$214/day for private room |
| Rate Increase | Annually; usually 1% |
| Reimbursement | Medicare, Medicaid, Private pay, Veterans |

## PORTRAIT

The budget-conscious individual who desires peace and quiet will find a good choice in Senior Care Beltline. This facility is well-tended and serene despite nearby construction on the same busy street. There is limited parking for visiting friends and family.

Residents' small semi-private rooms feature petite windows and shared closets. One resident, who has lived at Senior Care for several months, cheerfully described how she moved to this more affordable facility after her private funding ran out. She chose to have a reclining chair in her room rather than a bed, as there isn't room for both. Her wall space was completely covered with photographs, prompting her to relate stories about her family and cats.

Staff turnover is low; many have worked at Senior Care for years. Staff and residents interact with obvious affection. A social worker informed us that residents are most active in the morning. Fewer activities are held in the afternoons, when most residents tend to relax in their rooms.

The shiny linoleum hallways have serviceable handrails. Easily accessible racks of clean linen and wheelchairs line the halls, interspersed with sitting areas, med carts and cleaning carts. The lighting is artificial but adequate. There are two paved outdoor patios; one is a designated smoking area. Potted plants add a hint of green in lieu of flowerbeds. Iron chairs and a concrete bench form the patio seating area.

## VERANDA PRESTON HOLLOW A/D

11409 North Central Expressway
Dallas, TX 75243

(214) 363-5100
www.verandaprestonhollow.com

**TOTAL GOVERNMENT DEFICIENCIES: 5** — Reviewed on: September 1, 2005

| Environmental | Nutrition and Dietary | Administration Rights |
|---|---|---|
| 3 | 1 | 1 |

* IMPORTANT: REVIEW DETAILS OF EACH DEFICIENCY AT WWW.MEDICARE.GOV

**GILBERT GUIDE OBSERVATIONS**

| | | | |
|---|---|---|---|
| Administration & Staff | g g g | Dietary & Food Selection | g g g |
| Facility Aesthetics | g g | Activities | g g g |
| Facility Condition & Safety | g g g | Alzheimer's & Dementia Capabilities | g g g g |
| Residents | g g g | Access to Medical Care | g g g |

### DETAILS

Year Built: 2001
Current Mgmt. Since: 2003
No. of Floors: 2
Resident Capacity: 142
Facility Type: Long-term care, Short-term rehab, Alzheimer's unit

### SPECIAL

Special diets accommodated
Proximity to Emergency Svcs.: Less than 8 miles

### STAFF

Caregiver Training: Dementia, Family communication, Pain management, Patient transfers, Stress management, Universal precautions, Wound care
Criminal Background Check: Yes
Principal Staff Language(s): English
Other Staff Language(s): Spanish

### FACILITY FEATURES

Activities/Recreation
Beauty/Barber Shop ($)
Guest Meals
Private Dining Room
Private Visiting Room
Separate Therapy Room
24-hour Security
Whirlpool Baths

### ROOM FEATURES

Cable TV Ready
Space for personal items
Shared & Private Bathrooms
Telephone Ready

### COSTS

PRICES MAY INCREASE. PLEASE CALL FOR MOST CURRENT INFORMATION.

| | |
|---|---|
| Shared Room | $131–$156/day |
| Private Room | $176/day |

| | |
|---|---|
| Respite Stays | \$131–\$156/day for shared room<br>\$176/day for private room |
| Rate Increase | Annually; usually 4% |
| Reimbursement | Medicare, Medicaid, LTCI, HMO, Private pay |

**PORTRAIT**

Veranda Preston Hollow is an upscale facility located next to Central Expressway, a major Dallas thoroughfare. The skilled nursing area is housed on the third and fourth floors of the large brick building it shares with its sister assisted living unit. The lobby boasts several luxurious amenities, including a library, a grand piano and a cappuccino bar. Recessed fixtures spread soft lighting along the wide hallways. Expansive windows feature beautiful views of the walkways and flowers along the landscaped grounds. An elevator provides access to the upper floors.

Comfortable furniture and a big-screen TV furnish the third floor common area. A beverage bar offers coffee, tea and juice outside. the somewhat institutional dining room. Chairs, nightstands, armoires and hospital beds furnish residents' rooms on the fourth floor. Some of the rooms boast parquet floors. We were surprised and delighted to see a resident that we'd known from many years ago! She was as cheerful as ever and seemed to be enjoying her stay at Veranda Preston Hollow.

## THE VILLA AT MOUNTAIN VIEW

2918 Duncanville Road
Dallas, TX 75211

(214) 467-7090
(214) 657-1465

**TOTAL GOVERNMENT DEFICIENCIES: 6** Reviewed on: June 24, 2005

| Environmental | Pharmacy Service |
|---|---|
| 2 | 4 |

* IMPORTANT: REVIEW DETAILS OF EACH DEFICIENCY AT WWW.MEDICARE.GOV

**GILBERT GUIDE OBSERVATIONS**

| | | | |
|---|---|---|---|
| Administration & Staff | g g g | Dietary & Food Selection | g g g |
| Facility Aesthetics | g g g | Activities | g g g |
| Facility Condition & Safety | g g g | Access to Medical Care | g g |
| Residents | g g g | | |

THE VILLA AT MOUNTAIN VIEW (CONTINUED)

## DETAILS

Year Built: 1997
Current Mgmt. Since: 1997
No. of Floors: 1
Resident Capacity: 120
Facility Type: Long-term care

## SPECIAL

Special diets accommodated
Proximity to Emergency Svcs.: 9–15 Miles

## STAFF

Caregiver Training: Ethics, Family communication, Grief, Pain management, Patient transfers, Stress management, Transition issues, Universal precautions, Wound care
Criminal Background Check: Yes
Principal Staff Language(s): English
Other Staff Language(s): Spanish

## FACILITY FEATURES

Activities/Recreation
Beauty/Barber Shop ($)
Guest Meals ($)
Outside Patio/Gardens
Separate Therapy Room ($)
24-hour Security

## ROOM FEATURES

Cable TV Ready
Space for personal items
Shared Bathrooms
Telephone Ready

## COSTS

PRICES MAY INCREASE. PLEASE CALL FOR MOST CURRENT INFORMATION.

| | |
|---|---|
| Shared Room | $109.70/day |
| Rate Increase | Annually |
| Reimbursement | Medicare, Medicaid, LTCI, Private pay |

## PORTRAIT

The Villa at Mountainview is situated on a bustling street in southwestern Dallas. A white picket fence surrounds the red brick building, enclosing a portion of thick grass and shade trees. Despite the unremarkable appearance of the interior, the facility shines thanks to the friendly and attentive staff. They addressed each resident by name as we toured the home. The residents were subdued as they watched television or rested in their rooms. While all of the rooms are semi-private, residents may obtain special permission for a private room.

Handrails provide support in the broad hallways, where a handful of residents sat peacefully as they watched staff and visitors come and go. Fluorescent lighting and immaculate white walls and floors contribute to the facility's bright atmosphere. The spacious dining room features an outdoor area, where residents may dine and listen to the activity on busy Duncanville Road.

## WALNUT PLACE A/D

5515 Glen Lakes Drive
Dallas, TX 75231
(214) 361-8923

**TOTAL GOVERNMENT DEFICIENCIES: 8** Reviewed on: January 28, 2005

| Administration | Environmental | Nutrition and Dietary | Pharmacy Service |
|---|---|---|---|
| 1 | 2 | 1 | 2 |
| **Quality Care** | **Resident Rights** | | |
| 1 | 1 | | |

* IMPORTANT: REVIEW DETAILS OF EACH DEFICIENCY AT WWW.MEDICARE.GOV

**GILBERT GUIDE OBSERVATIONS**

| | | | |
|---|---|---|---|
| Administration & Staff | g g g g g | Dietary & Food Selection | g g g g |
| Facility Aesthetics | g g g g | Activities | g g g g g |
| Facility Condition & Safety | g g g | Alzheimer's & Dementia Capabilities | g g g g g |
| Residents | g g g | Access to Medical Care | g g g g g |

### DETAILS

Year Built: 1980
Year Remodeled: 2003
Current Mgmt. Since: 1980
No. of Floors: 3
Resident Capacity: 210
Facility Type: Long-term care, Short-term rehab, Alzheimer's unit

### SPECIAL

Special diets accommodated
Proximity to Emergency Svcs.: Less than 8 miles

### STAFF

Caregiver Training: Dementia, Ethics, Family communication, Grief, Pain management, Patient transfers, Stress management, Transition issues, Universal precautions, Validation therapy, Wound care
Criminal Background Check: Yes
Principal Staff Language(s): English
Other Staff Language(s): Cantonese, Mandarin, Spanish

### FACILITY FEATURES

Activities/Recreation
Beauty/Barber Shop ($)
Chapel Services
Guest Meals ($)
Outside Patio/Gardens
Private Dining Room
Private Visiting Room
Separate Therapy Room
24-hour Security

### ROOM FEATURES

Cable TV Ready
Space for personal items
Shared & Private Bathrooms
Telephone Ready

WALNUT PLACE (CONTINUED)

## COSTS

PRICES MAY INCREASE. PLEASE CALL FOR MOST CURRENT INFORMATION.

| | |
|---|---|
| Shared Room | $130/day |
| Private Room | $175–$200/day |
| Respite Stays | $130/day for shared room<br>$175–$200/day for private room |
| Rate Increase | Annually; usually 4% |
| Reimbursement | Medicare, LTCI, Private pay |

## PORTRAIT

Walnut Place is set back from the street—most passersby don't even realize it's there—which is unfortunate, for it is a true gem. Walnut Place offers specialized care for Alzheimer's patients in addition to regular nursing care. Due to its urban location, the facility doesn't have enough property for an outdoor area; instead, the building has a wonderful atrium at its center. One excellent feature of the facility is the onsite pharmacy, which is staffed by a full-time pharmacist.

Even those who reside at Walnut Place briefly, for short-term rehab, remember the staff with affection. The activity director postponed her vacation to throw a huge birthday party for one resident who turned 100. The director not only coordinated the party, she also decorated the room and helped clean up afterward. An annual employee Halloween costume contest helps employees and residents get into the spirit of the season.

Several large birdcages containing different varieties of birds contribute to the cheery environment. The lobby features fresh cut flowers. The building's first three floors completely encircle the atrium. Some residents walk this circle for exercise, and use the opportunity to visit with each other. Artificial light brightens the spacious hallways. The halls in the nursing area are somewhat darker than the rest. Two dining areas reduce crowding; they are also used for activities. Many Thursday mornings feature a "pie bake," the results of which are eaten in the afternoons.

Residents' sunny rooms face outside or into the atrium. Many contain two closets, giving residents in the semi-private rooms additional storage space. The secured Alzheimer's unit is located on the fifth floor. Walnut Place has a unique tradition with regard to residents' furnishings. When a resident passes away, the family takes the furnishings they want. The unwanted furniture is then auctioned off to the employees. The proceeds go to the "sunshine fund," which is used to send flowers to employees when they are ill.

## Windsor Place Nursing Center

2537 West Pleasant Run Road (972) 228-8029
Lancaster, TX 75146

---

**TOTAL GOVERNMENT DEFICIENCIES: 4** Reviewed on: March 3, 2005

| Deficiencies Reported Between Inspections | Mistreatment | Nutrition and Dietary | Resident Rights |
|---|---|---|---|
| 1 | 1 | 1 | 1 |

* IMPORTANT: REVIEW DETAILS OF EACH DEFICIENCY AT WWW.MEDICARE.GOV

**GILBERT GUIDE OBSERVATIONS**

| | | | |
|---|---|---|---|
| Administration & Staff | g g g | Dietary & Food Selection | g g g |
| Facility Aesthetics | g g g | Activities | g g g |
| Facility Condition & Safety | g g g | Access to Medical Care | g g g g |
| Residents | g g g | | |

### DETAILS

Year Built: 1997
Current Mgmt. Since: 1997
No. of Floors: 1
Resident Capacity: 111
Facility Type: Long-term care

### SPECIAL

Special diets accommodated
Proximity to Emergency Svcs.: Less than 8 miles

### STAFF

Caregiver Training: Dementia, Ethics, Family communication, Grief, Pain management, Patient transfers, Stress management, Transition issues, Universal precautions, Validation therapy, Wound care
Criminal Background Check: Yes
Principal Staff Language(s): English
Other Staff Language(s): Spanish

### FACILITY FEATURES

Activities/Recreation
Beauty/Barber Shop ($)
Chapel Services
Guest Meals ($)
Separate Therapy Room
24-hour Security

### ROOM FEATURES

Cable TV Ready
Space for personal items
Shared Bathrooms
Telephone Ready

### COSTS

PRICES MAY INCREASE. PLEASE CALL FOR MOST CURRENT INFORMATION.

| | |
|---|---|
| Shared Room | $116/day |
| Rate Increase | Annually; usually $2/day |
| Reimbursement | Medicare, Medicaid, LTCI, Private pay |

WINDSOR PLACE NURSING CENTER (CONTINUED)

**PORTRAIT**

Upon entering Windsor Place Nursing Center, visitors are greeted in a cozy reception area. Despite meager furniture accommodations, the area features a lovely marble fireplace that frequently attracts resident gatherings.

Residents' rooms are fairly institutional, fully furnished, and feature a small TV and additional storage for personal items. The spacious dining area doubles as the main common room. Residents navigate through broad hallways, which are equipped with handrails. Adequate florescent lighting is prevalent throughout. Immaculate floors and a neatly kept facility restate Windsor's classic appeal.

Staff and residents have a pleasant rapport with one another. Although Windsor Place is without frills, its caring staff is the driving force of the operation. It was obvious to us that while management cuts decorative corners, they seem focused on genuine concern and care of their residents.

## Winters Park

3737 North Garland Road
Garland, TX 75044

(972) 495-7000
www.wphcsnf.com

**TOTAL GOVERNMENT DEFICIENCIES: 11** Reviewed on: September 30, 2005

| Administration | Mistreatment | Pharmacy Service |
|---|---|---|
| 2 | 1 | 4 |
| **Quality Care** | **Resident Rights** | |
| 3 | 1 | |

* IMPORTANT: REVIEW DETAILS OF EACH DEFICIENCY AT WWW.MEDICARE.GOV

**GILBERT GUIDE OBSERVATIONS**

| | | | |
|---|---|---|---|
| Administration & Staff | g g g g | Dietary & Food Selection | g g g g g |
| Facility Aesthetics | g g g g | Activities | g g |
| Facility Condition & Safety | g g g g g | Access to Medical Care | g g g |
| Residents | g g g g | | |

**DETAILS**

Year Built: 2004
Current Mgmt. Since: 2004
No. of Floors: 1
Resident Capacity: 132
Facility Type: Long-term care

**SPECIAL**

Special diets accommodated
Proximity to Emergency Svcs.: Less than 8 miles

## STAFF

Caregiver Training: Ethics, Family communication, Pain management, Patient transfers, Stress management, Transition issues, Universal precautions, Validation therapy, Wound care
Criminal Background Check: Yes
Principal Staff Language(s): English
Other Staff Language(s): Spanish

## FACILITY FEATURES

Activities/Recreation
Beauty/Barber Shop ($)
Guest Meals
Outside Patio/Gardens
Private Dining Room
Separate Therapy Room
24-hour Security
Wanderguard
Whirlpool Baths

## ROOM FEATURES

Cable TV Ready
Space for personal items
Shared Bathrooms
Telephone Ready

## COSTS

PRICES MAY INCREASE. PLEASE CALL FOR MOST CURRENT INFORMATION.

| | |
|---|---|
| Shared Room | $125–$135/day |
| Private Room | $210/day if available |
| Rate Increase | Periodically |
| Reimbursement | Medicare, Medicaid, Private pay |

## PORTRAIT

Located in the midst of a vibrant urban village complete with shopping and dining possibilities, Winters Park is pristine and welcoming. All four halls converge at the nurses' desk in the lobby. Fresh flower arrangements and plentiful magazines make the well-lit space homey.

The residents' rooms are spacious and comfortably accommodate reclining chairs, beds, nightstands, dressers and TVs. Large windows and cheerful wallpaper brighten every room. Excellent natural lighting and the clearly visible nursing station at the confluence of the hallways make the facility easy to navigate. The extra-wide hallways are equipped with handrails.

Winters Park residents were engaging and sociable, and seemed very much at home. Conversation punctuated by frequent laughter among residents was the order of the day when we visited. The main dining room is bright and spacious, with a multitude of windows. The tables are set widely apart to allow for wheelchair mobility and for staff to hand-deliver meals. A smaller dining area affords privacy for residents who require feeding assistance. A third dining room is employed for conferences and family meetings.

The physical therapy room features state-of-the-art training equipment. Another room, designated for music therapy, has a piano. There are two gazebos in the backyard for residents to enjoy in agreeable weather. Both are wheelchair and walker friendly. All doors leading outside are locked.

The staff is very accommodating. They believe that Winters Park is a home first and a facility second. One example of this occurred on our visit when an aide accommodated a resident's request to work on the parallel bars in the therapy room although it was nearly dinnertime and the room was locked.

## IN-HOME CARE PROVIDERS

# A C O Alternative Care Opportunity Healthcare

8600 Thackery, Suite 1201
Dallas, TX 75225
(469) 547-8586

SEE CHAPTER 1 FOR A DESCRIPTION OF IN-HOME CARE SERVICES.

### DETAILS

Years in Business: 2
Home Health Services Provided: Yes
Care Visits Provided Within a Facility: No
Dementia Care Provided: Yes
Will Replace Caregiver Within 48 Hours Upon Request: Yes

### CAREGIVERS

RN on Staff: Yes
Hiring Qualifications: 5 years of experience, Criminal background check, CNA certification, 3 references required
Caregiver Training: Dementia, Ethics, Family communication, Grief, Patient transfers, Stress management
Frequency of Caregiver Training: Initial formal training program, Monthly
Language(s) Spoken: English

### AVAILABILITY

Service Availability: 24/7
On-call Supervisor Availability: 24/7

### COSTS

PRICES MAY INCREASE. PLEASE CALL FOR MOST CURRENT INFORMATION.

Hourly: Call for rates
Minimum Hours per Day: None
Minimum Days per Week: None
Sliding Fee Schedule Available: No

### UNIQUE QUALITIES

Trust is important to ACO, so the staff works diligently to establish close bonds between families and caregivers. They assess clients' needs and develop individualized care plans based on these assessments. If ACO staff feel they do not have the resources to meet a certain client's needs, they do not hesitate to refer the client elsewhere. This clearly shows their dedication to ensuring that clients receive the best care possible.

## Anchor Home Health Services

310 Crooked Creek
Garland, TX 75043

(972) 279-1846

---

SEE CHAPTER 1 FOR A DESCRIPTION OF IN-HOME CARE SERVICES.

### DETAILS

Years in Business: 6 months
Home Health Services Provided: Yes
Care Visits Provided Within a Facility: No
Dementia Care Provided: No
Will Replace Caregiver Within 48 Hours Upon Request: Yes

### CAREGIVERS

RN on Staff: Yes
Hiring Qualifications: 2 years of experience, DMV check, TB test, Criminal background check, CNA certification, 3 references required
Caregiver Training: Dementia, Ethics, Family communication, Grief, Patient transfers, Stress management
Frequency of Caregiver Training: Initial formal training program, Semiannual
Language(s) Spoken: English

### AVAILABILITY

Service Availability: 24/7
On-call Supervisor Availability: 24/7

### COSTS

PRICES MAY INCREASE. PLEASE CALL FOR MOST CURRENT INFORMATION.

Rate: Call for rates
Minimum Hours per Day: None
Minimum Days per Week: None
Sliding Fee Schedule Available: No

### UNIQUE QUALITIES

Anchor Home Health Services takes great pride in the care they offer; they put clients' needs ahead of all else. They believe in establishing close relationships with clients and their families. Anchor Home is certified by Medicare and Medicaid.

## Angels of Hands Home Health Agency

630 Blue Chalk Drive (972) 230-2828
Cedar Hill, TX 75104

SEE CHAPTER 1 FOR A DESCRIPTION OF IN-HOME CARE SERVICES.

### DETAILS

Years in Business: 2
Home Health Services Provided: Yes
Care Visits Provided Within a Facility: Yes
Dementia Care Provided: No
Will Replace Caregiver Within 48 Hours Upon Request: Yes

### CAREGIVERS

RN on Staff: Yes
Hiring Qualifications: 6 months of experience, DMV check, TB test, Criminal background check, CNA certification, 1 reference required
Caregiver Training: Dementia, Ethics, Family communication, Grief, Patient transfers, Stress management
Frequency of Caregiver Training: Initial formal training program, Monthly
Language(s) Spoken: English, Sign Language, Spanish

### AVAILABILITY

Service Availability: 24/7
On-call Supervisor Availability: 24/7

### COSTS

PRICES MAY INCREASE. PLEASE CALL FOR MOST CURRENT INFORMATION.

Rate: Call for rates
Minimum Hours per Day: None
Minimum Days per Week: None
Sliding Fee Schedule Available: No

### UNIQUE QUALITIES

The owner of this agency, an experienced nurse, treats clients as if they were family. The staff of skilled caregivers focuses on prolonging clients' independence so that they may continue to stay with their loved ones rather than move to a long-term care facility.

## Aspen Home Care

1000 Nora Lane
Desoto, TX 75115
(214) 500-6009

SEE CHAPTER I FOR A DESCRIPTION OF IN-HOME CARE SERVICES.

### DETAILS

Years in Business: 1
Home Health Services Provided: Yes
Care Visits Provided Within a Facility: Yes
Dementia Care Provided: No
Will Replace Caregiver Within 48 Hours Upon Request: Yes

### CAREGIVERS

RN on Staff: Yes
Hiring Qualifications: 2 years of experience, TB test, Criminal background check, CNA certification, 3 references required
Caregiver Training: Dementia, Ethics, Family communication, Grief, Patient transfers, Stress management
Frequency of Caregiver Training: Initial formal training program, Semiannual
Language(s) Spoken: English, Spanish

### AVAILABILITY

Service Availability: 24/7
On-call Supervisor Availability: 24/7

### COSTS

PRICES MAY INCREASE. PLEASE CALL FOR MOST CURRENT INFORMATION.

Rate: Call for rates
Minimum Hours per Day: None
Minimum Days per Week: None
Sliding Fee Schedule Available: No

### UNIQUE QUALITIES

Aspen Home Care fights to prolong the independence of its clients. The caregivers strive to provide compassionate, nonintrusive care. An experienced nurse supervises the care. The agency accepts Medicare and Medicaid.

## Beacon Home Health Services

1000 Nora Lane (972) 223-0074
Desoto, TX 75115

SEE CHAPTER 1 FOR A DESCRIPTION OF IN-HOME CARE SERVICES.

### DETAILS

Years in Business: 9
Home Health Services Provided: No
Care Visits Provided Within a Facility: Yes
Dementia Care Provided: No
Will Replace Caregiver Within 48 Hours Upon Request: Yes

### CAREGIVERS

RN on Staff: Yes
Hiring Qualifications: TB test, Criminal background check, CNA certification, 3 references required
Caregiver Training: Dementia, Ethics, Family communication, Grief, Patient transfers, Stress management
Frequency of Caregiver Training: Initial formal training program, Semiannual
Language(s) Spoken: English, Spanish

### AVAILABILITY

Service Availability: 24/7
On-call Supervisor Availability: 24/7

### COSTS

PRICES MAY INCREASE. PLEASE CALL FOR MOST CURRENT INFORMATION.

Rate: $15.50/hour
Live-In: $372/day
Sleepover: $186/night
Minimum Hours per Day: 4
Minimum Days per Week: None
Sliding Fee Schedule Available: No

### UNIQUE QUALITIES

The goal of Beacon Home is to provide excellent care at a cost that is lower than average. The agency's management and caregivers listen carefully to clients' needs to maximize their independence and comfort. Beacon Home works hard to establish trust and friendship between clients and caregivers.

## Care Solutions Home Health LLC

1144 North Plano Road, Suite 11 (214) 646-6275
Richardson, Dallas 75081

SEE CHAPTER 1 FOR A DESCRIPTION OF IN-HOME CARE SERVICES.

### DETAILS

Years in Business: 1
Home Health Services Provided: No
Care Visits Provided Within a Facility: Yes
Dementia Care Provided: No
Will Replace Caregiver Within 48 Hours Upon Request: Yes

### CAREGIVERS

RN on Staff: No
Hiring Qualifications: 1 year of experience, Criminal background check, 2 references required
Caregiver Training: Dementia, Ethics, Family communication, Grief, Patient transfers, Stress management
Frequency of Caregiver Training: Initial formal training program, Monthly
Language(s) Spoken: English, Spanish

### AVAILABILITY

Service Availability: 24/7
On-call Supervisor Availability: 24/7

### COSTS

PRICES MAY INCREASE. PLEASE CALL FOR MOST CURRENT INFORMATION.

Rate: $18–$25/hour
Live-In: $215/day
Minimum Hours per Day: 4
Minimum Days per Week: None
Sliding Fee Schedule Available: No

### UNIQUE QUALITIES

Care Solutions' management believes it is important for clients and caregivers to be compatible, so they place clients accordingly. They try to create an atmosphere of fun for their clients, and to encourage mental and physical stimulation through daily activities. Caregivers attend continuing education classes on a monthly basis.

## Comfort Home Health Care, Inc.

410 West Main Street, Suite 102 (972) 203-1010
Mesquite, TX 75149

SEE CHAPTER 1 FOR A DESCRIPTION OF IN-HOME CARE SERVICES.

### DETAILS

Years in Business: 3
Home Health Services Provided: Yes
Care Visits Provided Within a Facility: Yes
Dementia Care Provided: No
Will Replace Caregiver Within 48 Hours Upon Request: Yes

### CAREGIVERS

RN on Staff: Yes
Hiring Qualifications: 1 year of experience, Criminal background check, 2 references required
Caregiver Training: Ethics, Family communication, Grief, Patient transfers, Stress management, Transition
Frequency of Caregiver Training: Initial formal training program, Quarterly
Language(s) Spoken: English, Spanish

### AVAILABILITY

Service Availability: 24/7
On-call Supervisor Availability: 24/7

### COSTS

PRICES MAY INCREASE. PLEASE CALL FOR MOST CURRENT INFORMATION.

Rate: Call for rates
Minimum Hours per Day: None
Minimum Days per Week: None
Sliding Fee Schedule Available: No

### UNIQUE QUALITIES

Comfort Home Health has an experienced nurse on staff who handles patients' needs. The management is in constant communication with caregivers in the field. The agency accepts Medicaid and Medicare.

## Custom Caregivers LLC

111 Jolly Way
Waxahachie, TX 75165

(972) 938-0703
www.customcaregivers.com

SEE CHAPTER 1 FOR A DESCRIPTION OF IN-HOME CARE SERVICES.

### DETAILS

Years in Business: 1½
Home Health Services Provided: No
Care Visits Provided Within a Facility: Yes
Dementia Care Provided: Yes
Will Replace Caregiver Within 48 Hours Upon Request: Yes

### CAREGIVERS

RN on Staff: No
Hiring Qualifications: 2 years of experience, DMV check, TB test, Criminal background check, CNA certification, 3 references required
Caregiver Training: Dementia, Ethics, Family communication, Grief, Patient transfers, Transition issues
Frequency of Caregiver Training: Initial formal training program, Semiannual
Language(s) Spoken: English

### AVAILABILITY

Service Availability: 24/7
On-call Supervisor Availability: 24/7

### COSTS

PRICES MAY INCREASE. PLEASE CALL FOR MOST CURRENT INFORMATION.

Rate: Call for rates
Minimum Hours per Day: 4
Minimum Days per Week: None
Sliding Fee Schedule Available: No

### UNIQUE QUALITIES

The goal of Custom Caregivers is to enhance clients' quality of life through companionship, as well as assistance with the activities of daily living. The agency prioritizes close relationships with clients and their families. It offers a cognitive retention therapy program for early-to-midstage dementia clients, including those with Alzheimer's. Custom Caregivers primarily serves an Ellis County population, but will consider prospective clients from neighboring counties.

## Grace Healthcare Services

12959 Jupiter Road, Suite 230 (214) 221-8585
Dallas, TX 75238

SEE CHAPTER 1 FOR A DESCRIPTION OF IN-HOME CARE SERVICES.

### DETAILS

Years in Business: 4
Home Health Services Provided: Yes
Care Visits Provided Within a Facility: Yes
Dementia Care Provided: Yes
Will Replace Caregiver Within 48 Hours Upon Request: Yes

### CAREGIVERS

RN on Staff: Yes
Hiring Qualifications: 2 years of experience, TB test, Criminal background check, CNA certification, 2 references required
Caregiver Training: Dementia, Ethics, Family communication, Patient transfers
Frequency of Caregiver Training: Initial formal training program, Monthly
Language(s) Spoken: English, Spanish

### AVAILABILITY

Service Availability: 24/7
On-call Supervisor Availability: 24/7

### COSTS

PRICES MAY INCREASE. PLEASE CALL FOR MOST CURRENT INFORMATION.

Rate: Call for rates
Minimum Hours per Day: None
Minimum Days per Week: None
Sliding Fee Schedule Available: No

### UNIQUE QUALITIES

Grace Healthcare Services works hard to build strong relationships with clients and their families. One of the agency's top priorities is to maintain clients' dignity. Grace Healthcare caregivers attend monthly continuing education sessions.

## Heaven at Home

4141 Blue Lake Circle
Dallas, TX 75244

(972) 245-1515
(866) 381-0500
www.heavenathomecare.com

SEE CHAPTER 1 FOR A DESCRIPTION OF IN-HOME CARE SERVICES.

### DETAILS

Years in Business: Unknown
Home Health Services Provided: No
Care Visits Provided Within a Facility: Yes
Dementia Care Provided: Yes
Will Replace Caregiver Within 48 Hours Upon Request: Yes

### CAREGIVERS

RN on Staff: Yes
Hiring Qualifications: 3 years of experience, DMV check, TB test, Criminal background check, CNA certification, 3 references required
Caregiver Training: Dementia, Ethics, Family communication, Grief, Patient transfers, Stress management
Frequency of Caregiver Training: Initial formal training program, Monthly
Language(s) Spoken: English

### AVAILABILITY

Service Availability: 24/7
On-call Supervisor Availability: 24/7

### COSTS

PRICES MAY INCREASE. PLEASE CALL FOR MOST CURRENT INFORMATION.

Rate: $14.95–$17.95/hour
Live-In: $175–$225/day
Sleepover: $125–$135/night
Minimum Hours per Day: 4
Minimum Days per Week: 3
Sliding Fee Schedule Available: No

### UNIQUE QUALITIES

Heaven at Home's objective is to help clients stay safely at home, thereby preserving their dignity and independence. To that end, the caregivers address the concerns of clients as well their families, and work closely with home health care and hospice services. Heaven at Home does not require a long-term commitment from its clients.

## Home Health Specialties

8500 North Stemmons Freeway, Suite 6070 (214) 689-2002
Dallas, TX 75247

SEE CHAPTER 1 FOR A DESCRIPTION OF IN-HOME CARE SERVICES.

### DETAILS

Years in Business: 30
Home Health Services Provided: Yes
Care Visits Provided Within a Facility: Yes
Dementia Care Provided: Yes
Will Replace Caregiver Within 48 Hours Upon Request: Yes

### CAREGIVERS

RN on Staff: Yes
Hiring Qualifications: 1 year of experience, TB test, Criminal background check, CNA certification, 2 references required
Caregiver Training: Dementia, Ethics, Family communication, Grief, Patient transfers, Transition issues
Frequency of Caregiver Training: Initial formal training program, Monthly, Annually
Language(s) Spoken: English, Spanish

### AVAILABILITY

Service Availability: 24/7
On-call Supervisor Availability: 24/7

### COSTS

PRICES MAY INCREASE. PLEASE CALL FOR MOST CURRENT INFORMATION.

Rate: Call for rates
Minimum Hours per Day: None
Minimum Days per Week: None
Sliding Fee Schedule Available: Yes

### UNIQUE QUALITIES

Home Health Specialties boasts thirty years of homecare experience in the Dallas area. The agency offers services that range from pediatrics to geriatrics. The therapy program is staffed by full-time professionals who specialize in speech, physical and occupational therapies. They pride themselves on smoothly transitioning clients from one program to another as necessary.

## Homewatch Caregivers

1700 Alma Drive, Suite 242
Plano, TX 75075

(972) 422-1156
(800) 777-9770
www.homewatchcaregivers.com

SEE CHAPTER 1 FOR A DESCRIPTION OF IN-HOME CARE SERVICES.

### DETAILS

Years in Business: 20
Home Health Services Provided: No
Care Visits Provided Within a Facility: Yes
Dementia Care Provided: Yes
Will Replace Caregiver Within 48 Hours Upon Request: Yes

### CAREGIVERS

RN on Staff: Yes
Hiring Qualifications: 2 years of experience, Criminal background check, 3 references required
Caregiver Training: Dementia, Ethics, Family communication, Grief, Patient transfers, Stress management
Frequency of Caregiver Training: Initial formal training program, Quarterly
Language(s) Spoken: English

### AVAILABILITY

Service Availability: 24/7
On-call Supervisor Availability: 24/7

### COSTS

PRICES MAY INCREASE. PLEASE CALL FOR MOST CURRENT INFORMATION.

Rate: Call for rates
Minimum Hours per Day: None
Minimum Days per Week: None
Sliding Fee Schedule Available: No

### UNIQUE QUALITIES

Homewatch Caregivers' excellent reputation is built on twenty years of experience. Its services include mentally stimulating activities that are designed to maintain clients' dignity and independence. The agency employs an open-door policy to promote peace of mind in clients and their families. Caregivers undergo training on a continual basis. Homewatch does not require money or deposits up front.

## In Home Care

8700 North Stemmons Freeway, Suite 4070 (214) 920-9296
Dallas, TX 75247

SEE CHAPTER I FOR A DESCRIPTION OF IN-HOME CARE SERVICES.

### DETAILS

Years in Business: 18
Home Health Services Provided: Yes
Care Visits Provided Within a Facility: Yes
Dementia Care Provided: No
Will Replace Caregiver Within 48 Hours Upon Request: Yes

### CAREGIVERS

RN on Staff: Yes
Hiring Qualifications: 5 years of experience, DMV check, TB test, Criminal background check, CNA certification, 4 references required
Caregiver Training: Dementia, Ethics, Family communication, Grief, Patient transfers, Stress management
Frequency of Caregiver Training: Initial formal training program, Monthly
Language(s) Spoken: English, Spanish

### AVAILABILITY

Service Availability: 24/7
On-call Supervisor Availability: 24/7

### COSTS

PRICES MAY INCREASE. PLEASE CALL FOR MOST CURRENT INFORMATION.

Rate: Call for rates
Minimum Hours per Day: None
Minimum Days per Week: None
Sliding Fee Schedule Available: No

### UNIQUE QUALITIES

In Home Care believes in educating their clients in addition to caring for them. The agency conducts evaluations to assess clients' needs and recommends other services they might find beneficial. In Home Care offers its caregivers a monthly continuing education program. This agency is Medicare- and Medicaid-certified.

## Paradigm Home Health Services

6033 Melody Lane, Suite 141
Dallas, TX 75231
(214) 378-8484

SEE CHAPTER 1 FOR A DESCRIPTION OF IN-HOME CARE SERVICES.

### DETAILS

Years in Business: 21
Home Health Services Provided: No
Care Visits Provided Within a Facility: Yes
Dementia Care Provided: Yes
Will Replace Caregiver Within 48 Hours Upon Request: Yes

### CAREGIVERS

RN on Staff: Yes
Hiring Qualifications: 1 year of experience, DMV check, TB test, Criminal background check, CNA certification, 4 references required
Caregiver Training: Dementia, Ethics, Family communication, Grief, Patient transfers, Stress management
Frequency of Caregiver Training: Initial formal training program, Monthly
Language(s) Spoken: English, French, Spanish

### AVAILABILITY

Service Availability: 24/7
On-call Supervisor Availability: 24/7

### COSTS

PRICES MAY INCREASE. PLEASE CALL FOR MOST CURRENT INFORMATION.

Rate: Call for rates
Minimum Hours per Day: None
Minimum Days per Week: None
Sliding Fee Schedule Available: No

### UNIQUE QUALITIES

Paradigm has provided homecare for over two decades. The administrator makes regular home visits to ensure that clients' needs are being met. Paradigm specializes in caring for people with dementia. The agency provides a monthly continuing education program to its caregivers.

## Primestaff Home Health Agency

3906 Lemmon, Suite 212
Dallas, TX 75219
(214) 599-9083
www.domestic-agency.com

SEE CHAPTER I FOR A DESCRIPTION OF IN-HOME CARE SERVICES.

### DETAILS

Years in Business: 26
Home Health Services Provided: No
Care Visits Provided Within a Facility: Yes
Dementia Care Provided: Yes
Will Replace Caregiver Within 48 Hours Upon Request: Yes

### CAREGIVERS

RN on Staff: Yes
Hiring Qualifications: 4 years of experience, DMV check, TB test, Criminal background check, CNA certification, 3 references required
Caregiver Training: Dementia, Ethics, Family communication, Grief, Patient transfers, Transition issues
Frequency of Caregiver Training: Initial formal training program
Language(s) Spoken: English, Spanish

### AVAILABILITY

Service Availability: 24/7
On-call Supervisor Availability: 24/7

### COSTS

PRICES MAY INCREASE. PLEASE CALL FOR MOST CURRENT INFORMATION.

Rate: $15.50–$18.50/hour
Live-In: $200/day
Minimum Hours per Day: 4
Minimum Days per Week: None
Sliding Fee Schedule Available: Yes

### UNIQUE QUALITIES

Primestaff has been in operation for twenty-six years. The caregivers take an individualized approach to client care. The agency offers personal assistance, home management and companionship services, and makes a concerted effort to keep its rates competitive.

## Total Health Care

3333 Knoll Crest Lane (972) 222-1234
Mesquite, TX 75181

SEE CHAPTER 1 FOR A DESCRIPTION OF IN-HOME CARE SERVICES.

### DETAILS

Years in Business: 3
Home Health Services Provided: Yes
Care Visits Provided Within a Facility: Yes
Dementia Care Provided: Yes
Will Replace Caregiver Within 48 Hours Upon Request: Yes

### CAREGIVERS

RN on Staff: Yes
Hiring Qualifications: 1 year of experience, Criminal background check, CNA certification, 3 references required
Caregiver Training: Dementia, Ethics, Family communication, Grief, Patient transfers, Stress management
Frequency of Caregiver Training: Initial formal training program, Monthly
Language(s) Spoken: English, Spanish

### AVAILABILITY

Service Availability: 24/7
On-call Supervisor Availability: 24/7

### COSTS

PRICES MAY INCREASE. PLEASE CALL FOR MOST CURRENT INFORMATION.

Rate: Call for rates
Minimum Hours per Day: None
Minimum Days per Week: None
Sliding Fee Schedule Available: No

### UNIQUE QUALITIES

Total Health Care customizes care plans to suit each client's individual needs. The agency arranges transportation, as needed, to maintain clients' independence. Total Health Care is certified by both Medicare and Medicaid.

## Trinity Home Health Care

400 South Zang Boulevard, Suite 610 (214) 942-3200
Dallas, TX 75208

SEE CHAPTER 1 FOR A DESCRIPTION OF IN-HOME CARE SERVICES.

### DETAILS

Years in Business: 14
Home Health Services Provided: Yes
Care Visits Provided Within a Facility: Yes
Dementia Care Provided: Yes
Will Replace Caregiver Within 48 Hours Upon Request: Yes

### CAREGIVERS

RN on Staff: Yes
Hiring Qualifications: 2 years of experience, DMV check, TB test, Criminal background check, CNA certification, 3 references required
Caregiver Training: Dementia, Ethics, Grief, Patient transfers, Stress management, Transition issues
Frequency of Caregiver Training: Initial formal training program, Quarterly
Language(s) Spoken: English, French, Hindi, Sign Language, Spanish

### AVAILABILITY

Service Availability: 24/7
On-call Supervisor Availability: 24/7

### COSTS

PRICES MAY INCREASE. PLEASE CALL FOR MOST CURRENT INFORMATION.

Rate: Call for rates
Minimum Hours per Day: None
Minimum Days per Week: None
Sliding Fee Schedule Available: No

### UNIQUE QUALITIES

Trinity boasts a neuropathy program and anodyne therapy, which is used to reduce pain and increase circulation. Trinity has extensive experience in caring for clients with congestive heart failure. The caregiving staff is impressively multilingual. Trinity is Medicare and Medicaid certified.

## ADULT DAY CARE CENTERS

### SCENARIO ADULT RESTORATIVE NURSING AND DAY CENTER

3120 West Northwest Highway (214) 351-1212
Dallas, TX 75220

---

**GILBERT GUIDE OBSERVATIONS** gggg

#### DETAILS

Owner/Affiliation: Elizabeth Perez
Years in Business: 20
License/Certification: Texas Department of Human Services, Veterans Administration
Business Hours: Monday–Friday, 6:30am–6:30pm
Transportation provided ($)
Conditions Accepted: Alzheimer's/Dementia, Developmental disabilities, HIV/AIDS, Incontinence, Limited mobility, Mental illness, Stroke, Traumatic brain injury, Vision/Hearing impairment

#### SPECIAL

Special diets accommodated
Wheelchair accessible
Proximity to Emergency Svcs.: Under 8 miles

#### STAFF

Staff/Patient Ratio: 1:8
Criminal Background Check: Yes
Language(s) Spoken: English, Spanish

#### COSTS

PRICES MAY INCREASE. PLEASE CALL FOR MOST CURRENT INFORMATION.

Daily Costs: $40
Reimbursement: Medicaid, SSI

#### PORTRAIT

Although this facility commands a spectacular view of Bachman Lake through its multitude of expansive windows, its truly outstanding assets are the owner and her dedicated staff. The owner is familiar with Medicaid and SSI benefits and is happy to help potential clients obtain funding to attend the program. The staff is committed to providing the best care for their clients, which includes helping people with special needs, such as dementia and mental disabilities. The low staff turnover at this facility indicates great stability within the team.

The goal of the program is to maintain or improve clients' levels of functioning. Participants do well with Scenario's disciplined schedule of care. The staff can assist with physicians' orders ranging from weight control regimes to administering medication. The programming includes a comprehensive spectrum of activities that boasts hand-eye coordination and music therapy. History, science, geography and travel are all popular discussion topics. The administrative offices are located in the loft, which provides a good vantage point for staff to observe participants. The large rooms below have ample space for activities, which is where participants spend their time. One of the special features of this program is that it provides both breakfast and lunch.

### ADULT DAY HEALTH CARE CENTERS

## NEW HORIZONS AT C.C. YOUNG A/D

4829 Lawther Drive
Dallas, TX 75214

(214) 827-8080
www.ccyoung.org

---

**GILBERT GUIDE OVERALL OBSERVATIONS** g g g g

### DETAILS

Owner/Affiliation: C.C. Young
Years in Business: 70
License/Certification: Texas Department of Aging and Disability Services
Business Hours: Monday–Friday, 7:00am–6:00pm
Conditions Accepted: Alzheimer's/Dementia, Incontinence, Limited mobility, Stroke

### SPECIAL

Special diets accommodated
Wheelchair accessible
Proximity to Emergency Svcs.: Under 8 miles
Onsite Care: Nursing, Occupational therapy, Physical therapy, Speech therapy

### STAFF

Staff/patient ration: 1:8
Criminal Background Check: No
Language(s) spoken: English, Spanish

### COSTS

PRICES MAY INCREASE. PLEASE CALL FOR MOST CURRENT INFORMATION.

Daily Costs: $47
Reimbursement: LTCI, SSI

### PORTRAIT

New Horizons at C.C. Young is situated on a twenty-acre campus overlooking the north shore of White Rock Lake. Thick woods lie just within the gated park-like community. The interior is immaculate and well maintained.

Participants enjoy a breakfast and lunch service as well as morning and afternoon snacks.

NEW HORIZONS AT C.C. YOUNG (CONTINUED)

The kitchen prepares appetizing selections such as herb-baked chicken with rice and cheesy herbed fish with Alfredo noodles. Sandwiches and fruit are offered as light snacks. The varied activities calendar includes current events discussions, "mind challenges," sewing, woodworking, painting, music classes, theater, and arts and crafts. Mainstays such as bingo, game boards and puzzles are available as well. The common area is sparsely furnished, allowing participants ample room to move about during fitness instruction and other activities. The staff keeps an open-door policy with the participants, encouraging them to ask questions, voice concerns and suggest activities. The interaction between the two groups was warm and pleasant. The environment was lively, and everyone seemed involved in one activity or another. One group crafted holiday decorations during our visit.

New Horizons offers additional services such as physical, occupational and speech therapies, wound care, X-rays, routine lab work, podiatry care and minor dental work-all are performed onsite. Participants and caregivers are encouraged to take advantage of New Horizon's overnight respite care.

## GERIATRIC CARE MANAGERS

### Dallas Care Connection

Carol K. Franzen, MS, LMSW
P.O. Box 815848
Dallas, TX 75381

(972) 242-0901
cfranzen@dallascareconnection.com
www.dallascareconnection.com

SEE CHAPTER 1 FOR A DESCRIPTION OF GERIATRIC CARE MANAGER SERVICES.

#### DETAILS

Years of GCM Experience: 21
Degree(s) Held: Licensed Master Social Worker
Member of National Association of Professional Geriatric Care Managers
Language(s) Spoken: English

#### SERVICES

Staff on Call: 24/7
Client References Provided: Yes
Areas of Practice: Assessment, Care management, Counseling, Education, Family/Professional liaison
Assistance with Medicare/Medicaid Process: Yes

#### COSTS

PRICES MAY INCREASE. PLEASE CALL FOR MOST CURRENT INFORMATION.

Assessment: Call for rates
Hourly: Call for rates

#### UNIQUE QUALITIES

With over twenty years of case management experience behind her, Carol K. Franzen is highly skilled in assisting seniors and people with disabilities. Carol has provided case management services in the Dallas-Fort Worth area since 1985. Not surprisingly, other local care managers have referred a number of challenging cases to Dallas Care Connection; Carol's familiarity with long-term care services in the area is a great strength.

## Kay Paggi, LPC, NCGC, CMC

1134 Wilderness Trail
Richardson, TX 75080

(972) 839-0065
kay@kaypaggi.com
www.kaypaggi.com

SEE CHAPTER 1 FOR A DESCRIPTION OF GERIATRIC CARE MANAGER SERVICES.

### DETAILS

Years of GCM Experience: 10
Degree(s) Held: Certified Care Manager, Licensed Professional Counselor
Member of National Association of Professional Geriatric Care Managers
Language(s) Spoken: English

### SERVICES

Staff on Call: 24/7
Client References Provided: Yes
Areas of Practice: Assessment, Care management, Counseling, Education, Family/Professional liaison
Assistance with Medicare/Medicaid Process: Yes

### COSTS

PRICES MAY INCREASE. PLEASE CALL FOR MOST CURRENT INFORMATION.

Hourly: $70

### UNIQUE QUALITIES

Kay Paggi is the only National Certified Gerontological Counselor (NCGC) in the North Texas area. Her thorough care assessments include asking her elderly clients how they perceive aging, how they cared for their own parents, and what their expectations are for the final stage of life. This information guides her care recommendations. Kay counsels adult children privately and facilitates discussion and support groups for adults who are caring for their parents. Some of the topics include information on end-of-life care and purchasing long-term care insurance.

## Kilgore, Lenheiser & Associates, LLC

Cheryl Lenheiser, LMSW-ACP
G201 PMB 224, 700 North Pearl Street
Dallas, TX 75201

(972) 679-2766
cheryl@klacaremanagers.com
www.klacaremanagers.com

SEE CHAPTER 1 FOR A DESCRIPTION OF GERIATRIC CARE MANAGER SERVICES.

### DETAILS

Years of GCM Experience: 5
Degree(s) Held: Licensed Master Social Worker
Member of National Association of Professional Geriatric Care Managers
Language(s) Spoken: English

### SERVICES

Staff on Call: 24/7
Client References Provided: Yes
Areas of Practice: Assessment, Care management, Counseling, Education, Family/Professional liaison
Assistance with Medicare/Medicaid Process: Yes

### COSTS

PRICES MAY INCREASE. PLEASE CALL FOR MOST CURRENT INFORMATION.

Assessment: Call for rates
Hourly: Call for rates

### UNIQUE QUALITIES

Kilgore, Lenheiser & Associates offers comprehensive service, including around-the-clock availability during emergency situations.

## SeniorLink

Molly Shomer, LMSW
P.O. Box 700291
Dallas, TX 75370

(972) 395-7823
mshomer@eldercareteam.com
www.eldercareteam.com

SEE CHAPTER 1 FOR A DESCRIPTION OF GERIATRIC CARE MANAGER SERVICES.

### DETAILS

Years of GCM Experience: 15
Degree(s) Held: Licensed Master Social Worker
Member of National Association of Professional Geriatric Care Managers
Language(s) Spoken: English, German

### SERVICES

Staff on Call: 24/7
Client References Provided: Yes
Areas of Practice: Assessment, Care management, Counseling, Education, Family/Professional liaison
Assistance with Medicare/Medicaid Process: Yes

### COSTS

PRICES MAY INCREASE. PLEASE CALL FOR MOST CURRENT INFORMATION.

Assessment: Call for rates
Hourly: $95

### UNIQUE QUALITIES

SeniorLink founder Molly Shomer educates clients and their families to advocate for themselves in order to preserve their independence. Clients and their families are taught how to use established resources and how to preserve the funds they already possess. Molly's goal is to coach her clients until they no longer require her services.

#### HOSPICE PROVIDERS

## Aleita Healthcare

8204 Elmbrook Drive, #206
Dallas, TX 75247

(214) 689-3100
www.alietahealthcare.com

SEE CHAPTER 1 FOR A DESCRIPTION OF HOSPICE SERVICES.

### DETAILS

Affiliation: None
Licensed By: Texas Department of Health Services
Medicare certified

### CARE

At-home Care Provided: Yes
Inpatient Care Provided: Yes
Caregivers trained, supervised, and monitored
Supervisor on call 24/7
Language(s) Spoken: English, Spanish

### UNIQUE QUALITIES

Aleita Healthcare's continuous evolvement with the technologically advanced healthcare industry is what sets it apart from other hospices. The team of medical professionals, which includes doctors and a nurse practitioner, organizes patient information through electronic charting. This efficient system allows staff more time to devote to patients. The staff cares for patients as if they were family, making this final stage of life as comfortable a transition as possible.

## Autumn Journey Hospice

5347 Spring Valley Road
Dallas, TX 75254

(972) 233-0525
www.autumnjourneyhospice.com

SEE CHAPTER 1 FOR A DESCRIPTION OF HOSPICE SERVICES.

### DETAILS

Affiliation: None
Licensed By: Texas Department of Health Services
Medicare certified

### CARE

At-home Care Provided: Yes
Inpatient Care Provided: No
Caregivers trained, supervised, and monitored
Supervisor on call 24/7
Language(s) Spoken: English, Spanish

### UNIQUE QUALITIES

Autumn Journey is locally owned and operated. The agency's staff has a combined experience of over twenty years in hospice and palliative care. Its focus on both areas of care enables its employees to devote more time to patients. Every client can expect one-on-one attention from the hospice team. Autumn Journey aims to make the experience as intimate and compassionate as possible.

## Harris Hospice, Inc.

3001 LBJ Freeway, Suite 105
Dallas, TX 75234

(972) 852-2273

SEE CHAPTER 1 FOR A DESCRIPTION OF HOSPICE SERVICES.

### DETAILS

Affiliation: Texas New Mexico Hospice Organization/NHPCO
Licensed By: Texas Department of Health Services
Medicare certified

### CARE

At-home Care Provided: Yes
Inpatient Care Provided: Yes
Caregivers trained, supervised, and monitored
Supervisor on call 24/7
Language(s) Spoken: English, Spanish

### UNIQUE QUALITIES

Somewhat unusual for a hospice agency, Harris Hospice is owned and operated by medical professionals. The driving force behind their care is a steadfast belief in enhancing clients' quality of life by not focusing on death. Instead, they emphasize life by filling patients' final days with enjoyment, making them as meaningful as possible.

## Heartland Home Health Care And Hospice

8700 Stemmons Freeway, Suite 144
Dallas, TX 75247
(214) 630-9070
www.hcr-manorcare.com

SEE CHAPTER 1 FOR A DESCRIPTION OF HOSPICE SERVICES.

### DETAILS

Affiliation: HCR Manorcare
Licensed By: Texas Department of Health Services
Medicare certified

### CARE

At-home Care Provided: Yes
Inpatient Care Provided: No
Caregivers trained, supervised, and monitored
Supervisor on call 24/7
Language(s) Spoken: English, Spanish

### UNIQUE QUALITIES

Heartland clients rely on hospice care administered by highly experienced staff of caregivers. The medical director is also certified in palliative care. The agency emphasizes a holistic approach to hospice care not only for the body, but for the mind and spirit as well.

## Twinber Hospice Care

1925 East Beltline Road, Suite 214
Carrollton, TX 75006
(469) 385-7765
www.twinberinc.com

SEE CHAPTER 1 FOR A DESCRIPTION OF HOSPICE SERVICES.

### DETAILS

Affiliation: None
Licensed By: Texas Department of Health Services
Medicare certified

### CARE

At-home Care Provided: Yes
Inpatient Care Provided: No
Caregivers trained, supervised, and monitored
Supervisor on call 24/7
Language(s) Spoken: English, Spanish

### UNIQUE QUALITIES

Twinber Hospice Care is a Christian-based organization that strives to provide excellent patient care by focusing on life. The agency's unconditional client support is driven by the belief that disease and illness are indiscriminate. Twinber offers financial support to its clients.

## Vitas Healthcare Of Texas, LP

8585 North Stemmons Freeway, Suite 700 (972) 661-2004
Dallas, TX 75247 www. vitas.com

SEE CHAPTER 1 FOR A DESCRIPTION OF HOSPICE SERVICES.

### DETAILS

Affiliation: None
Licensed By: Texas Department of Health Services
Medicare certified

### CARE

At-home Care Provided: Yes
Inpatient Care Provided: Yes
Caregivers trained, supervised, and monitored
Supervisor on call 24/7
Language(s) Spoken: English, Spanish

### UNIQUE QUALITIES

Vitas Healthcare has been caring for the terminally ill for over twenty-five years; it operates hospice agencies across the country. Guided by this experience, Vitas Healthcare of Texas LP accommodates patients with high acuity illnesses and offers twenty-four hour care. Vitas has special arrangements with local health facilities that allows patients to receive necessary outside treatment and then return to the comfort of home, where their hospice care then continues. Part of the Vitas philosophy dictates that hospice care involves more than simple clinical decisions; it strives to involve patients and their families in the end-of-life care plan.

# FORT WORTH

CONTINUING CARE RETIREMENT COMMUNITIES

## Lakewood Village

5100 Randol Mill Road
Fort Worth, Texas 76112

(817) 451-8001, (817) 429-4198
www.christiancarecenters.org

### GILBERT GUIDE OBSERVATIONS

| | | | |
|---|---|---|---|
| Administration & Staff | g g g g | Residents | g g g g |
| Facility Aesthetics | g g g g g | Dietary & Food Selection | g g g |
| Facility Condition & Safety | g g g g | Activities | g g g g |

### DETAILS

Year Built: 1983
Year Remodeled: 2005
Current Mgmt. Since: 1983
No. of Floors: 2
Resident Capacity: 150 (IND), 34 (AL), 48 (SNF)

### SPECIAL

Mild dementia care provided
Diets Accommodated: Diabetic, Low-fat, Low-salt
Proximity to Emergency Svcs.: 9–15 Miles
Nearby shopping and entertainment
Pets allowed

### STAFF

Nurse/LVN/LPN: Onsite 24/7
Caregiver Training: Dementia, Ethics, Family communication, Grief, Patient transfers, Stress management, Transition issues, Validation therapy
Criminal Background Check: Yes
Principal Staff Language(s): English
Other Staff Language(s): Spanish

### FACILITY FEATURES

Activities/Recreation
Beauty/Barber Shop ($)
Chapel Services
Computer/Internet Access
Facility Parking ($)
Fitness Room/Gym
Guest Meals ($)
Outside Patio/Gardens
Overnight Guest Room ($)
Pharmaceutical Service ($)
Private Dining Room
Room Service ($)
Transportation to MD Appointments, Scheduled Outings
24-hour Security

### ROOM FEATURES

Cable TV Ready ($)
Emergency Call System
Grab Bars
Kitchenette
Private Bathrooms
Telephone Ready
Temperature Controls

## COSTS

PRICES MAY INCREASE. PLEASE CALL FOR MOST CURRENT INFORMATION.

| | |
|---|---|
| Studio Apt. | No entrance fee; See Portrait for details |
| One Bedroom Apt. | No entrance fee; See Portrait for details |
| Two Bedroom Apt. | No entrance fee; See Portrait for details |
| Costs of Care | Included in monthly rate |
| Rate Increase | Annually; usually 4% |
| Reimbursement | LTCI, Private pay, Veterans |
| Application Fee | $500 |

## PORTRAIT

Lakewood Village is situated on an expansive forty-six acres of wooded areas and lush green foliage. The outdoor area boasts a covered porch overlooking a private lake, where residents gather for barbeques. The picturesque refuge also features abundant trails and garden paths.

The interior is wallpapered in neutral colors. Furniture throughout the building is contemporary yet comfortable. Residents' rooms are bright and spacious. Each has a grand view of the wooded grounds. Although the property is located in an urban area, the atmosphere seems rural. The dining room, also used for scheduled activities, is elegantly furnished with cherrywood tables and chairs. Residents gather in the common room for musical performances by fellow residents as well as outside musical guests. An abundance of windows allow for plentiful natural light throughout the building. The hallways are spacious enough to accommodate residents who use wheelchairs.

Lakewood Village residents enjoy independence. The onsite Health Care Center provides quality care from caregivers who residents know and trust. The staff organizes various field trips including weekly shopping trips to Kohl's and ice cream outings to Ben & Jerry's. Other mainstays at Lakewood are morning fitness classes, book clubs and Bible study. Expressing her love for this community, one resident exclaimed, "What a wonderful blessing from God. We are enjoying a new environment, a new community and a new beginning—another spring in life!" The interaction we witnessed between residents echoes this sentiment.

Lakewood Village is unique in that management has eliminated the comprehensive entrance fee, instead having residents pay monthly rates according to the level of care they require and the size of the unit they choose. Independent living apartments range from $980 to $2,813; add $340 per month for double occupancy units. The rates for assisted living units range from $1,700 to $2,870 per month with an added $500 to $700 for double occupancy units; residents' level of care is determined through a thorough care assessment prior to admission. Lastly, skilled nursing facility units are rented for shared or private occupancy at a daily rate of $120 to $200.

## Trinity Terrace

1600 Texas Street
Fort Worth, TX 76102

(817) 338-2426
(800) 841-0561
www.retirement.org/tt

---

**GILBERT GUIDE OBSERVATIONS**

| | | | |
|---|---|---|---|
| Administration & Staff | g g g | Residents | g g g g g |
| Facility Aesthetics | g g g g g | Dietary & Food Selection | g g g g |
| Facility Condition & Safety | g g g | Activities | g g g |

### DETAILS

Year Built: 1985
Year Remodeled: 2006
Current Mgmt. Since: 1995
No. of Floors: 15
Resident Capacity: 180

### SPECIAL

Diets Accommodated: Diabetic, Low-fat, Low-salt, Renal
Proximity to Emergency Svcs.: Under 8 miles
Nearby shopping and entertainment
Pets allowed

### STAFF

Nurse/LVN/LPN: Onsite 24/7
Caregiver Training: Ethics, Family communication, Grief, Patient transfers, Stress management, Transition issues, Validation therapy
Criminal Background Check: Yes
Principal Staff Language(s): English
Other Staff Language(s): Spanish

### FACILITY FEATURES

Activities/Recreation
Beauty/Barber Shop ($)
Computer/Internet Access
Facility Parking
Fitness Room/Gym
Guest Meals ($)
Outside Patio/Gardens
Overnight Guest Room ($)
Pharmaceutical Service
Private Dining Room
Separate Therapy Room
Transportation to MD Appointments, Personal Outings ($), Scheduled Outings
24-hour Security

### ROOM FEATURES

Cable TV Ready ($)
Emergency Call System
Furnished
Grab Bars
Kitchenette
Private Bathrooms
Telephone Ready ($)
Temperature Controls

### COSTS

PRICES MAY INCREASE. PLEASE CALL FOR MOST CURRENT INFORMATION.

| | |
|---|---|
| Studio Apt. | $45,100–$65,200 entrance fee, $1,441–$2,084/month |

| | |
|---|---|
| One Bedroom Apt. | $75,400–$139,800 entrance fee, $1,673–$3,075/month<br>Double occupancy add $75,400–$139,800 entrance fee, $2,200–$3,602/month |
| Two Bedroom Apt. | $111,600–$185,800 entrance fee, $2,625–$3,845/month<br>Double occupancy add $111,600–$185,800 entrance fee, $3,152–$4,372/month |
| Costs of Care | Included in entrance fee and monthly rate |
| Rate Increase | Annually; usually 3.5% |
| Reimbursement | LTCI, Private pay, Veterans |
| Pet Deposit | $500 |

**PORTRAIT**

Trinity Terrace offers an impressive array of services to its residents. On top of independent living, assisted living and skilled nursing care, the facility offers physical, respiratory, occupational and speech therapies. Residents may also take advantage of temporary stays in the facility's health care center without an increase in their monthly fees. The highly professional staff is very attentive to residents' needs. Trinity Terrace enjoys a long-standing reputation of excellence built on being the sole CCRC in Tarrant County. As one might expect, there is normally a wait list. Staff members informed us that plans are underway to construct a new tower housing sixty-six apartments, an auditorium, an indoor pool and various other amenities.

The tall, tan building encompasses an entire city block just west of Fort Worth's dynamic downtown area. The garden terrace atop the large garage is a popular area for residents to view the city skyline and admire the Trinity River, which flows nearby. The facility boasts a woodworking shop and a hobby room as well as an arts and crafts room. The in-house TV station offers residents the opportunity to volunteer their time and talents. Activities include book and poetry readings. Residents' apartments come in a range of sizes, from 385 square foot studios to 1,310 square foot two-bedroom units. Sunlight streams into the rooms through floor-to-ceiling windows and sliding glass doors that open onto balconies. Marble countertops add style to the bathrooms, all of which feature convenient handheld showerheads.

The foyer is bright thanks to expansive windows and shiny wood floors. Residents and guests enjoy a number of seating areas, each upholstered in various patterns. Tan is the unifying color in the common areas, which are illuminated by a combination of wall sconces and fluorescent lighting. Residents often drink their morning coffee in the common area they refer to as the "socializing" room. A loveseat, couch and coffee table furnish the inviting area. Tables and wall decorations adorn the hallways, which are wide enough to accommodate wheelchair users. Residents take in the stunning view from the upscale dining room, where they feast on a variety of cuisines—some of the favorites are French and Mexican.

ASSISTED LIVING FACILITIES

## Ashwood Retirement & Assisted Living

7501 Glenview Drive
North Richland Hills, TX 76180

(817) 804-3100, (817) 681-2454
www.stonegateseniorcare.com

---

### GILBERT GUIDE OBSERVATIONS

| | | | |
|---|---|---|---|
| Administration & Staff | g g g g | Residents | g g g g g |
| Facility Aesthetics | g g g | Dietary & Food Selectiong | g g g |
| Facility Condition & Safety | g g g | Activities | g g g |

### DETAILS

Year Built: Unknown
Year Remodeled: Ongoing
Current Mgmt. Since: 2000
No. of Floors: 1
Resident Capacity: 120

### SPECIAL

Mild dementia care provided
Diets Accommodated: Low-fat, Low-salt
Proximity to Emergency Svcs.: Under 8 miles
Nearby shopping and entertainment
Some pets allowed

### STAFF

Nurse/LVN/LPN: 40 hours/week, On call 24/7
Caregiver Training: Dementia, Ethics, Grief, Patient transfers, Stress management, Transition issues
Criminal Background Check: Yes
Principal Staff Language(s): English
Other Staff Language(s): Spanish

### FACILITY FEATURES

Activities/Recreation
Beauty/Barber Shop ($)
Chapel Services
Computer/Internet Access
Facility Parking
Guest Meals ($)
Outside Patio/Gardens
Pharmaceutical Service ($)
Room Service ($)
Separate Therapy Room
Transportation to MD Appointments, Scheduled Outings
24-hour Security

### ROOM FEATURES

Cable TV Ready
Emergency Call System
Grab Bars
Kitchenette
Private Bathrooms
Telephone Ready
Temperature Controls

### COSTS

PRICES MAY INCREASE. PLEASE CALL FOR MOST CURRENT INFORMATION.

| | |
|---|---|
| Studio Apt. | $1,295–$2,195/month |
| One Bedroom Apt. | $2,495/month |
| | Double occupancy add $500/month |

| | |
|---|---|
| Two Bedroom Apt. | $3,700/month |
| Costs of Care | $450–$900/month based on individual need |
| Rate Increase | Annually; usually 3% |
| Reimbursement | LTCI, Private pay, Veterans |
| Security Deposit | $500 |
| Pet Deposit | $500 |

### PORTRAIT

Ashwood Retirement and Assisted Living is housed in a former hospital. Due to its past use, the facility's hallways, which are lined with benches, are exceptionally wide. A combination of large windows and fluorescent lighting brightens the interior. Faded upholstery covers the comfortable furniture in the numerous common areas. One room holds the library, and another area features a piano used for Sunday religious services.

Dark wooden tables and chairs furnish the large dining area, where meals are served restaurant-style. Fruit and other snacks are available all day. We noted residents eating salad, pot roast with asparagus, and chocolate pie as they enjoyed the view of one of the facility's two large patios. Oak trees shade each secured patio. Walkways crisscross the areas; some lead to patio tables and umbrellas. Feeding the outdoor birds is such a popular pastime that it prompted residents to develop a feeding schedule, as the birds were being overfed. Other activities include piano sing-alongs, religious services, and lessons on navigating the internet. Ashwood hosts a monthly birthday party for all residents whose birthdays occur that month.

We noticed much laughter and friendly chatting among residents and staff members. One resident informed us that she maintains her youth and beauty through frequent walks in the facility's hallways—and suggested we join her in order to trim our bellies!

## BARTON HOUSE I & II A/D

6939 River Park Circle
Fort Worth, TX 76117

(817) 731-1440
www.uncommoncare.com

### GILBERT GUIDE OBSERVATIONS

| | | | |
|---|---|---|---|
| Administration & Staff | g g g g g | Dietary & Food Selection | g g g g |
| Facility Aesthetics | g g g g | Activities | g g g g |
| Facility Condition & Safety | g g g g g | Alzheimer's & Dementia Capabilities | g g g g g |
| Residents | g g g g g | | |

### DETAILS

Year Built: 1996
Current Mgmt. Since: 1996

### SPECIAL

Alzheimer's/Dementia Only Facility
Diets Accommodated: Diabetic, Low-fat, Low-salt

BARTON HOUSE I & II (CONTINUED)

DETAILS (CONTINUED)

No. of Floors: 1
Resident Capacity: 40

SPECIAL (CONTINUED)

Proximity to Emergency Svcs.: Under 8 miles
Nearby shopping and entertainment
Pets allowed

## STAFF

Nurse/LVN/LPN: 40 hours/week, On call 24/7
Caregiver Training: Dementia, Ethics, Family communication, Grief, Patient transfers, Stress management, Transition issues, Validation therapy
Criminal Background Check: Yes
Principal Staff Language(s): English

## FACILITY FEATURES

Activities/Recreation
Beauty/Barber Shop ($)
Guest Meals
Outside Patio/Gardens
24-hour Security

## ROOM FEATURES

Cable TV Ready
Emergency Call System
Grab Bars
Kitchenette
Private Bathrooms
Telephone Ready

## COSTS

PRICES MAY INCREASE. PLEASE CALL FOR MOST CURRENT INFORMATION.

| | |
|---|---|
| Alzheimer's Unit | $4,100/month for private room |
| Costs of Care | Included in monthly rate |
| Rate Increase | Annually; usually 2–3% |
| Reimbursement | Private pay |
| Entrance Fee | $1,500 |
| Pet Deposit | $300 |

## PORTRAIT

Barton House I and II are prominent brick structures in a quiet cul-de-sac. Both buildings are homey with manicured grounds featuring trees, shrubbery and green grass. The foyer smells of calming lavender and is comfortably furnished with chairs and sofas. The interior walls are washed in muted tones and complemented by fresh flowers and decorative antiques. Upon entering, we observed residents socializing in this homelike common area.

Residents' rooms are spacious and all have windows. Although the furniture is supplied by Barton, residents and their families are encouraged to decorate to suit their tastes. Individual displays mounted outside residents' doors help patients with dementia recognize their rooms. The dining room is a popular spot for socializing and activities. Fragrant smells wafted from the kitchen, piquing delightful curiosity from passersby. The kitchen staff prepares four meals and two snacks every day.

The outdoor patio is appropriately furnished for casual dining and social visits. The groomed landscape is etched with lovely walkways throughout. Residents are encouraged to plant and garden. The short hallways are wide and free of clutter. The soft artificial lighting is dimmed during evening hours to prepare residents for bedtime. Residents and staff interact warmly with one another. Management and staff emphasize open communication with residents and their families, making sure everyone is well informed on residents' behalf.

## Bethesda Home

5417 Altamesa Boulevard
Fort Worth, TX 76123

(817) 292-8886
www.BACBloom.com

**GILBERT GUIDE OBSERVATIONS**

| | | | |
|---|---|---|---|
| Administration & Staff | g g g | Residents | g g g g |
| Facility Aesthetics | g g g g g | Dietary & Food Selection | g g g g |
| Facility Condition & Safety | g g g g g | Activities | g g g g |

### DETAILS

Year Built: 2000
Current Mgmt. Since: 2000
No. of Floors: 1
Resident Capacity: 120

### SPECIAL

Mild dementia care provided
Diets Accommodated: Diabetic, Low-fat, Low-salt
Proximity to Emergency Svcs.: Under 8 miles
Nearby shopping and entertainment
Pets allowed

### STAFF

Nurse/LVN/LPN: 40 hours/week, On call 24/7
Caregiver Training: Dementia, Ethics, Family communication, Grief, Patient transfers, Stress management, Transition issues
Criminal Background Check: Yes
Principal Staff Language(s): English
Other Staff Language(s): Russian, Sign Language

### FACILITY FEATURES

Activities/Recreation
Beauty/Barber Shop ($)
Chapel Services
Computer/Internet Access
Facility Parking
Guest Meals ($)
Outside Patio/Gardens
Overnight Guest Room ($)
Pharmaceutical Service ($)
Private Dining Room
Room Service ($)
Transportation
24-hour Security

### ROOM FEATURES

Cable TV Ready
Grab Bars
Kitchenette
Private Bathrooms
Telephone Ready
Temperature Controls

BETHESDA HOME (CONTINUED)

## COSTS

PRICES MAY INCREASE. PLEASE CALL FOR MOST CURRENT INFORMATION.

| | |
|---|---|
| Studio Apt. | $2,160–$2,400/month |
| One Bedroom Apt. | $2,750/month |
| Two Bedroom Apt. | $3,100/month |
| Respite Stays | Call for private room rates |
| Costs of Care | $200–$600/month based on individual need |
| Rate Increase | Every 6 months; usually 2% |
| Reimbursement | LTCI, Private pay |
| Security Deposit | $500 |
| Pet Deposit | $500 |

## PORTRAIT

The stucco building that houses Bethesda Gardens resembles an apartment complex. Parking areas surround the facility, which is located in a developing neighborhood of Fort Worth. High windows create a light and spacious atmosphere. The facility emits such a homey feeling that it was easy to imagine living there! The furnishings are marked by comfort and good taste. Handrails line the hallways, which feature sitting areas.

Residents' apartments have nameplates, doorbells and locking front doors that create a sense of privacy. Residents furnish their owns apartments, and enjoy walk-in closets with plentiful storage space. Some apartments boast individual covered patios. From there, they can view the facility's gardens, where a number of the residents utilize their green thumbs.

Residents are served restaurant-style service in the expansive dining area. Bethesda Gardens features a small private kitchen as well as a private dining area that residents and their families reserve for special occasions. Religious services are held in the on-site chapel throughout the week. Other popular pastimes include playing cards and board games, as well as going on outings. We overheard residents and staff cheerfully catching up on each other's lives.

## Broadway Plaza at Cityview

5301 Bryant Irvin Road
Fort Worth, TX 76132

(817) 346-9407, (817) 219-5434
www.arclp.com

---

### GILBERT GUIDE OBSERVATIONS

| | | | |
|---|---|---|---|
| Administration & Staff | g g g | Residents | g g g |
| Facility Aesthetics | g g g | Dietary & Food Selection | g g g |
| Facility Condition & Safety | g g g | Activities | g g g |

### DETAILS

Year Built: 1988
Year Remodeled: 2000
Current Mgmt. Since: 1989
No. of Floors: 3
Resident Capacity: 40

### SPECIAL

Diets Accommodated: Diabetic, Low-fat, Low-salt, Renal
Proximity to Emergency Svcs.: Under 8 miles
Nearby shopping and entertainment
No pets allowed

### STAFF

Nurse/LVN/LPN: Onsite 24/7
Caregiver Training: Ethics, Family communication, Grief, Patient transfers, Stress management, Transition issues, Validation therapy
Criminal Background Check: Yes
Principal Staff Language(s): English
Other Staff Language(s): Spanish

### FACILITY FEATURES

Activities/Recreation
Beauty/Barber Shop ($)
Facility Parking
Guest Meals ($)
Outside Patio/Gardens
Overnight Guest Room ($)
Pharmaceutical Service
Separate Therapy Room
Transportation to MD Appointments, Scheduled Outings

### ROOM FEATURES

Cable TV Ready ($)
Emergency Call System
Kitchenette
Private Bathrooms
Telephone Ready ($)
Temperature Controls

### COSTS

PRICES MAY INCREASE. PLEASE CALL FOR MOST CURRENT INFORMATION.

| | |
|---|---|
| Studio Apt. | $2,899–$3,856/month |
| Costs of Care | $200–$1,000/month based on individual need |
| Rate Increase | Annually; usually 4% |
| Reimbursement | LTCI, Private pay |
| Entrance Fee | $1,500 |
| Pet Deposit | $350 |

BROADWAY PLAZA AT CITYVIEW (CONTINUED)

### PORTRAIT

Bordered by manicured lawns and grand cedar trees, Broadway Plaza at Cityview is a staple in this hillside community of townhouses and villa-like apartments. Assisted living residents occupy the first floor, while residents of the skilled nursing facility reside on the second and third floors. Through the north entrance is a long hallway leading to the reception area—an elegant setting with chairs upholstered in pretty floral patterns, artificial potted plants, paintings of townscapes and cottages, and rich window treatments that pop against muted walls.

Residents' rooms each have one window. The rooms range from small to medium in size. The dining area is a cozy arrangement of mahogany tables draped in blue linen. Lovely sconces lend a soft ambience as residents enjoy restaurant-style meal service. A sample menu features meatloaf, grilled vegetables and tossed salad. Both common areas are furnished with loveseats and chairs.

The outdoor area is a picturesque retreat. The stone birdbath and bench underneath the towering cedar tree are centerpieces of the blossoming garden. Huge windows at the end of each of the broad hallways flood the interior with light. Fluorescent lighting brightens the rest of the facility.

Broadway Plaza residents are lively and fairly independent; most need only moderate assistance. The event calendar has few scheduled activities, which is perhaps a reflection of the amount of time residents spend with friends and loved ones. Weekly craft activities and shopping trips are two of the popular offerings on the schedule.

## THE BROADWAY PLAZA AT WESTOVER HILLS A/D

6201 Plaza Parkway
Fort Worth, TX 76116

(817) 989-1174, (817) 994-4579
www.arclp.com

---

**GILBERT GUIDE OBSERVATIONS**

| | | | |
|---|---|---|---|
| Administration & Staff | g g g | Dietary & Food Selection | g g g |
| Facility Aesthetics | g g g g | Activities | g g g |
| Facility Condition & Safety | g g g g | Alzheimer's & Dementia Capabilities | g g g g |
| Residents | g g g | | |

### DETAILS

Year Built: 2000
Year Remodeled: Ongoing
Current Mgmt. Since: 2000
No. of Floors: 3
Resident Capacity: 31

### SPECIAL

Diets Accommodated: Diabetic, Low-salt
Proximity to Emergency Svcs.: Under 8 miles
Nearby shopping and entertainment
Some pets allowed

### STAFF

Nurse/LVN/LPN: 40 hours/week, On call 24/7
Caregiver Training: Dementia, Ethics, Grief, Stress management, Transition issues
Criminal Background Check: Yes
Principal Staff Language(s): English
Other Staff Language(s): Spanish

### FACILITY FEATURES

Activities/Recreation
Beauty/Barber Shop ($)
Chapel Services
Computer/Internet Access
Facility Parking
Guest Meals ($)
Outside Patio/Gardens
Pharmaceutical Service ($)
Room Service ($)
Separate Therapy Room
Transportation
24-hour Security

### ROOM FEATURES

Cable TV Ready ($)
Emergency Call System
Grab Bars
Kitchenette
Private Bathrooms
Telephone Ready
Temperature Controls

### COSTS

PRICES MAY INCREASE. PLEASE CALL FOR MOST CURRENT INFORMATION.

| | |
|---|---|
| One Bedroom Apt. | $2,000–$4,000/month |
| Alzheimer's Unit | Call for private/shared room rates |
| Respite Stays | Call for shared room rates |
| Costs of Care | Call for rates |
| Rate Increase | Annually; usually 2–5% |
| Reimbursement | LTCI, Private pay |
| Entrance Fee | $1,000 |
| Pet Deposit | $500 |

### PORTRAIT

The Broadway Plaza is a magnificent building at the corner of Plaza Parkway, easily accessible to Interstate 30. The red brick facility is surrounded by young oak trees, colorful blossoms and trimmed hedges. The entryway is a grand two-story room furnished with cherrywood tables and dark blue and floral-print sofas. The fireplace is flanked by built-in bookshelves.

Residents' moderately sized rooms have plenty of closet space. Residents decorate and paint the rooms to suit their tastes. Each has two large windows. The dining room features a lovely view of the patio. Brass and crystal chandeliers illuminate an elegant display of white linen tablecloths and maroon and floral-print upholstered chairs. The kitchen staff prepares mouthwatering entrées such as beef lasagna, Italian vegetables, fresh tossed salad, garlic bread and strawberry rhubarb pie. The common areas located at both ends of the halls are furnished with plush sofas and chairs. We observed many residents visiting and socializing in these areas. A group of women fresh from the beauty salon looked lovely.

BROADWAY PLAZA AT WESTOVER HILLS (CONTINUED)

Recessed lighting, along with natural light, gives the building a soft glow. Residents take full advantage of comfortable rest spots in the halls. The outdoor area is lush with greenery.

One tour guide informed us that resident participation is very high at Broadway Plaza. Residents enjoy a calendar chock-full of events that include morning exercise classes, dominoes, bridge, bingo, Scrabble, movie nights, scenic drives and outings to the grocery store. The atmosphere is decidedly warm and inviting.

## Castle Rock Assisted Living

5519 South Collins Street
Arlington, TX 76018
(817) 557-2221

### GILBERT GUIDE OBSERVATIONS

| | | | |
|---|---|---|---|
| Administration & Staff | g g g g | Residents | g g g g g |
| Facility Aesthetics | g g g g g | Dietary & Food Selection | g g g g g |
| Facility Condition & Safety | g g g g g | Activities | g g g |

### DETAILS

Year Built: 2001
Current Mgmt. Since: 2001
No. of Floors: 1
Resident Capacity: 57

### SPECIAL

Mild dementia care provided
Diets Accommodated: Diabetic, Low-fat, Low-salt
Proximity to Emergency Svcs.: Under 8 miles
Nearby shopping and entertainment
Pets allowed

### STAFF

Nurse/LVN/LPN: 40 hours/week, On call 24/7
Caregiver Training: Dementia, Ethics, Family communication, Grief, Patient transfers, Stress management, Transition issue
Criminal Background Check: Yes
Principal Staff Language(s): English
Other Staff Language(s): Spanish

### FACILITY FEATURES

Activities/Recreation
Beauty/Barber Shop ($)
Chapel Services
Computer/Internet Access
Private Dining Room
Transportation
24-hour Security

### ROOM FEATURES

Grab Bars
Kitchenette
Private Bathrooms
Telephone Ready
Temperature Controls

### COSTS

PRICES MAY INCREASE. PLEASE CALL FOR MOST CURRENT INFORMATION.

| | |
|---|---|
| Studio Apt. | $1,800–$1,990/month |
| One Bedroom Apt. | $2,255/month |
| Two Bedroom Apt. | $2,368/month |
| Costs of Care | $295–$590/month based on individual need |
| Rate Increase | Annually; usually 2–3% |
| Reimbursement | LTCI, Private pay |
| Entrance Fee | $1,000 |
| Pet Deposit | $300 |

### PORTRAIT

A brick building houses Castle Rock, a family-owned business. The facility has abundant parking and is located next to the Arlington Airport. Crown moldings, wood columns, and archways embellish the brightly lit common areas, which are decorated in green and beige. Handrails line the wide, uncluttered hallways. Residents' rooms are moderately sized and feature windows, as well as walk-in showers with padded seats.

Meals are served restaurant-style in the elegant dining area, where social occasions also take place. Residents surf the web on computers in the library. Shopping excursions to major retailers such as Target are also popular. Other activities include watching movies and playing board games. Residents enjoy access to a whirlpool bath. The outdoor barbecue area has ample seating for residents and their guests. A gazebo overlooks walkways meandering through trimmed grass and shrubs. We noticed several residents conversing easily with staff members during our visit to Castle Rock.

## THE COURTYARDS AT RIVER PARK

3201 River Park Drive
Fort Worth, TX 76116

(817) 732-4436
www.elderlycareinc.com

---

**GILBERT GUIDE OBSERVATIONS**

| | | | |
|---|---|---|---|
| Administration & Staff | g g g | Residents | g g g g |
| Facility Aesthetics | g g g g | Dietary & Food Selection | g g g g |
| Facility Condition & Safety | g g g g | Activities | g g g g |

### DETAILS

Year Built: 1987
Year Remodeled: 2005
Current Mgmt. Since: 1987
No. of Floors: 3
Resident Capacity: 100

### SPECIAL

Mild dementia care provided
Diets Accommodated: Diabetic, Low-fat, Low-salt
Proximity to Emergency Svcs.: Under 8 miles
Nearby shopping and entertainment
Pets allowed

THE COURTYARDS AT RIVER PARK (CONTINUED)

## STAFF

Nurse/LVN/LPN: 24 hours/week, On call 24/7
Caregiver Training: Dementia, Ethics, Family communication, Grief
Criminal Background Check: Yes
Principal Staff Language(s): English
Other Staff Language(s): Spanish

## FACILITY FEATURES

Activities/Recreation
Beauty/Barber Shop ($)
Chapel Services
Computer/Internet Access
Guest Meals
Overnight Guest Room ($)
Pharmaceutical Service
Private Dining Room ($)
Room Service
Transportation
24-hour Security

## ROOM FEATURES

Cable TV Ready ($)
Emergency Call System
Grab Bars
Kitchenette
Shared & Private Bathrooms
Telephone Ready ($)
Temperature Controls

## COSTS

PRICES MAY INCREASE. PLEASE CALL FOR MOST CURRENT INFORMATION.

| | |
|---|---|
| Studio Apt. | $1,875–$1,950/month |
| One Bedroom Apt. | $2,380/month |
| Costs of Care | $175–$300/month based on individual need |
| Rate Increase | Annually; usually 2–3% |
| Reimbursement | LTCI, Private pay, Veterans |
| Security Deposit | $300 |
| Pet Deposit | $200 |

## PORTRAIT

The Courtyards at River Park seems far from civilization. Visitors can easily imagine they are vacationing in a national forest—towering pine and oak trees dwarf shrubs and flowers across the five-acre campus. Abundant outdoor seating areas allow residents to take in the view.

The residents love playing bingo and board games. They also frequent shopping areas and join in community events. Scheduled activities at the facility include exercise, religious services and watching guest performances. The facility features a craft room. Residents and their guests enjoy using the swimming pool. We saw a handful of residents as they interacted pleasantly with staff members, who addressed them by their first names.

Mellow lighting and the green and beige color scheme contribute to a homey atmosphere. Group meetings and card games take place in the spacious lounge area, which is warmed by a fireplace. The wide hallways are clear and lined with handrails. Residents' large rooms offer beautiful views of the campus. The dining room is easily accessible from all residents' rooms. The menu lists homemade meals, such as fried chicken, mashed potatoes, mixed vegetables, and fruit pie. Residents may also choose from healthy alternatives such as vegetables and salads.

## Covenant Place Burleson

611 Northeast Alsbury Boulevard
Burleson, TX 76028

(817) 447-4477, (817) 454-2372
www.covenantplaceburleson.com

### GILBERT GUIDE OBSERVATIONS

| | | | |
|---|---|---|---|
| Administration & Staff | g g g g | Residents | g g g |
| Facility Aesthetics | g g g g g | Dietary & Food Selection | g g g |
| Facility Condition & Safety | g g g | Activities | g g g |

### DETAILS

Year Built: 1997
Year Remodeled: Ongoing
Current Mgmt. Since: 1997
No. of Floors: 1
Resident Capacity: 80

### SPECIAL

Mild dementia care provided
Diets Accommodated: Diabetic, Low-fat, Low-salt
Proximity to Emergency Svcs.: Under 8 miles
Nearby shopping and entertainment
No pets allowed

### STAFF

Nurse/LVN/LPN: On call 24/7
Caregiver Training: Dementia, Ethics, Family communication, Grief, Patient transfers, Stress management, Transition issues, Validation therapy
Criminal Background Check: Yes
Principal Staff Language(s): English
Other Staff Language(s): Spanish

### FACILITY FEATURES

Activities/Recreation
Beauty/Barber Shop ($)
Chapel Services
Fitness Room/Gym
Guest Meals ($)
Outside Patio/Gardens
Pharmaceutical Service ($)
Private Dining Room ($)
Transportation to MD Appointments, Scheduled Outings
24-hour Security

### ROOM FEATURES

Cable TV Ready ($)
Emergency Call System
Private Bathrooms
Telephone Ready ($)
Temperature Controls

COVENANT PLACE BURLESON (CONTINUED)

## COSTS

PRICES MAY INCREASE. PLEASE CALL FOR MOST CURRENT INFORMATION.

| | |
|---|---|
| Studio Apt. | $2,075–$2,195/month |
| One Bedroom Apt. | $2,325–$2,450/month<br>Double occupancy add $400/month |
| Two Bedroom Apt. | $2,675–$2,695/month<br>Double occupancy add $400/month |
| Costs of Care | Included in monthly rate |
| Rate Increase | Annually; usually 3% |
| Reimbursement | LTCI, Private pay, Veterans |
| Entrance Fee | $1,000 |
| Pet Deposit | $500 |

## PORTRAIT

The exterior of Covenant Place evokes a Southern mansion; the portico at the entrance is supported by large white columns. The yard features manicured shrubs and a lawn bordered by colorful flowers. The interior is equally grand, with an elegant formal dining room as well as a luxurious private dining room, including a cherrywood table dressed in linen. Residents may reserve the private dining room for meals and special events. Carpeting helps to reduce noise within the facility. The light tan wallpaper and off-white paint in the hallways softens the fluorescent lighting. The wide hallways are lined with handrails. The facility is immaculate.

Residents' rooms, although moderate in size, seem upscale. Each has ample closet space and expansive windows that let in natural light. There are abundant common areas throughout the facility. The activity room contains a variety of board games, books and puzzles, and the library is lined with books. Covenant Place boasts four courtyards, located at different ends of the building, each with manicured grass and trees; all have comfortable patio furniture.

We noted a very professional atmosphere from the moment we began our tour. Covenant Place management clearly runs a right ship; the staff were all involved in various tasks with residents. They know each resident by name. It is apparent that much thought has gone into the menu, which features hearty favorites including chicken fried steak, mashed potatoes, vegetables and apple pie. Coffee and snacks are available all day. Weekly shopping and restaurant outings are a highlight of the activities calendar, which also lists bingo, shopping, movies and Bible study.

## EDEN TERRACE & MEMORY CARE UNIT A/D

2500 Woodside Drive
Arlington, TX 76016

(817) 457-9710
www.sunriseseniorliving.com

### GILBERT GUIDE OBSERVATIONS

| | | | |
|---|---|---|---|
| Administration & Staff | g g g g g | Dietary & Food Selection | g g g g g |
| Facility Aesthetics | g g g g g | Activities | g g g g g |
| Facility Condition & Safety | g g g g g | Alzheimer's & Dementia Capabilities | g g g g g |
| Residents | g g g g | | |

### DETAILS

Year Built: 2000
Current Mgmt. Since: Unknown
No. of Floors: 1
Resident Capacity: 50 (AL), 29 (ALZ)

### SPECIAL

Diets Accommodated: Diabetic, Low-fat, Low-salt
Proximity to Emergency Svcs.: Under 8 miles
Nearby shopping and entertainment
Pets allowed

### STAFF

Nurse/LVN/LPN: Onsite 24/7
Caregiver Training: Dementia, Ethics, Family communication, Grief, Stress management, Transition issues, Validation therapy
Criminal Background Check: Yes
Principal Staff Language(s): English

### FACILITY FEATURES

Activities/Recreation
Beauty/Barber Shop ($)
Chapel Services
Facility Parking
Guest Meals
Outside Patio/Gardens
Pharmaceutical Service
Private Dining Room
Separate Therapy Room
Transportation to MD Appointments, Scheduled Outings
24-hour Security

### ROOM FEATURES

Cable TV Ready
Emergency Call System
Grab Bars
Private Bathrooms
Telephone Ready ($)
Temperature Controls

### COSTS

PRICES MAY INCREASE. PLEASE CALL FOR MOST CURRENT INFORMATION.

| | |
|---|---|
| Studio Apt. | $76/day |
| One Bedroom Apt. | $81/day |
| | Double occupancy add $27/day |
| Alzheimer's Unit | $69/day for shared room |
| | $76–$81/day for private room |
| Costs of Care | $600–$1,100/month based on individual need |

EDEN TERRACE & MEMORY CARE UNIT (CONTINUED)

| | |
|---|---|
| Rate Increase | Annually; usually 2–3% |
| Reimbursement | LTCI, Private pay, Veterans |
| Entrance Fee | $1,500 |
| Pet Deposit | $500 |

**PORTRAIT**

Eden Terrace is easily accessible from Interstates 30 and 20, just minutes away from Arlington Memorial Hospital and the Medical Center of Arlington. A lovely medley of flowering shrubs and young trees surround a stone table near the entrance. The homelike lobby is furnished with wicker rockers and chairs upholstered in a floral pattern. A well-stocked coffee bar is available to both residents and visitors. The facility's south wing houses the secured Alzheimer's unit, which has a capacity of thirty residents. The specialized unit has its own dining area and common areas, to facilitate familiarity and comfort for residents with dementia.

Residents' rooms are moderately sized and have spacious walk-in closets. Residents with Alzheimer's display knickknacks and pictures outside their rooms to jog their memories. Meals are served restaurant-style. During our visit, the kitchen staff prepared an appetizing selection of beef barley soup, barbeque pork ribs, chicken fried steak, mashed potatoes and coleslaw. The common areas feature different entertainment mediums: one boasts a sixty-inch TV and a fireplace; the other, a piano.

The outdoor courtyard is a blossoming scene of flowers and trees set among garden paths. Residents are encouraged to garden in the raised planters. The spacious hallways have furnished rest spots for impromptu visits among residents. The event calendar is varied and features quilting and traveling clubs, fitness instruction, arts and crafts, outings and worship sessions. Stimulating activities for residents with Alzheimer's include mental games such as "dream driving" and music memories. The staff and residents appear very comfortable with one another. We observed a very attentive and professional staff during our visit.

## FOUNTAINS OF HULEN A/D

6617 Dan Danciger Pond (817) 423-0226
Fort Worth, TX 76133

---

**GILBERT GUIDE OBSERVATIONS**

| | | | |
|---|---|---|---|
| Administration & Staff | g g g g g | Dietary & Food Selection | g g g g |
| Facility Aesthetics | g g g | Activities | g g g g |
| Facility Condition & Safety | g g g | Alzheimer's & Dementia Capabilities | g g g |
| Residents | g g g g g | | |

## DETAILS

Year Built: 1980s
Year Remodeled: 2000
Current Mgmt. Since: 2000
No. of Floors: 1
Resident Capacity: 30 (AL), 17 (ALZ)

## SPECIAL

Diets Accommodated: Diabetic, Low-fat, Low-salt, Renal
Proximity to Emergency Svcs.: Under 8 miles
Nearby shopping and entertainment
Pet visits allowed

## STAFF

Nurse/LVN/LPN: 10 hours/week, On call 24/7
Caregiver Training: Dementia, Ethics, Family communication, Grief, Patient transfers, Stress management, Transition issues, Validation therapy
Criminal Background Check: Yes
Principal Staff Language(s): English
Other Staff Language(s): Spanish, Tagalog

## FACILITY FEATURES

Activities/Recreation
Beauty/Barber Shop
Chapel Services
Facility Parking
Guest Meals
Outside Patio/Gardens
Pharmaceutical Service ($)
Separate Therapy Room
Transportation
24-hour Security

## ROOM FEATURES

Cable TV Ready
Emergency Call System
Furnished
Shared Bathrooms
Telephone Ready

## COSTS

PRICES MAY INCREASE. PLEASE CALL FOR MOST CURRENT INFORMATION.

| | |
|---|---|
| One Bedroom Apt. | $2,300/month |
| Alzheimer's Unit | $2,500/month for shared room |
| Costs of Care | Included in monthly rate |
| Rate Increase | Periodically |
| Reimbursement | Private pay, SSI |
| Application Fee | $500 (portion applied to rent/security deposit) |

## PORTRAIT

Fountains of Hulen and its sister Alzheimer's facility rest on peaceful Dan Danciger Road in Fort Worth. A number of nursing homes, hospitals and doctors' offices are also in the vicinity. The exterior is well-maintained and surrounded by a beautiful lawn. During our tour, a delicious aroma wafted from the kitchen, adding to the homey atmosphere. The kitchen staff takes a health-conscious approach to the food they serve. Fried food, which can be difficult to digest, is not a part of the menu. The Filipino chef takes pride in serving her native dishes.

The common areas are comfortably furnished and feature fresh flowers. The lighting throughout is soft and adequate. The hallways and other common areas are very tidy. The

FOUNTAINS OF HULEN (CONTINUED)

dining room is an appropriate size for the number of residents, and features very comfortable seating. Residents enjoy relaxing in the solarium.

Residents of the assisted living facility laughed and conversed together during our visit. Alzheimer's residents seemed to be reserved, for the most part, although we did witness a few of them socializing. The staff conducts many one-on-one activities with residents. The atmosphere is inviting. It is plain to see that staff and residents genuinely care for one another; they were interacting warmly and referred to each other by name. One resident told us that our tour guide was like a daughter to her.

Residents can choose to decorate their rooms or to use furniture supplied by the facility. Each room features generously sized windows. Residents seem to enjoy the outdoor patio, where they are welcome to garden with plants of their choosing, or to simply relax.

## GREENBRIAR MANSION AT CITYVIEW

7865 Oakmont Boulevard (817) 292-0792
Fort Worth, TX 76132

**GILBERT GUIDE OBSERVATIONS**

| | | | |
|---|---|---|---|
| Administration & Staff | g g g | Residents | g g g |
| Facility Aesthetics | g g g g | Dietary & Food Selection | g g g |
| Facility Condition & Safety | g g g | Activities | g g g |

### DETAILS

Year Built: 2002
Current Mgmt. Since: 1995
No. of Floors: 1
Resident Capacity: 16

### SPECIAL

Diets Accommodated: Low-fat
Proximity to Emergency Svcs.: Under 8 miles
Nearby shopping and entertainment
Pets allowed

### STAFF

Nurse/LVN/LPN: None on staff
Caregiver Training: Ethics, Family communication, Grief, Transition issues
Criminal Background Check: Yes
Principal Staff Language(s): English

### FACILITY FEATURES

Activities/Recreation
Guest Meals ($)
Pharmaceutical Service
Private Dining Room
Transportation to MD Appointments, Scheduled Outings

### ROOM FEATURES

Cable TV Ready ($)
Emergency Call System
Kitchenette
Private Bathrooms
Telephone Ready
Temperature Controls

### COSTS

PRICES MAY INCREASE. PLEASE CALL FOR MOST CURRENT INFORMATION.

| | |
|---|---|
| One Bedroom Apt. | $1,900/month |
| Respite Stays | $65/day for private room |
| Costs of Care | Included in monthly rate |
| Rate Increase | Annually; usually 3% |
| Reimbursement | Private pay |
| Pet Deposit | $300 |

### PORTRAIT

Perhaps it is because Greenbriar Mansion has such a small resident population that it fosters friendly intimacy among the group. We observed the staff and manager cheerfully attending to residents' needs and smiling constantly during our tour. The facility offers three daily activities, including bingo and cards. Residents take part in weekly outings to local destinations such as the library.

The facility boasts pretty views of the surrounding urban neighborhood from its position atop a grassy hill. Vividly hued flowers decorate the manicured lawn surrounding the pink brick building, where four columns support an attractive portico. The tastefully appointed entryway is full of rich color, from the maroon carpeting to the Queen Anne furniture upholstered in purple. Dark wooden accents offer a pleasing contrast to the entryway's white walls and columns. Lamps cast mellow light throughout the facility. Windows brighten the broad hallways. Residents enjoy large, sunny rooms with royal blue carpet and painted baseboards.

A vaulted ceiling commands attention in the spacious dining room. Expansive windows and recessed fixtures spill light onto the linen-draped tables. A baby grand piano and floral arrangements add sophisticated elements to the room. Daily snacks include fresh vegetables and fruit. Hearty favorites such as meatloaf, mashed potatoes and green beans are staples on the menu.

## Heritage Square

500 South Beach Street
Fort Worth, TX 76105
(817) 534-0013

---

### GILBERT GUIDE OBSERVATIONS

| | | | |
|---|---|---|---|
| Administration & Staff | g g g g g | Residents | g g g g g |
| Facility Aesthetics | g g g | Dietary & Food Selection | g g g g g |
| Facility Condition & Safety | g g g g g | Activities | g g g |

### DETAILS

Year Built: 1987
Current Mgmt. Since: 1987
No. of Floors: 2
Resident Capacity: 80

### SPECIAL

Mild dementia care provided
Diets Accommodated: Diabetic, Low-fat, Low-salt
Proximity to Emergency Svcs.: Under 8 miles
Nearby shopping and entertainment
Pets allowed

### STAFF

Nurse/LVN/LPN: 8 hours/week
Caregiver Training: Dementia, Ethics, Family communication, Grief, Patient transfers, Stress management, Transition issues
Criminal Background Check: Yes
Principal Staff Language(s): English
Other Staff Language(s): Spanish

### FACILITY FEATURES

Activities/Recreation
Beauty/Barber Shop ($)
Chapel Services
Facility Parking
Guest Meals ($)
Outside Patio/Gardens
Transportation
24-hour Security

### ROOM FEATURES

Cable TV Ready
Emergency Call System
Grab Bars
Kitchenette
Shared & Private Bathrooms
Telephone Ready
Temperature Controls

### COSTS

PRICES MAY INCREASE. PLEASE CALL FOR MOST CURRENT INFORMATION.

| | |
|---|---|
| Shared Room | $1,450/month |
| Private Room | $1,650/month |
| Respite Stays | $1,450/month for shared room |
| Costs of Care | Included in monthly rate |
| Rate Increase | Annually |
| Reimbursement | CBA, CCAD, Private pay |
| Pet Deposit | $300 (refundable) |

## PORTRAIT

As we approached Heritage Square, we were greeted by a group of friendly residents who welcomed us to their facility. The crisp white interior and shiny linoleum floors create a bright and spacious feel. The H-shaped layout accommodates several seating areas, nestled in each hallway. Residents' generously sized rooms feature ample closet space. Each has a lovely seating area flushed with natural light. Double occupancy rooms are available on the second floor.

The dining area has all the charm of an old saloon. At one end is a stage; at the other, an extensive bar with ample seating. The horizontal mirror behind the bar rounds out the authentic setting. Circular dining tables are frequently used for playing cards during activity hours. Live piano entertainment in the dining hall is another welcomed pastime. Heritage Square residents, who impressed us as being especially active, enjoy the cafeteria-style meals. An old-fashioned porch swing and playful swing set beckon residents to spend time outdoors. Ceiling fans provide a gentle breeze over the furnished patio.

All staff is cross-trained in different facets of care to ensure efficiency. Most of the residents are recipients of Community Based Alternatives (CBA) and Community Care for the Aged and Disabled (CCAD) awards. The staff and management foster a warm environment where residents appear comfortable and content. A recent bus trip to Oklahoma was a wonderful bonding activity for both groups. From the smiling faces that greeted us to the helpful staff, it is plain to see that Heritage Square is a happy home to everyone!

# JAMES L. WEST ALZHEIMER CENTER A/D

1111 Summit Avenue
Fort Worth, TX 76102

(817) 877-1199 x107
www.jameslwest.com

---

**GILBERT GUIDE OBSERVATIONS**

| | | | |
|---|---|---|---|
| Administration & Staff | g g g g g | Dietary & Food Selection | g g g g g |
| Facility Aesthetics | g g g g g | Activities | g g g g |
| Facility Condition & Safety | g g g g g | Alzheimer's & Dementia Capabilities | g g g g g |
| Residents | g g g g | | |

## DETAILS

Year Built: 1991
Current Mgmt. Since: 1991
No. of Floors: 5
Resident Capacity: 350

## SPECIAL

Alzheimer's/Dementia Only Facility
Diets Accommodated: Diabetic, Low-fat, Low-salt, Renal
Proximity to Emergency Svcs.: Under 8 miles
Nearby shopping and entertainment
No pets allowed

JAMES L. WEST ALZHEIMER CENTER (CONTINUED)

## STAFF

Nurse/LVN/LPN: Onsite 24/7
Caregiver Training: Dementia, Ethics, Family communication, Stress management
Criminal Background Check: Yes
Principal Staff Language(s): English
Other Staff Language(s): Japanese, Spanish

## FACILITY FEATURES

Activities/Recreation
Beauty/Barber Shop ($)
Chapel Services
Facility Parking
Guest Meals ($)
Outside Patio/Gardens
Private Dining Room
Separate Therapy Room
Transportation
24-hour Security

## ROOM FEATURES

Cable TV Ready
Emergency Call System
Grab Bars
Private Bathrooms
Telephone Ready

## COSTS

PRICES MAY INCREASE. PLEASE CALL FOR MOST CURRENT INFORMATION.

| | |
|---|---|
| Alzheimer's Unit | $2,000–$3,500/month for shared room<br>$3,000–$4,300/month for private room |
| Costs of Care | Included in monthly rate |
| Rate Increase | Annually; usually 2% |
| Reimbursement | Private pay |
| Security Deposit | $500 |

## PORTRAIT

A great location and wonderful amenities make James L. West a standout. The center is housed in a red brick building with white trim, only four miles from Harris Methodist Hospital and minutes from the newly revitalized downtown area. Conveniently, residents may purchase items ranging from fresh produce to antique vases at the shopping center on the premises.

The facility projects a comfortable atmosphere. Five large, well-furnished common areas per floor provide excellent opportunities for residents to congregate and socialize. Residents can often be found reading in one of the facility's libraries. The halls are lined with handrails. Frosted windows flood the facility with soft, natural light. This, coupled with an abundance of lush plants and indoor trees, gives the impression of being in nature. The facility boasts a 10,000 square foot garden, with a walkway, water fountain and a red brick gazebo. During our visit, the weather was gorgeous and we saw numerous residents in the garden. Several commented that it was their favorite part of the facility. Charming statues of people reading newspapers adorn some of the benches; additional statues of children playing are also featured in the garden.

Appetizing scents drifted from the spacious buffet-style dining rooms on our visit. Feeding assistance is available for residents who request help. Residents' rooms are spacious and bright; some have a view of downtown or wheelchair-accessible bathrooms.

We were pleased to note the residents interacting with each other and staff. Bingo, exercise, games, music therapy, sing-alongs, shopping excursions, ladies' tea, and trips to the zoo are a sample of the wide offering of activities. The facility welcomes volunteer entertainers, and also hosts Pet Day, when animals are brought in to spend time with the residents.

## Manor Care Health Services A/D

2129 Skyline Drive
Fort Worth, TX 76114

(817) 626-1956
(817) 797-3047

---

### GILBERT GUIDE OBSERVATIONS

| | | | |
|---|---|---|---|
| Administration & Staff | g g g g g | Dietary & Food Selection | g g g g |
| Facility Aesthetics | g g g g | Activities | g g g g g |
| Facility Condition & Safety | g g g g | Alzheimer's & Dementia Capabilities | g g g g g |
| Residents | g g g g | | |

### DETAILS

Year Built: 1981
Year Remodeled: 2004
Current Mgmt. Since: 2001
No. of Floors: 1
Resident Capacity: 100

### SPECIAL

Diets Accommodated: Diabetic, Low-fat, Low-salt
Proximity to Emergency Svcs.: 9–15 Miles
Pet visits allowed

### STAFF

Nurse/LVN/LPN: Onsite 24/7
Caregiver Training: Dementia, Family communication, Stress management
Criminal Background Check: Yes
Principal Staff Language(s): English

### FACILITY FEATURES

Activities/Recreation
Beauty/Barber Shop ($)
Facility Parking
Guest Meals
Outside Patio/Gardens
Private Dining Room
Separate Therapy Room
Transportation to MD Appointments ($), Scheduled Outings
24-hour Security

### ROOM FEATURES

Cable TV Ready
Emergency Call System
Grab Bars
Shared & Private Bathrooms
Telephone Ready

MANOR CARE HEALTH SERVICES (CONTINUED)

## COSTS

PRICES MAY INCREASE. PLEASE CALL FOR MOST CURRENT INFORMATION.

| | |
|---|---|
| Shared Room | $3,223/month |
| Private Room | Up to $3,500/month |
| Alzheimer's Unit | $3,223/month for shared room |
| Costs of Care | $300–$800/month based on individual need |
| Rate Increase | Annually; usually 3% |
| Reimbursement | Private pay |
| Entrance Fee | $1,100 |
| Security Deposit | $350 |

## PORTRAIT

Manor Care Health Services is housed in two well-maintained older buildings; the assisted living facility and the Alzheimer's are next door to one another. The yard was full of Halloween spirit when we visited, thanks to residents' handmade decorations. Rocking chairs rest on the patio, under handy ceiling fans.

A receptionist welcomes visitors at the greeting station, which has new carpet and fresh paint. The furniture is worn, but is clean and well-maintained. The soothing color scheme, which combines dark shades and soft pastels, is punctuated by bright flower arrangements. The facility has a bright, airy atmosphere. A Halloween party was taking place on the day of our visit. Several animated residents and staff were in costume. The staff enjoyed entertaining the residents with music and games. Regular field trips include outings to a bingo hall, where residents are monitored by staff. A delicious aroma emanated from the kitchen as the chefs prepared dinner. Several large tables in the dining area were set with pretty floral arrangements. The common areas are spotless and a variety of board games are available. The spacious hallways are equipped with handrails. Residents are welcome to decorate and paint their rooms, which are small to moderately sized. Each has a bed, nightstand and dresser.

The outdoor area is attractively landscaped with bushes, trees and miniature rose gardens. We were delighted to watch residents on the lawn playing baseball with foam bats and balls. A tall fence encloses the area, beyond which lies a beautiful, fragrant cedar forest.

## Meadow View

2815 Medlin Drive
Arlington, TX 76015

(817) 465-9596

### GILBERT GUIDE OBSERVATIONS

| | | | |
|---|---|---|---|
| Administration & Staff | g g g | Residents | g g g |
| Facility Aesthetics | g g g | Dietary & Food Selection | g g g |
| Facility Condition & Safety | g g g | Activities | g g g |

### DETAILS

Year Built: 1990
Current Mgmt. Since: 1990
No. of Floors: 1
Resident Capacity: 80

### SPECIAL

Diets Accommodated: Diabetic, Low-fat, Low-salt
Proximity to Emergency Svcs.: Under 8 miles
Nearby shopping and entertainment
Pet visits allowed

### STAFF

Nurse/LVN/LPN: On call 24/7
Caregiver Training: Dementia, Ethics, Family communication, Grief, Patient transfers, Transition issues
Criminal Background Check: Yes
Principal Staff Language(s): English
Other Staff Language(s): Spanish

### FACILITY FEATURES

Activities/Recreation
Beauty/Barber Shop ($)
Facility Parking
Guest Meals ($)
Outside Patio/Gardens
Overnight Guest Room ($)
Private Dining Room
Transportation to MD Appointments ($), Personal Outings ($), Scheduled Outings ($)
24-hour Security

### ROOM FEATURES

Cable TV Ready ($)
Emergency Call System
Grab Bars
Kitchenette
Shared Bathrooms
Telephone Ready ($)
Temperature Controls

### COSTS

PRICES MAY INCREASE. PLEASE CALL FOR MOST CURRENT INFORMATION.

| | |
|---|---|
| Studio Apt. | $1,200–$1,490/month |
| Costs of Care | Based on individual assessment |
| Rate Increase | Annually; usually 2% |
| Reimbursement | Private pay |

MEADOW VIEW (CONTINUED)

### PORTRAIT

Neighborhood renovations at the time of our visit did not upset the quiet atmosphere on Medlin Drive, where Meadowview sits. A brick building surrounded by flowers houses the facility. Artificial plants provide touches of green throughout the well-lit home. Handrails line the wide, clutter-free hallways. White walls in the hallways and residents' rooms create a somewhat institutional feel. Residents' rooms are sunny, moderately sized and furnished by the residents. The dining room doubles as an activities area.

Residents socialized comfortably in the common areas while we visited. They enjoy manicures, bingo, cooking, arts and crafts, and performances by entertainers such as the Singing Angels. Outdoor seating areas allow residents to view the garden, which features paths and manicured trees. Staff members were friendly during our visit to Meadowview.

## OAK PARK ASSISTED LIVING

4242 Bryant Irvin Road
Fort Worth, TX 76109

(817) 763-0088
www.provident.org

---

**GILBERT GUIDE OBSERVATIONS**

| | | | |
|---|---|---|---|
| Administration & Staff | g g g g | Residents | g g g |
| Facility Aesthetics | g g g g | Dietary & Food Selection | g g g g g |
| Facility Condition & Safety | g g g g g | Activities | g g g g |

### DETAILS

Year Built: 1986
Year Remodeled: 2000
Current Mgmt. Since: Unknown
No. of Floors: 3
Resident Capacity: 150

### SPECIAL

Mild dementia care provided
Diets Accommodated: Diabetic, Low-fat, Low-salt
Proximity to Emergency Svcs.: Under 8 miles
Nearby shopping and entertainment
Pets allowed

### STAFF

Nurse/LVN/LPN: 40 hours/week, On call 24/7
Caregiver Training: Dementia, Ethics, Family communication, Grief, Patient transfers, Stress management, Transition issues
Criminal Background Check: Yes
Principal Staff Language(s): English
Other Staff Language(s): Spanish

## FACILITY FEATURES

Activities/Recreation
Chapel Services
Facility Parking
Guest Meals ($)
Outside Patio/Gardens
Overnight Guest Room ($)
Transportation
24-hour Security

## ROOM FEATURES

Cable TV Ready
Emergency Call System
Grab Bars
Kitchenette
Private Bathrooms
Telephone Ready
Temperature Controls

## COSTS

PRICES MAY INCREASE. PLEASE CALL FOR MOST CURRENT INFORMATION.

| | |
|---|---|
| Studio Apt. | $1,900–$1,925/month |
| One Bedroom Apt. | $2,000–$2,700/month |
| | Double occupancy add $550/month |
| Respite Stays | $95/day for private room |
| Costs of Care | Starting at $25/month based on individual need |
| Rate Increase | Annually; usually 3–4% |
| Reimbursement | LTCI, Private pay |
| Application Fee | $500 |
| Pet Deposit | $500 |

## PORTRAIT

Oak Park, a stucco building with a somewhat institutional air, enjoys privacy from passers-by on Bryant Irvin Road due to its screen of large trees. The covered loading area attached to the front of the building is flanked by shrubbery. An upscale Fort Worth neighborhood provides the backdrop to the facility. Inside, floral borders highlight the beige décor. Residents enjoy abundant and comfortable seating areas both inside the facility and outside on the patios. Wheelchair users have ample room in the hallways, which are lined with handrails. Residents have several size options to choose from when they select a room, all of which have a window. The bathrooms feature practical touches such as raised toilet seats and walk-in showers.

Meals are served restaurant-style in the spacious dining area. The facility boasts a "satellite" dining room, which is used by residents who desire privacy. Activities also take place in the dining area. Staff members post a monthly events calendar, which lists exercise, bingo, scenic drives and shopping trips. The residents assist staff members in producing a monthly publication. We noticed pleasant interaction between the two groups.

## Tandy Village A/D

2601 Tandy Avenue
Fort Worth, TX 76103

(817) 535-1253

### GILBERT GUIDE OBSERVATIONS

| | | | |
|---|---|---|---|
| Administration & Staff | g | Dietary & Food Selection | g g g g g |
| Facility Aesthetics | g g | Activities | g g |
| Facility Condition & Safety | g g g | Alzheimer's & Dementia Capabilities | g g g |
| Residents | g g g g | | |

### DETAILS

Year Built: 1922
Year Remodeled: 1984
Current Mgmt. Since: December 2005
No. of Floors: 1
Resident Capacity: 120

### SPECIAL

Diets Accommodated: None
Proximity to Emergency Svcs.: Under 8 miles
Nearby shopping and entertainment
Pets allowed

### STAFF

Nurse/LVN/LPN: 40 hours/week
Caregiver Training: Dementia, Ethics, Family communication, Grief, Patient transfers, Stress management, Transition issues
Criminal Background Check: Yes
Principal Staff Language(s): English
Other Staff Language(s): Spanish

### FACILITY FEATURES

Activities/Recreation
Beauty/Barber Shop ($)
Chapel Services
Facility Parking
Guest Meals
Outside Patio/Gardens
Transportation

### ROOM FEATURES

Cable TV Ready
Emergency Call System
Grab Bars
Kitchenette
Shared & Private Bathrooms
Telephone Ready
Temperature Controls

### COSTS

PRICES MAY INCREASE. PLEASE CALL FOR MOST CURRENT INFORMATION.

| | |
|---|---|
| Shared Room | $1,400–$2,400/month |
| Private Room | $1,800–$3,000/month |
| Respite Stays | $75/day for shared room |
| Costs of Care | Included in monthly rate |
| Rate Increase | Annually |
| Reimbursement | Private pay |
| Security Deposit | $350 |
| Pet Deposit | $300 |

### PORTRAIT

Tandy Village is one of the few Dallas facilities that accepts recipients funded through the Community Based Alternatives (CBA) and Community Care for the Aged and Disabled (CCAD) programs. The facility, a former school, is a quiet retreat in an outlying downtown neighborhood. Floor-to-ceiling windows allow natural light to flood the interior. All windows are covered with a mesh screen to soften the glare, a thoughtful feature that aids residents with visual deficiencies. A playful and cheery environment, the interior is fashioned into a town square where street signs direct residents to their respective halls.

Both single and double occupancy rooms are available. The double occupancy rooms are divided by a wall, allowing maximum privacy. All rooms feature private closets and additional storage space. Aside from the tiled kitchenette, each room is fully carpeted. The secured Alzheimer's unit houses sixteen rooms with similar accommodations. The several spacious common areas are perfect for social visits and weekly activities. One popular common area is "The Village"; an ice cream parlor, a museum, a library and a big-screen TV are among its main attractions! A stage in "The Village" is used for live performances. Two entrées are featured daily. Snacks, assorted juices and coffee are available around the clock. Residents in the Alzheimer's unit have a separate dining area. One good-humored resident accompanied us on part of our tour, entertaining us with pleasant conversation before sauntering off in another direction.

## TANGLEWOOD OAKS A/D

2698 South Hulen Street
Fort Worth, TX 76109

(817) 922-9559
www.emeritus.com

---

**GILBERT GUIDE OBSERVATIONS**

| | | | |
|---|---|---|---|
| Administration & Staff | g g g g g | Dietary & Food Selection | g g g g |
| Facility Aesthetics | g g g g | Activities | g g g g |
| Facility Condition & Safety | g g g g g | Alzheimer's & Dementia Capabilities | g g g g g |
| Residents | g g g g | | |

### DETAILS

Year Built: 1994
Year Remodeled: 2004
Current Mgmt. Since: 2002
No. of Floors: 1
Resident Capacity: 116

### SPECIAL

Diets Accommodated: Diabetic, Low-fat, Low-salt
Proximity to Emergency Svcs.: Under 8 miles
Nearby shopping and entertainment
Pets allowed

TANGLEWOOD OAKS (CONTINUED)

### STAFF

Nurse/LVN/LPN: 40 hours/week, On call 24/7
Caregiver Training: Dementia, Ethics, Family communication, Grief, Patient transfers, Stress management, Transition issues, Validation therapy
Criminal Background Check: Yes
Principal Staff Language(s): English
Other Staff Language(s): German, Spanish

### FACILITY FEATURES

Activities/Recreation
Beauty/Barber Shop
Chapel Services
Computer/Internet Access
Facility Parking
Fitness Room/Gym
Guest Meals
Outside Patio/Gardens
Overnight Guest Room ($)
Pharmaceutical Service ($)
Private Dining Room
Room Service ($)
Separate Therapy Room
Transportation to MD Appointments ($), Personal Outings, Scheduled Outings
24-hour Security

### ROOM FEATURES

Cable TV Ready
Emergency Call System
Grab Bars
Kitchenette
Private Bathrooms
Telephone Ready ($)
Temperature Controls

### COSTS

PRICES MAY INCREASE. PLEASE CALL FOR MOST CURRENT INFORMATION.

| | |
|---|---|
| Studio Apt. | $2,315–$2,765/month |
| One Bedroom Apt. | $3,165–$3,615/month<br>Double occupancy add $220/month |
| Two Bedroom Apt. | $5,000/month |
| Alzheimer's Unit | $3,250/month for shared room<br>$5,000/month for private room |
| Respite Stays | $125/day for private room (ALZ) |
| Costs of Care | Included in monthly rate |
| Rate Increase | Annually; usually 3% |
| Reimbursement | LTCI, Private pay, Veterans |
| Entrance Fee | $7,500 |
| Pet Deposit | $500 |

### PORTRAIT

Tanglewood Oaks is tucked away on South Hulen Street in a bustling, upscale area of Fort Worth, amid neighboring office buildings. The gray brick facility is surrounded by a manicured landscape of trees, shrubs and pink and purple flowers. A combination of artificial and fresh floral arrangements pops against the green and beige color palette inside. The facility is furnished with pristine, comfortable furniture. White paneling lines the walls of the expansive hallways. Staff and family members decorate residents' sunny, moderately sized rooms. Mouthwatering aromas of chicken fried steak, vegetables and freshly baked pie wafted from the kitchen into the homey dining area during our visit, where green linen dresses the tables. The meals at Tanglewood Oaks are designed to meet a variety of dietary needs and preferences, from diabetic to vegetarian.

Residents enjoy sitting in the gazebo or strolling on the paved walkways that curve beneath towering oaks in the inner courtyard. Small groups and one-on-one interaction between staff members and residents form the core of the activities program, which features arts and crafts, picnics and outings to the zoo, among others. Staff members collaborate with residents' families on individual care plans. Tanglewood Oaks also offers respite care.

## Whitley Place

800 Whitley Road
Keller, TX 76248

(817) 379-0795
www.cathedralrock.com

---

**GILBERT GUIDE OBSERVATIONS**

| | | | |
|---|---|---|---|
| Administration & Staff | g g g | Residents | g g |
| Facility Aesthetics | g g g | Dietary & Food Selection | g g |
| Facility Condition & Safety | g g g | Activities | g g g |

### DETAILS

Year Built: 1989
Year Remodeled: 1996
Current Mgmt. Since: 2001
No. of Floors: 1
Resident Capacity: 65

### SPECIAL

Mild dementia care provided
Diets Accommodated: Diabetic, Low-fat, Low-salt
Proximity to Emergency Svcs.: 9–15 Miles
Nearby shopping and entertainment
Pets allowed

### STAFF

Nurse/LVN/LPN: 40 hours/week, On call 24/7
Caregiver Training: Ethics, Family communication, Patient transfers, Transition issues, Validation therapy
Criminal Background Check: Yes
Principal Staff Language(s): English

### FACILITY FEATURES

Activities/Recreation
Beauty/Barber Shop ($)
Facility Parking
Guest Meals ($)
Outside Patio/Gardens

### ROOM FEATURES

Cable TV Ready ($)
Emergency Call System
Kitchenette
Private Bathrooms
Telephone Ready ($)

WHITLEY PLACE (CONTINUED)

**FACILITY FEATURES** (CONTINUED)
Pharmaceutical Service
Private Dining Room
Room Service
Transportation
24-hour Security

**ROOM FEATURES** (CONTINUED)
Temperature Controls

## COSTS

PRICES MAY INCREASE. PLEASE CALL FOR MOST CURRENT INFORMATION.

| | |
|---|---|
| Studio Apt. | $1,975–$2,150/month |
| One Bedroom Apt. | $2,375–$2,500/month<br>Double occupancy add $600/month |
| Two Bedroom Apt. | $3,000/month<br>Double occupancy add $600/month |
| Costs of Care | $200–$800/month based on individual need |
| Rate Increase | Annually; usually 3% |
| Reimbursement | LTCI, Private pay, SSI, Veterans |
| Entrance Fee | $400 |
| Pet Deposit | $250 (refundable) |

## PORTRAIT

Whitley Place, housed in a brick structure with a shingled roof, blends well into the residential area near Highway 377. Expansive lawns flank the building. Residents stroll along the concrete pathway that curves around the facility. The covered entrance is convenient when entering and exiting in inclement weather.

Dark blue carpet covers the floor of the large foyer and contrasts with the off-white walls. Antique lamps and wood furniture upholstered in red and white plaid generate a country atmosphere in the common areas. Sconces and artificial lighting brighten the facility. The hallways are broad enough to allow two wheelchair users to pass one another with ease. Residents' rooms vary in size from small to spacious and feature large windows. Each bathroom is equipped with a walk-in shower. Some rooms have direct access to the inner courtyard.

Residents spend a great deal of time in the common areas, which are gender-specific, where they watch TV and play games. Many exercise daily. They also enjoy special events, such as performances by the Glenview Baptist Ukulele Band. For the most part, staff members leave the residents in peace, but they are available when needed. The central courtyard features a grill, a picnic area and a wooden gazebo. Multicolored shrubbery decorates the manicured lawn. Young and mature trees provide shade.

Whitley Place chefs prepare homestyle meals such as spaghetti and meatballs, squash, wedge salad and strawberry shortcake. Residents snacked on fruit cocktail and crackers on the day of our tour. Residents often submit recipes to the cooks, the results of which are then served at lunch. Generously sized tables made of light wood add a bright element to the cozy dining area.

### SKILLED NURSING FACILITIES

## Broadway Plaza at Cityview

5301 Bryant Irvin Road
Fort Worth, TX 76132

(817) 346-9407, (877) 219-5434
www.arclp.com

---

**TOTAL GOVERNMENT DEFICIENCIES: 0** Reviewed on: November 12, 2004

No Deficiencies

* IMPORTANT: REVIEW DETAILS OF EACH DEFICIENCY AT WWW.MEDICARE.GOV

**GILBERT GUIDE OBSERVATIONS**

| | | | |
|---|---|---|---|
| Administration & Staff | g g g | Dietary & Food Selection | g g g g |
| Facility Aesthetics | g g g | Activities | g g g |
| Facility Condition & Safety | g g g | Access to Medical Care | g g g |
| Residents | g g g | | |

### DETAILS

Year Built: 1988
Year Remodeled: 2000
Current Mgmt. Since: 1989
No. of Floors: 3
Resident Capacity: 122
Facility Type: Long-term care, Short-term rehab

### SPECIAL

Special diets accommodated
Proximity to Emergency Svcs.: Less than 8 miles

### STAFF

Caregiver Training: Ethics, Family communication, Grief, Pain management, Patient transfers, Stress management, Transition issues, Universal precautions, Validation therapy, Wound care
Criminal Background Check: Yes
Principal Staff Language(s): English
Other Staff Language(s): Spanish

### FACILITY FEATURES

Beauty/Barber Shop
Guest Meals ($)
Outside Patio/Gardens
Separate Therapy Room
Whirlpool Baths

### ROOM FEATURES

Cable TV Ready
Space for personal items
Shared & Private Bathrooms
Telephone Ready ($)

BROADWAY PLAZA AT CITYVIEW (CONTINUED)

### COSTS

PRICES MAY INCREASE. PLEASE CALL FOR MOST CURRENT INFORMATION.

| | |
|---|---|
| Shared Room | $133/day |
| Private Room | $190/day |
| Rate Increase | Annually; usually 4% |
| Reimbursement | Medicare, Medicaid, LTCI, HMO, Private pay, SSI, Veterans |

### PORTRAIT

Broadway Plaza's skilled nursing facility is located at the rear of an expansive gated compound. The stately brick building is outlined by manicured shrubs and towering oak and cedar trees. The SNF occupies the second and third floors, which are lined with blue carpeting and wallpapered in neutral shades. Artificial plants and hanging pastoral prints spruce up the otherwise simple décor.

Residents' rooms have a somewhat institutional feel, although large windows allow lots of light and add cheer to the space. Each floor has a cozy dining area that doubles as an activity room, where residents enjoy playing board games and working on puzzles. For outdoor enjoyment, residents gather on the furnished back patio. A stone birdbath attracts much activity from the facility's winged neighbors—delightful entertainment for bird lovers!

The hallways are spacious enough to accommodate residents in hospital beds. Natural light radiates throughout the facility. At the time of our visit, many of the residents were busy with daily therapies. The majority of the staff has been at Broadway Plaza for several years, adding reliability and consistency to the homey environment.

## GARDEN TERRACE ALZHEIMER'S CENTER OF EXCELLENCE A/D

7500 Oakmont Boulevard
Fort Worth, TX 76132

(817) 346-8080
www.gardenterrace.net

**TOTAL GOVERNMENT DEFICIENCIES: 2** — Reviewed on: December 9, 2004

| Mistreatment | Resident Rights |
|---|---|
| 1 | 1 |

* IMPORTANT: REVIEW DETAILS OF EACH DEFICIENCY AT WWW.MEDICARE.GOV

**GILBERT GUIDE OBSERVATIONS**

| | | | |
|---|---|---|---|
| Administration & Staff | g g g g | Dietary & Food Selection | g g g |
| Facility Aesthetics | g g g g | Activities | g g g g |
| Facility Condition & Safety | g g g g g | Alzheimer's & Dementia Capabilities | g g g g g |
| Residents | g g g g | Access to Medical Care | g g g g |

**DETAILS**

Year Built: 1998
Current Mgmt. Since: 1998
No. of Floors: 1
Resident Capacity: 120
Facility Type: Long-term care, Short-term rehab, Alzheimer's unit

**SPECIAL**

Special diets accommodated
Proximity to Emergency Svcs.: Under 8 miles

**STAFF**

Caregiver Training: Dementia, Ethics, Family communication, Grief, Pain management, Patient transfers, Stress management, Transition issues, Universal precautions, Validation therapy, Wound care
Criminal Background Check: Yes
Principal Staff Language(s): English

**FACILITY FEATURES**

Activities/Recreation
Beauty/Barber Shop ($)
Chapel Services
Guest Meals
Outside Patio/Gardens
Private Dining Room
Private Visiting Room
Separate Therapy Room ($)
24-hour Security
Wanderguard
Whirlpool Baths

**ROOM FEATURES**

Space for personal items
Shared Bathrooms

**COSTS**

PRICES MAY INCREASE. PLEASE CALL FOR MOST CURRENT INFORMATION.

| | |
|---|---|
| Dementia Unit | $143–$154/day for shared room<br>$174/day for private room |
| Respite Stays | Call for rates and availability for shared room |
| Rate Increase | Annually |
| Reimbursement | Medicare, LTCI, Private pay |

**PORTRAIT**

Garden Terrace is a short distance from Benbrook Lake, neighboring parks, shopping centers and medical facilities. The lobby is a comfortable gathering place that boasts a grand view of the patio. Although the building has a somewhat institutional look, its soft interior color scheme of earth tones provides a warm and homey contrast.

Residents' furnished rooms are spacious and get plenty of natural light. Residents add their own decorative knickknacks. Each floor is secured and comes with its own recreational and dining room. The dining room is adequately sized to accommodate residents on each floor. The building is brightened by an abundance of windows and lovely glass chandeliers. The hallways are broad and neat. During our visit, the halls were festively adorned with Halloween decorations. The garden patio is furnished for outdoor rest and relaxation.

GARDEN TERRACE ALZHEIMER'S CENTER OF EXCELLENCE (CONTINUED)

The Garden Terrace staff specializes in Alzheimer's and dementia care. The facility is divided into five units—Medicare, hospice, high functioning, behavioral, and hospice for residents with Alzheimer's. Residents benefit from respite care as well as inpatient and outpatient therapy services.

## Immanuel's Healthcare

4515 Village Creek Road
Fort Worth, TX 76119

(817) 451-8704
www.immanuels.com

**TOTAL GOVERNMENT DEFICIENCIES: 1** — Reviewed on: May 11, 2005

| Mistreatment |
|---|
| 1 |

* IMPORTANT: REVIEW DETAILS OF EACH DEFICIENCY AT WWW.MEDICARE.GOV

**GILBERT GUIDE OBSERVATIONS**

| | | | |
|---|---|---|---|
| Administration & Staff | g g g g | Dietary & Food Selection | g g g |
| Facility Aesthetics | g g g g g | Activities | g g g g |
| Facility Condition & Safety | g g g g g | Access to Medical Care | g g g |
| Residents | g g g g | | |

### DETAILS

Year Built: 2004
Current Mgmt. Since: 2004
No. of Floors: 1
Resident Capacity: 84
Facility Type: Long-term care

### SPECIAL

Special diets accommodated
Proximity to Emergency Svcs.: 9–15 Miles

### STAFF

Caregiver Training: Dementia, Ethics, Pain management, Patient transfers, Stress management, Universal precautions, Validation therapy
Criminal Background Check: Yes
Principal Staff Language(s): English

## FACILITY FEATURES

Activities/Recreation
Beauty/Barber Shop ($)
Chapel Services
Facility Parking
Guest Meals
Outside Patio/Gardens
Private Dining Room
Private Visiting Room
Separate Therapy Room
24-hour Security
Wanderguard
Whirlpool Baths

## ROOM FEATURES

Cable TV Ready
Space for personal items
Shared & Private Bathrooms
Telephone Ready ($)

## COSTS

PRICES MAY INCREASE. PLEASE CALL FOR MOST CURRENT INFORMATION.

| | |
|---|---|
| Shared Room | $115/day |
| Private Room | $130/day |
| Rate Increase | Periodically |
| Reimbursement | Medicare, Medicaid, LTCI, Private pay |

## PORTRAIT

Immanuel's Health Care is the house that faith built. The thirty-eight member congregation of the local World Baptist Missionary Church raised $4.4 million to construct Immanuel's, making it East Fort Worth's first new SNF in over thirty-five years. It is owned and operated by a nonprofit corporation. The management team worked together prior to the opening of the facility. During our visit, we noted the warm interaction between residents and staff.

Immanuel's sits on a quiet section of Village Creek Road. The brick exterior is immaculate, as are the grounds, which include ample parking. Warm earth tones and soft lighting pervade the facility. Silk flowers add spots of bright color throughout. The wide hallways are equipped with handrails and feature comfortable seating areas. Residents personalize their rooms with their own furnishings. The rooms are bright and moderately sized.

Schoolchildren from the neighboring church were entertaining the residents in the activities area when we visited. In addition to the main dining room, there are two private dining rooms, which may be reserved for events such as birthday parties and family dinners. Residents use the spacious chapel in the center of the facility for worship and community events. Services are held several times a week. Plans to build an affiliated school and church are in the works.

## Interlochen Health and Rehab

2645 West Randol Mill Road
Arlington, TX 76012
(817) 277-6789

**TOTAL GOVERNMENT DEFICIENCIES: 19** — Reviewed on: August 5, 2005

| Administration | Environmental | Mistreatment | Nutrition and Dietary |
|---|---|---|---|
| 4 | 3 | 1 | 1 |
| **Pharmacy Service** | **Quality Care** | **Resident Assessment** | **Resident Rights** |
| 2 | 2 | 4 | 2 |

* IMPORTANT: REVIEW DETAILS OF EACH DEFICIENCY AT WWW.MEDICARE.GOV

**GILBERT GUIDE OBSERVATIONS**

| | | | |
|---|---|---|---|
| Administration & Staff | g g g g g | Dietary & Food Selection | g g g g |
| Facility Aesthetics | g g g | Activities | g g g g |
| Facility Condition & Safety | g g g | Access to Medical Care | g g g g g |
| Residents | g g g g | | |

### DETAILS

Year Built: 1975
Year Remodeled: 2006
Current Mgmt. Since: 2003
No. of Floors: 1
Resident Capacity: 120
Facility Type: Long-term care, Short-term rehab

### SPECIAL

Special diets accommodated
Proximity to Emergency Svcs.: Under 8 miles

### STAFF

Caregiver Training: Dementia, Ethics, Family communication, Grief, Pain management, Patient transfers, Stress management, Transition issues, Universal precautions, Wound care
Criminal Background Check: Yes
Principal Staff Language(s): English
Other Staff Language(s): Spanish

### FACILITY FEATURES

Activities/Recreation
Beauty/Barber Shop
Chapel Services
Guest Meals
Outside Patio/Gardens
Private Visiting Room
Separate Therapy Room
24-hour Security
Wanderguard
Whirlpool Baths

### ROOM FEATURES

Cable TV Ready
Space for personal items
Shared & Private Bathrooms
Telephone Ready

## COSTS

PRICES MAY INCREASE. PLEASE CALL FOR MOST CURRENT INFORMATION.

| | |
|---|---|
| Shared Room | $115/day |
| Private Room | $175/day |
| Respite Stays | $115/day for shared room |
| Rate Increase | Annually; usually 2–3% |
| Reimbursement | Medicare, Medicaid, LTCI, HMO, Private pay, SSI, Veterans |

## PORTRAIT

Interlochen rests against a hillside in residential Arlington, amid trees and shrubs. Artificial plants complement the green and beige walls in the entry, which features comfortable furniture. The garden areas, hallways, floors and residents' rooms were all undergoing an extensive remodel at the time of our visit. Management hopes that the remodel will make the facility a bit more homey. Sunlight warms residents' moderately sized rooms. The furnished rooms boast satellite TV and extra space for personal belongings.

The dining area doubles as an activities area. Feeding assistance is provided in smaller dining rooms. Near the dining area is the facility's therapy room, an important element of rehabilitative therapy. The wide hallways are softly lit, in keeping with the rest of the facility. Staff members interacted warmly with residents and actively encouraged residents as they assisted them in performing activities of daily living. We found the management team friendly and helpful.

## Life Care Center of Haltom

2936 Markum Drive
Fort Worth, TX 76117

(817) 831-0545
www.lcca.com

**TOTAL GOVERNMENT DEFICIENCIES: 10** — Reviewed on: July 28, 2005

| Administration | Nutrition and Dietary | Pharmacy Service | Quality Care |
|---|---|---|---|
| 1 | 1 | 1 | 1 |

| Resident Assessment | Resident Rights |
|---|---|
| 1 | 5 |

* IMPORTANT: REVIEW DETAILS OF EACH DEFICIENCY AT WWW.MEDICARE.GOV

**GILBERT GUIDE OBSERVATIONS**

| | | | |
|---|---|---|---|
| Administration & Staff | g g g g g | Dietary & Food Selection | g g g |
| Facility Aesthetics | g g g g g | Activities | g g g g |
| Facility Condition & Safety | g g g g g | Access to Medical Care | g g g g |
| Residents | g g g g | | |

### DETAILS

Year Built: 1962
Year Remodeled: 2003
Current Mgmt. Since: 2000
No. of Floors: 1
Resident Capacity: 144
Facility Type: Long-term care, Short-term rehab

### SPECIAL

Special diets accommodated
Proximity to Emergency Svcs.: Under 8 miles

### STAFF

Caregiver Training: Dementia, Ethics, Family communication, Pain management, Patient transfers, Transition issues, Universal precautions, Validation therapy
Criminal Background Check: Yes
Principal Staff Language(s): English
Other Staff Language(s): Spanish

### FACILITY FEATURES

Activities/Recreation
Chapel Services
Facility Parking
Guest Meals ($)
Outside Patio/Gardens
Private Dining Room
Private Visiting Room
Separate Therapy Room
24-hour Security
Wanderguard

### ROOM FEATURES

Cable TV Ready ($)
Space for personal items
Shared Bathrooms
Telephone Ready ($)

## COSTS

PRICES MAY INCREASE. PLEASE CALL FOR MOST CURRENT INFORMATION.

| | |
|---|---|
| Shared Room | $128/day |
| Respite Stays | $123/day for shared room |
| Rate Increase | Annually; usually 1–3% |
| Reimbursement | Medicare, Medicaid, HMO, Private pay, SSI, Veterans |

## PORTRAIT

Life Care Center of Haltom is an outstanding facility that offers wound and respite care in addition to anodyne, speech, physical and occupational therapies. The energetic staff members exude friendliness and professionalism. Oak trees encircle the stately beige building, which neighbors a pharmacy. Retail establishments, including grocery and clothing stores, line nearby Belknap Street. The area is predominantly residential.

The home is immaculate. A trio of hallways connects the reception area to the activities area and residents' rooms. Soothing wallpaper in brown and beige stripes covers the walls. Furnishings are upholstered in a royal combination of purple and gold. Pastoral paintings and artificial trees add hints of nature to the rooms. Quaint paintings of cottages and forests accent the pretty floral wallpaper in the wide hallways. The bottom half of the walls, beneath the handrails, complement the floral design with a rich brown color. Residents' rooms are spotless and bright, in keeping with the rest of the home. A bed and a nightstand furnish each of the rooms, which also boast two closets. The bathrooms abound with practical considerations such as raised sinks and toilets, walk-in showers and linen closets.

The dining room features intimate groupings of four seats to each table, providing ample space for wheelchair users. Gold chandeliers and sunshine fill the room with mellow light. Residents and their families frequently share meals in the private dining area. Residents enjoy watching television and listening to the radio in the spacious activity room, which also hosts chess matches and card games. Fluorescent lighting brightens the rest of the home. A sunroom opens to the inner courtyard, where a gazebo and walkways tempt residents to spend time among the flowers, shrubs and oak trees. Residents socialized extensively with one another during our time at the facility.

## Renaissance Park Multi Care Center

4252 Bryant Irvin Road
Fort Worth, TX 76109

(817) 738-2975
www.renaissancepark-fw.com

**TOTAL GOVERNMENT DEFICIENCIES: 11** — Reviewed on: November 18, 2005

| Administration | Deficiencies Reported Between Inspections | Environmental | Mistreatment |
|---|---|---|---|
| 2 | 1 | 2 | 1 |
| **Nutrition and Dietary** | **Pharmacy Service** | **Quality Care** | **Resident Rights** |
| 1 | 1 | 2 | 1 |

* IMPORTANT: REVIEW DETAILS OF EACH DEFICIENCY AT WWW.MEDICARE.GOV

**GILBERT GUIDE OBSERVATIONS**

| | | | |
|---|---|---|---|
| Administration & Staff | g g g g g | Dietary & Food Selection | g g g g |
| Facility Aesthetics | g g g g | Activities | g g g g g |
| Facility Condition & Safety | g g g g | Access to Medical Care | g g g g |
| Residents | g g g | | |

### DETAILS

Year Built: 1988
Year Remodeled: 2003
Current Mgmt. Since: Unknown
No. of Floors: 2
Resident Capacity: 120
Facility Type: Long-term care, Short-term rehab

### SPECIAL

Special diets accommodated
Proximity to Emergency Svcs.: Under 8 miles

### STAFF

Caregiver Training: Dementia, Ethics, Family communication, Grief, Pain management, Patient transfers, Stress management, Transition issues, Universal precautions, Validation therapy, Wound care
Criminal Background Check: Yes
Principal Staff Language(s): English
Other Staff Language(s): Spanish

### FACILITY FEATURES

Activities/Recreation
Beauty/Barber Shop ($)
Chapel Services
Guest Meals ($)
Outside Patio/Gardens
Private Dining Room
Private Visiting Room

### ROOM FEATURES

Cable TV Ready ($)
Space for personal items
Shared Bathrooms
Telephone Ready ($)

FACILITY FEATURES (CONTINUED)
Separate Therapy Room
24-hour Security
Whirlpool Baths

## COSTS

PRICZES MAY INCREASE. PLEASE CALL FOR MOST CURRENT INFORMATION.

| | |
|---|---|
| Shared Room | $115/day |
| Private Room | $178/day |
| Respite Stays | $115/day for shared room<br>$178/day for private room |
| Rate Increase | Annually |
| Reimbursement | Medicare, Medicaid, HMO, Private pay |

## PORTRAIT

Renaissance Park is located on bustling Bryant Irvin Road, near restaurants and shops. The stucco frame and well-maintained landscape make the attractive property blend right in with its affluent urban surroundings. The interior is wallpapered in muted colors and lined with new carpeting. During a recent remodel, management added contemporary furniture throughout the facility to counter the somewhat institutional environment.

Residents' rooms are moderately sized. Each has a window and is furnished with the essentials. The dining room and activity parlor are the main common areas. Residents and their loved ones reserve the private dining room for intimate gatherings. The outdoor area features comfortable patio furniture. Hallways are spacious and neat. Soft artificial lighting is used to accommodate the special needs of residents with dementia.

Renaissance Park staff encourages residents to be as independent as possible; the rehabilitation programs are vital to this effort. The rehabilitation department, staffed by Medicare-certified caregivers, provides speech and hearing therapy, physical therapy, respiratory and occupational therapy, and outpatient therapeutic services. Residents enjoy a full calendar of events, which includes cooking classes, dances, late night bingo, church services and wine and cheese socials. The staff believes that by actively participating in this community, residents will reach their full potential.

## Shady Grove Nursing Home

814 Weiler Boulevard (817) 654-3613
Fort Worth, TX 76112

---

**TOTAL GOVERNMENT DEFICIENCIES: 10** Reviewed on: April 7, 2005

| Administration | Environmental | Mistreatment | Nutrition and Dietary |
|---|---|---|---|
| 1 | 1 | 1 | 2 |
| **Quality Care** | **Resident Rights** | | |
| 2 | 3 | | |

* IMPORTANT: REVIEW DETAILS OF EACH DEFICIENCY AT WWW.MEDICARE.GOV

**GILBERT GUIDE OBSERVATIONS**

| | | | |
|---|---|---|---|
| Administration & Staff | g g g g | Dietary & Food Selection | g g g |
| Facility Aesthetics | g g g | Activities | g g g g |
| Facility Condition & Safety | g g g | Access to Medical Care | g g g g g |
| Residents | g g g | | |

### DETAILS

Year Built: 1970's
Current Mgmt. Since: 2002
No. of Floors: 1
Resident Capacity: 60
Facility Type: Long-term care, Short-term rehab

### SPECIAL

Special diets accommodated
Proximity to Emergency Svcs.: Under 8 miles

### STAFF

Caregiver Training: Dementia, Ethics, Family communication, Grief, Pain management, Patient transfers, Stress management, Transition issues, Universal precautions, Validation therapy, Wound care
Criminal Background Check: Yes
Principal Staff Language(s): English
Other Staff Language(s): Spanish

### FACILITY FEATURES

Activities/Recreation
Beauty/Barber Shop ($)
Chapel Services
Facility Parking
Guest Meals
Outside Patio/Gardens
Separate Therapy Room ($)
24-hour Security

### ROOM FEATURES

Cable TV Ready ($)
Space for personal items
Shared Bathrooms
Telephone Ready

### COSTS

PRICES MAY INCREASE. PLEASE CALL FOR MOST CURRENT INFORMATION.

| | |
|---|---|
| Shared Room | $75/day |
| Private Room | $125/day |
| Respite Stays | $75/day for shared room<br>$125/day for private room |
| Rate Increase | Periodically |
| Reimbursement | Medicare, Medicaid, Private pay, Veterans |

### PORTRAIT

Shady Grove Nursing Home, named for the large trees that surround it, is housed in a brick building on quiet Weiler Boulevard. St. Rita Catholic Church and St. Rita Catholic School are nearby. The church has a group of adults and children who volunteer at Shady Grove. The children engage in fun activities with the residents, such as bingo and arts and crafts, while the adults offer ministering, Bible study and other religious services.

Shady Grove's homelike ambiance is immediately apparent. It is very quiet and peaceful, somewhat atypical of a SNF. The home is clean and brightly lit, and the wide hallways are uncluttered. The comfortable dining area doubles as an activities area. Several staff members informed us that the food is excellent. We noted the great quantity of time staff spent with the residents. Their conversations were relaxed and comfortable. Shady Grove has a notably low staff turnover, which indicates high job satisfaction and stability.

Residents' spacious rooms easily accommodate personal items. Each room has a window that lets in sunlight. The spacious outdoor area is enclosed. Residents use the backyard for gardening and socializing.

## SOUTHWEST NURSING & REHAB

5300 Altamesa Boulevard
Fort Worth, TX 76133

(817) 346-1800
www.southwestnursingandrehab.com

---

**TOTAL GOVERNMENT DEFICIENCIES: 3** — Reviewed on: September 29, 2005

| Nutrition and Dietary | Pharmacy Service | Quality Care |
|---|---|---|
| 1 | 1 | 1 |

* IMPORTANT: REVIEW DETAILS OF EACH DEFICIENCY AT WWW.MEDICARE.GOV

**GILBERT GUIDE OBSERVATIONS**

| | | | |
|---|---|---|---|
| Administration & Staff | g g g | Dietary & Food Selection | g g g g |
| Facility Aesthetics | g g g g | Activities | g g g g |
| Facility Condition & Safety | g g g g | Access to Medical Care | g g g |
| Residents | g g g g | | |

SOUTHWEST NURSING & REHAB (CONTINUED)

### DETAILS

Year Built: 1980
Year Remodeled: 2000
Current Mgmt. Since: 2000
No. of Floors: 1
Resident Capacity: 160
Facility Type: Long-term care, Short-term rehab

### SPECIAL

Special diets accommodated
Proximity to Emergency Svcs.: Under 8 miles

### STAFF

Caregiver Training: Dementia, Ethics, Family communication, Grief, Pain management, Patient transfers, Stress management, Transition issues, Universal precautions, Validation therapy, Wound care
Criminal Background Check: Yes
Principal Staff Language(s): English
Other Staff Language(s): Spanish

### FACILITY FEATURES

Activities/Recreation
Beauty/Barber Shop
Guest Meals
Outside Patio/Gardens
Private Dining Room
Private Visiting Room
Separate Therapy Room
Whirlpool Baths

### ROOM FEATURES

Space for personal items
Shared Bathrooms
Telephone Ready ($)

### COSTS

PRICES MAY INCREASE. PLEASE CALL FOR MOST CURRENT INFORMATION.

| | |
|---|---|
| Shared Room | $110/day |
| Respite Stays | $110/day for shared room |
| Rate Increase | Annually; usually 4% |
| Reimbursement | Medicare, Medicaid, Private pay |

### PORTRAIT

Southwest sits on elevated ground above Alta Mesa Boulevard. Lush foliage of trees and trimmed shrubs deck the entrance to the facility. Neutral-colored walls of the interior complement the light brown squares in the tiled floor. Hanging prints of nature scenes adorn the walls.

Residents' rooms are clean and spacious, although somewhat institutional. The wide hallways are equipped with handrails. The building is brightened by a combination of natural and fluorescent lighting. The comfortably furnished dining room is also used for socials, dances and occasional performances by local children's singing groups. Residents gather and socialize in the activity parlor as well as the library. During our visit, many residents were chatting in the garden while relaxing on comfortable patio furniture. Everyone seemed to be enjoying the cool afternoon breeze.

Residents and staff interact warmly with each other. The monthly newsletter, produced jointly by residents and staff, alerts residents' families of upcoming events, monthly menus and care plan schedules. The goal to keep everyone informed has created a close-knit community. We found the staff very accommodating. At the time of our visit, residents and staff had raised over $1,000 for victims of Hurricane Katrina.

## VILLAGE CREEK NURSING HOME A/D

3825 Village Creek Road
Fort Worth, TX 76119

(817) 429-1991
www.villagecreeknursinghome.com

**TOTAL GOVERNMENT DEFICIENCIES: 6** Reviewed on: December 3, 2004

| Environmental | Quality Care | Resident Assessment |
|---|---|---|
| 3 | 2 | 1 |

* IMPORTANT: REVIEW DETAILS OF EACH DEFICIENCY AT WWW.MEDICARE.GOV

**GILBERT GUIDE OBSERVATIONS**

| | | | |
|---|---|---|---|
| Administration & Staff | g g g g | Dietary & Food Selection | g g g |
| Facility Aesthetics | g g g | Activities | g g g |
| Facility Condition & Safety | g g g | Alzheimer's & Dementia Capabilities | g g g |
| Residents | g g g | Access to Medical Care | g g g g |

### DETAILS

Year Built: 1970's
Year Remodeled: 2000
Current Mgmt. Since: 2000
No. of Floors: 1
Resident Capacity: 100
Facility Type: Long-term care, Short-term rehab, Alzheimer's unit

### SPECIAL

Special diets accommodated
Proximity to Emergency Svcs.: Less than 8 miles

### STAFF

Caregiver Training: Dementia, Ethics, Family communication, Grief, Pain management, Patient transfers, Universal precautions, Validation therapy, Wound care
Criminal Background Check: Yes
Principal Staff Language(s): English
Other Staff Language(s): Spanish

VILLAGE CREEK NURSING HOME (CONTINUED)

### FACILITY FEATURES

Activities/Recreation
Beauty/Barber Shop ($)
Chapel Services
Outside Patio/Gardens
Private Dining Room
Private Visiting Room
Separate Therapy Room
Whirlpool Baths

### ROOM FEATURES

Space for personal items
Shared Bathrooms
Telephone Ready ($)

### COSTS

PRICES MAY INCREASE. PLEASE CALL FOR MOST CURRENT INFORMATION.

| | |
|---|---|
| Shared Room | $90/day |
| Private Room | $90/day if available |
| Respite Stays | $90/day for shared room |
| Rate Increase | Periodically |
| Reimbursement | Medicare, Medicaid, LTCI, Private pay, SSI, Veterans |

### PORTRAIT

During our visit to Village Creek Nursing Home, the staff proudly introduced us to a gentleman who has lived there for almost twenty years. One of several residents who have a long history at the facility, he seemed quite happy with his surroundings. The staff and residents were pleasant and fell into easy conversation with one another. We admired photographs of a recent Juneteenth celebration, which depicted a large group of people smiling and dancing. The tables were festively decorated with red balloons and tablecloths, and the residents looked as though they had a marvelous time.

The facility has been well-maintained through a series of remodeling. Staff recently held a contest amongst themselves to redecorate the shower areas using color on the walls and shower curtains. The results added simple cheer. The lobby of Village Creek is furnished with comfortable chairs and sofas, beckoning residents and guests to relax and visit. Residents often enjoy people-watching on the facility's front porch. A secured wing featuring a dining area and common rooms houses the Alzheimer's unit. Village Creek competently addresses an impressively broad range of needs, from cancer and pain management to schizophrenia and multiple personality disorder.

**IN-HOME CARE PROVIDERS**

## Home Health Specialties

4239 Road to the Mall (817) 496-5400
North Richland Hills, TX 76180

SEE CHAPTER 1 FOR A DESCRIPTION OF IN-HOME CARE SERVICES.

### DETAILS

Years in Business: 30
Home Health Services Provided: Yes
Care Visits Provided Within a Facility: Yes
Dementia Care Provided: Yes
Will Replace Caregiver Within 48 Hours Upon Request: Yes

### CAREGIVERS

RN on Staff: Yes
Hiring Qualifications: 1 year of experience, TB test, Criminal background check, CNA certification, 2 references required
Caregiver Training: Dementia, Ethics, Family communication, Grief, Patient transfers, Transition issues
Frequency of Caregiver Training: Initial formal training program, Monthly
Language(s) Spoken: English, Spanish

### AVAILABILITY

Service Availability: 24/7
On-call Supervisor Availability: 24/7

### COSTS

PRICES MAY INCREASE. PLEASE CALL FOR MOST CURRENT INFORMATION.

Rate: Call for rates
Minimum Hours per Day: None
Minimum Days per Week: None
Sliding Fee Schedule Available: Yes

### UNIQUE QUALITIES

Home Health Specialties boasts thirty years of homecare experience in the Dallas area. The agency offers services that range from pediatrics to geriatrics. The therapy program is staffed by full-time professionals who specialize in speech, physical and occupational therapies. They pride themselves on smoothly transitioning clients from one program to another as necessary.

## ADULT DAY CARE CENTERS

### JAMES L. WEST ALZHEIMER CENTER A/D

1111 Summit Avenue
Fort Worth, TX 76102

(817) 536-8693
www.jameslwest.com

---

**GILBERT GUIDE OBSERVATIONS** gggggg

#### DETAILS

Owner/Affiliation: James L. and Eunice P. West Charitable Trust
Years in Business: 14
License/Certification: Texas Department of Aging and Disability Services, Texas Department of Human Services
Business Hours: Sunday–Saturday, 7:30am–6:00pm
Transportation provided ($)
Conditions Accepted: Alzheimer's/Dementia, HIV/AIDS, Incontinence, Limited mobility, Mental illness, Stroke, Vision/Hearing impairment

#### SPECIAL

Special diets accommodated
Wheelchair accessible
Proximity to Emergency Svcs.: Under 8 miles

#### STAFF

Staff/Patient Ratio: 1:5
Criminal Background Check: Yes
Language(s) Spoken: English, Japanese, Spanish

#### COSTS

PRICES MAY INCREASE. PLEASE CALL FOR MOST CURRENT INFORMATION.

Daily Costs: $46 with reservation; $52 without reservation; $30 for 4 hours
Reimbursement: Medicare, Medicaid

#### PORTRAIT

The quality of the James L. West adult day program is impressive. The kind staff exemplifies Southern hospitality. They enjoyed conversing with us during our visit, readily describing the activities and type of care provided in the program. We noted staff and participants interacting extensively, playing games, reading and talking with one another.

The day program and affiliated assisted living facility are both housed in a well-maintained brick building. The day care is secured. The large room is clean and divided by a row of potted plants. One side features comfortable sofas and a birdcage with parakeets. The other half is used for activities and meals. A separate rehabilitation room is used for exercise.

Mental stimulation and memory improvement exercise are among a few of the many activities. Word games, sing-alongs, cooking and reminiscing activities round out the mix. One favorite activity is storytime: participants begin telling a story in the morning and then break for lunch; afterward, everyone tries to recall the first part of the story.

### GERIATRIC CARE MANAGERS

## DALLAS CARE CONNECTION

Carol K. Franzen, MS, LMSW
P.O. Box 815848
Dallas, TX 75381

(972) 242-0901
cfranzen@dallascareconnection.com
www.dallascareconnection.com

SEE CHAPTER 1 FOR A DESCRIPTION OF GERIATRIC CARE MANAGER SERVICES.

### DETAILS

Years of GCM Experience: 21
Degree(s) Held: Licensed Master Social Worker
Member of National Association of Professional Geriatric Care Managers
Language(s) Spoken: English

### SERVICES

Staff on Call: 24/7
Client References Provided: Yes
Areas of Practice: Assessment, Care management, Counseling, Education, Family/Professional liaison
Assistance with Medicare/Medicaid Process: Yes

### COSTS

PRICES MAY INCREASE. PLEASE CALL FOR MOST CURRENT INFORMATION.

Assessment: Call for rates
Hourly: Call for rates

### UNIQUE QUALITIES

With over twenty years of case management experience behind her, Carol K. Franzen is highly skilled in assisting seniors and people with disabilities. Carol has provided case management services in the Dallas-Fort Worth area since 1985. Not surprisingly, other local care managers have referred a number of challenging cases to Dallas Care Connection; Carol's familiarity with long-term care services in the area is a great strength.

## Senior Assistance Resource Network

Jane Oderberg, MED, LMSW
4763 Barwick Drive, Suite 100
Fort Worth, TX 76132

(817) 263-5196, (817) 905-6166
jane@seniorassistance-fw.com
www.seniorassistance-fw.com

SEE CHAPTER 1 FOR A DESCRIPTION OF GERIATRIC CARE MANAGER SERVICES.

### DETAILS

Years of GCM Experience: 5
Degree(s) Held: Licensed Master Social Worker
Member of National Association of Professional Geriatric Care Managers
Language(s) Spoken: English

### SERVICES

Staff on Call: 24/7
Client References Provided: Yes
Areas of Practice: Assessment, Care management, Counseling, Education, Family/Professional liaison
Assistance with Medicare/Medicaid Process: Yes

### COSTS

PRICES MAY INCREASE. PLEASE CALL FOR MOST CURRENT INFORMATION.

Assessment: $240
Hourly: $65

### UNIQUE QUALITIES

Jane Oderberg's Senior Assistance Resource Network is a one-stop shop: she is equipped to handle all types of services, with the exception of homecare, for which she provides referrals. Jane works with clients and their families to find cost-effective solutions to maintain independence.

#### HOSPICE PROVIDERS

## Community Hospice Of Texas

301 Medpark Circle
Burleson, TX 76028

(817) 615-2150
www.chot.org

SEE CHAPTER 1 FOR A DESCRIPTION OF HOSPICE SERVICES.

### DETAILS

Affiliation: None
Licensed By: Texas Department of Health Services
Medicare certified

## CARE

At-home Care Provided: Yes
Inpatient Care Provided: Yes
Caregivers trained, supervised, and monitored
Supervisor on call 24/7
Language(s) Spoken: English, Spanish

## UNIQUE QUALITIES

The caregivers of Community Hospice feel they are "answering a calling." Because it is a community-owned nonprofit, the commitment to high-quality care exceeds the normal boundaries and extends to patients and their loved ones, as well as employees and the community at large. The organization provides care for more non-funded patients than any other hospice in the area. Community Hospice includes five homecare units and two inpatient units.

# NORTH DALLAS

ASSISTED LIVING FACILITIES

## Alterra Sterling House of Lewisville

965 Gardenridge Road
Lewisville, TX 75077

(972) 420-9600
www.assisted.com

**GILBERT GUIDE OBSERVATIONS**

| | | | |
|---|---|---|---|
| Administration & Staff | g g g g g | Residents | g g g g g |
| Facility Aesthetics | g g g g g | Dietary & Food Selection | g g g g |
| Facility Condition & Safety | g g g g g | Activities | g g g g |

### DETAILS

Year Built: 1996
Current Mgmt. Since: 1996
No. of Floors: 1
Resident Capacity: 42

### SPECIAL

Mild dementia care provided
Diets Accommodated: Diabetic, Low-fat, Low-salt
Proximity to Emergency Svcs.: Under 8 miles
Nearby shopping and entertainment
Pets allowed

### STAFF

Nurse/LVN/LPN: 80 hours/week, On-call 24/7
Caregiver Training: Dementia, Ethics, Family communication, Grief, Patient transfers, Stress management, Transition issues
Criminal Background Check: Yes
Principal Staff Language(s): English
Other Staff Language(s): Spanish

### FACILITY FEATURES

Activities/Recreation
Beauty/Barber Shop ($)
Chapel Services
Facility Parking
Guest Meals
Outside Patio/Gardens
Overnight Guest Room
Room Service ($)
Transportation
24-hour Security

### ROOM FEATURES

Cable TV Ready
Emergency Call System
Grab Bars
Kitchenette
Private Bathrooms
Telephone Ready
Temperature Controls

### COSTS

PRICES MAY INCREASE. PLEASE CALL FOR MOST CURRENT INFORMATION.

| | |
|---|---|
| Studio Apt. | $2,410/month |
| One Bedroom Apt. | $2,620–$2,830/month |
| Costs of Care | $58–$812/month based on individual need |
| Rate Increase | Annually; usually 3% |

| | |
|---|---|
| Reimbursement | LTCI, Private pay |
| Entrance Fee | $1,000 |
| Pet Deposit | $250 |

**PORTRAIT**

The director of Alterra Sterling House of Lewisville has implemented many positive changes since she began there in 2005; not only are there many new staff members, most of the residents are new as well (there were only fourteen when she took her post). We observed several of them creating table decorations for the monthly family night that includes a buffet and entertainment, courtesy of the director. The activity calendar listed a poetry workshop, a Super Bowl party and visits from a local Brownie troop and community choir. Residents enjoy craft projects, such as devising cards for Valentine's Day. The large sink and tile floor in the activity room make cleaning up after cooking and other messy projects a breeze. A traveling library makes regular stops so that residents may check out reading materials.

We came across a resident with mild dementia as she wandered about a broad hallway. Our guide, the director, greeted her by name and asked her to join our tour. The director then encouraged her to answer our questions about residents' rooms, making her feel useful. The sunny rooms feature walk-in closets with shelves, which the staff thoughtfully adjusts to each resident's height. All of the bathrooms have walk-in showers and additional storage space.

The appealing aroma of fresh coffee wafted from the charming dining room. Meals are served cafeteria-style through a window between the kitchen and dining areas. Expansive windows and archways give the dining room an airy quality. 1930s music played softly in the background as we took in the sunny living room. Birds preened in their cage while fish darted about the fish tank. A piano and fireplace add to the appeal. French doors open from the living area to a lovely sunroom furnished with wicker chairs and potted ferns. The square-shaped facility features a courtyard at its heart, where residents exercise along the pathways and seating areas invite quiet contemplation.

## Appletree Court Assisted Living

870 West Arapaho Road
Richardson, TX 75080

(972) 889-2300
www.appletreecourt.com

**GILBERT GUIDE OBSERVATIONS**

| | | | |
|---|---|---|---|
| Administration & Staff | g g g g g | Residents | g g g g g |
| Facility Aesthetics | g g g g g | Dietary & Food Selection | g g g g g |
| Facility Condition & Safety | g g g g g | Activities | g g g g |

APPLETREE COURT ASSISTED LIVING (CONTINUED)

### DETAILS

Year Built: 1999
Year Remodeled: 2003
Current Mgmt. Since: 1999
No. of Floors: 2
Resident Capacity: 106

### SPECIAL

Mild dementia care provided
Diets Accommodated: Diabetic, Low-fat, Low-salt
Proximity to Emergency Svcs.: Under 8 miles
Nearby shopping and entertainment
Pets allowed

### STAFF

Nurse/LVN/LPN: 40 hours/week
Caregiver Training: Dementia, Ethics, Family communication, Grief, Patient transfers, Stress management, Transition issues, Validation therapy
Criminal Background Check: Yes
Principal Staff Language(s): English
Other Staff Language(s): Spanish

### FACILITY FEATURES

Activities/Recreation
Beauty/Barber Shop
Computer/Internet Access
Facility Parking
Outside Patio/Gardens
Overnight Guest Room ($)
Private Dining Room
Transportation

### ROOM FEATURES

Cable TV Ready
Emergency Call System
Grab Bars
Kitchenette
Private Bathrooms
Telephone Ready ($)

### COSTS

PRICES MAY INCREASE. PLEASE CALL FOR MOST CURRENT INFORMATION.

| | |
|---|---|
| Studio Apt. | $2,370/month |
| One Bedroom Apt. | $2,830/month<br>Double occupancy add $750/month |
| Two Bedroom Apt. | $3,550/month |
| Respite Stays | $85/day for private room |
| Costs of Care | $2,370–$3,550/month based on individual need |
| Rate Increase | Every 3 years; usually 3% |
| Reimbursement | Private pay |
| Security Deposit | $750 (refundable) |
| Pet Deposit | $500 |

### PORTRAIT

Appletree Court is adjacent to Richardson Senior Health Clinic and Richardson Senior Center on West Arapaho Road. Mature trees and a flowered landscape surround the lovely brick home, which features a grand portico, stone columns and archways. The gazebo encircled by a white fence is a relaxing spot for reading or contemplation. Planters filled with blossoms reside on window sills. Comfortable rockers furnish the porch, where residents enjoy cookouts. Past the entrance is a plant-filled atrium with a lovely seating area.

Stone columns soar to the vaulted ceiling above the dining and activities room, where chandeliers shed light upon elegant china and linen-draped mahogany tables. Natural lighting is plentiful throughout the facility. Framed prints and oil paintings adorn the short hallways. Residents decorate their rooms, which range from moderately to generously sized. Mini-blinds hang from residents' windows.

Staff members are well acquainted with residents, who seem very much at home in Appletree Court. The dietary manager, who supervises residents' diets, relies on residents' opinions regarding menu options. Mouthwatering entrées such as barbecued ribs, pot roast and roasted chicken with vegetables are regular offerings, accompanied by a variety of low-sugar desserts. Popular activities among residents include exercise, singing and classes on dancing and cooking. Wine and cheese gatherings and guest musical performances are also widely attended, in addition to picnics and shopping trips. Each month residents are treated to a themed dinner that features decorations and entertainment.

## ATRIA CARROLLTON A/D

1825 Arbor Creek Drive
Carrollton, TX 75010

(972) 862-8700
(214) 725-8089
www.atriaseniorliving.com

---

**GILBERT GUIDE OBSERVATIONS**

| | | | |
|---|---|---|---|
| Administration & Staff | g g g g g | Dietary & Food Selection | g g g g g |
| Facility Aesthetics | g g g g g | Activities | g g g g |
| Facility Condition & Safety | g g g g g | Alzheimer's & Dementia Capabilities | g g g g g |
| Residents | g g g g g | | |

### DETAILS

Year Built: 2000
Current Mgmt. Since: 2000
No. of Floors: 3
Resident Capacity: 74

### SPECIAL

Diets Accommodated: Low-fat, Low-salt
Proximity to Emergency Svcs.: Under 8 miles
Nearby shopping and entertainment
Pets allowed

### STAFF

Nurse/LVN/LPN: 40 hours/week, On-call 24/7
Caregiver Training: Dementia, Ethics, Family communication, Grief, Patient transfers, Stress management, Transition issues, Validation therapy
Criminal Background Check: Yes
Principal Staff Language(s): English
Other Staff Language(s): Spanish

ATRIA CARROLLTON (CONTINUED)

**FACILITY FEATURES**

Activities/Recreation
Beauty/Barber Shop ($)
Chapel Services
Computer/Internet Access
Facility Parking
Fitness Room/Gym
Guest Meals ($)
Outside Patio/Gardens
Private Dining Room ($)
Separate Therapy Room
Transportation
24-hour Security

**ROOM FEATURES**

Cable TV Ready ($)
Emergency Call System
Furnished
Grab Bars
Kitchenette
Shared & Private Bathrooms
Telephone Ready
Temperature Controls

**COSTS**

PRICES MAY INCREASE. PLEASE CALL FOR MOST CURRENT INFORMATION.

| | |
|---|---|
| Studio Apt. | $3,095/month |
| One Bedroom Apt. | $3,395/month<br>Double occupancy add $995/month |
| Two Bedroom Apt. | $3,895/month |
| Alzheimer's Unit | $3,450–$5,250/month for shared room |
| Respite Stays | $110–$120/day for private room |
| Costs of Care | $325–$1,600/month based on individual need |
| Rate Increase | Annually; usually 5–9% |
| Reimbursement | LTCI, Private pay |
| Entrance Fee | $1,500 |
| Pet Deposit | $750 |

**PORTRAIT**

Located on bustling, tree-lined Arbor Creek Drive, Atria Carrollton is a red brick building with cheerful yellow siding and tall white columns. Ceiling fans generate a cool breeze over the wicker chairs on the veranda. Pink and white crepe myrtles, colorful pansies and tufts of monkey grass decorate the lawn. Barbecues in the outdoor courtyard are a popular event, perhaps in part because residents enjoy relaxing beneath the shade trees and near the marble fountain.

Yellow canaries and blue parakeets sing from their perches in the aviary, while tropical fish create vivid color in aquariums placed throughout the facility. Lithographs of Greek and Roman pottery hang from the walls. Comfortable, modern furnishings fit well with the color scheme of yellow, orange and green.

Decadent meals, such as grilled chicken with baby squash and fresh green beans, are served restaurant-style in the elegant dining room. White tablecloths dress the round oak tables; matching chairs are upholstered in maroon. Glass chandeliers hang from the ceiling. A selection of several menus includes hearty staples such as chicken noodle soup and ham sandwiches; the Weight Watcher selection lists low-fat options and smaller portions. Atria's residents are a happy, animated group with a variety of interests. Residents lunch at restaurants every other week. Outback Steak House is a favorite. Residents sponsor art bizarres that feature their paintings and other crafts; all proceeds benefit the Alzheimer's Association. During our tour, we noticed the staff smiling and sharing inside jokes with the residents.

A black baby grand sits in the library, which doubles as a common area. Large oak tables and blue and green couches furnish the other common areas. The wide hallways are equipped with dark wooden handrails. Sunlight supplements fluorescent lighting throughout the building. That, along with white window treatments and pale walls add a spacious air to residents' rooms. The rooms feature ample storage space. Residents proudly display their artwork and seasonal decorations on small shelves outside their doors.

## Atria Flower Mound

6051 Morris Road
Flower Mound, TX 75028

(972) 539-9444, (972) 809-8506
www.arvi.com

**GILBERT GUIDE OBSERVATIONS**

| | | | |
|---|---|---|---|
| Administration & Staff | g g g g | Residents | g g g |
| Facility Aesthetics | g g g | Dietary & Food Selection | g g g |
| Facility Condition & Safety | g g g | Activities | g g g |

### DETAILS

Year Built: 1998
Year Remodeled: Ongoing
Current Mgmt. Since: 1998
No. of Floors: 1
Resident Capacity: 78

### SPECIAL

Diets Accommodated: Diabetic, Low-fat, Low-salt, Renal
Proximity to Emergency Svcs.: Under 8 miles
Nearby shopping and entertainment
Some pets allowed

### STAFF

Nurse/LVN/LPN: 40 hours/week, On-call 24/7
Caregiver Training: Ethics, Family communication, Stress management
Criminal Background Check: Yes
Principal Staff Language(s): English
Other Staff Language(s): Spanish

### FACILITY FEATURES

Activities/Recreation
Beauty/Barber Shop ($)
Chapel Services
Facility Parking
Guest Meals ($)
Outside Patio/Gardens

### ROOM FEATURES

Cable TV Ready
Emergency Call System
Grab Bars
Kitchenette
Private Bathrooms
Telephone Ready

ATRIA FLOWER MOUND (CONTINUED)

**FACILITY FEATURES (CONTINUED)**

Pharmaceutical Service ($)
Room Service ($)
Transportation to MD Appointments, Personal Outings
24-hour Security

**ROOM FEATURES (CONTINUED)**

Temperature Controls

## COSTS

PRICES MAY INCREASE. PLEASE CALL FOR MOST CURRENT INFORMATION.

| | |
|---|---|
| Studio Apt. | $1,795–$4,195/month |
| Two Bedroom Apt. | $3,495–$4,695/month |
| Respite Stays | $125/day for private room |
| Costs of Care | Included in monthly rate |
| Rate Increase | Annually; usually 3–4% |
| Reimbursement | LTCI, Private pay, Veterans |
| Entrance Fee | $1,500 |
| Pet Deposit | $800 |

## PORTRAIT

A cheerful receptionist greeted us as we entered Atria Flower Mound, located on a busy street in a building of red brick and wood. The facility's entrance opens to the dining room. Two elegant chandeliers hang from the vaulted ceiling and shed mellow light onto the brick fireplace and hardwood floor. As we entered, residents were just finishing a breakfast of ham and cheese omelets, scrambled eggs, bacon and sausage. Several residents chatted with each other and staff members, who cleared the tables.

Residents are encouraged to decorate their rooms. Most rooms boast a private patio, enclosed by a white fence, where residents are fond of spending their time. Smoked glass and brass fixtures fill the facility, including the wide hallways, with soft light. A comfortably furnished common room features a snack bar that is open around the clock. Residents use this area to watch TV and play cards and board games. Atria Flower Mound News, a newsletter for residents, lists each month's activities, which include poker, Sunday Sundaes, conversational Spanish and Friday night movies. Oaks and flowering trees grow in the main patio area, where residents frequently have their families over to barbecue. Residents mentioned that they have been perhaps too successful in raising a family of finches in one of the activity rooms, as the finches "are reproducing like crazy!"

## AUTUMN LEAVES OF CARROLLTON A/D

1800 King Arthur Boulevard
Carrollton, TX 750101

(972) 492-7700
(877) 688-7700
www.autumnleavesliving.com

---

### GILBERT GUIDE OBSERVATIONS

| | | | |
|---|---|---|---|
| Administration & Staff | g g g | Dietary & Food Selection | g g g |
| Facility Aesthetics | g g g g | Activities | g g g g |
| Facility Condition & Safety | g g g g g | Alzheimer's & Dementia Capabilities | g g g |
| Residents | g g g | | |

### DETAILS

Year Built: 2002
Current Mgmt. Since: 2002
No. of Floors: 1
Resident Capacity: 44

### SPECIAL

Alzheimer's/Dementia Only Facility
Diets Accommodated: Diabetic, Low-fat, Low-salt
Proximity to Emergency Svcs.: Under 8 miles
Nearby shopping and entertainment
No pets allowed

### STAFF

Nurse/LVN/LPN: 20 hours/week, On-call 24/7
Caregiver Training: Dementia, Ethics, Family communication, Grief, Patient transfers, Stress management, Transition issues, Validation therapy
Criminal Background Check: Yes
Principal Staff Language(s): English
Other Staff Language(s): Spanish

### FACILITY FEATURES

Activities/Recreation
Beauty/Barber Shop
Chapel Services
Guest Meals
Outside Patio/Gardens
Separate Therapy Room
Transportation to MD Appointments
24-hour Security

### ROOM FEATURES

Cable TV Ready ($)
Emergency Call System
Furnished
Grab Bars
Kitchenette
Shared & Private Bathrooms
Temperature Controls

### COSTS

PRICES MAY INCREASE. PLEASE CALL FOR MOST CURRENT INFORMATION.

| | |
|---|---|
| Alzheimer's Unit | $3,550–$4,000/month for private room |
| Costs of Care | Included in monthly rate |
| Rate Increase | Every 2 years; usually 1–2% |
| Reimbursement | Private pay |

AUTUMN LEAVES OF CARROLLTON (CONTINUED)

**PORTRAIT**

Autumn Leaves sits upon a gentle slope. Laughter from the nearby preschool punctuates the otherwise quiet residential neighborhood. Water spouts from a fountain decorated with a statue of a young boy. The driveway encircles oaks and cypresses. Pansies and potted hibiscus grow around the covered entrance supported by white columns. Mauve bricks, white siding and maroon shutters create an attractive facade.

Cream and green-striped wallpaper matches the linen tablecloths in the dining area. The menu on the day of our visit featured ground meat with gravy, creamed corn and mashed potatoes. Snacks are offered around the clock. Expansive windows, supplemented by fluorescent lights, brighten the spacious common areas. Colorful couches and chairs comprise the comfortable, well-maintained furnishings. Landscape and floral prints adorn the walls. Handrails line the four expansive hallways. Each hallway has a theme to stimulate residents' memories; the themes are expressed through distinct colors, paper borders, and nautical knickknacks. Residents' rooms range from small to large. White walls and sparse furnishings lend a somewhat institutional air, although sunlight from the large windows adds warmth. Memory shelves and plaques with residents' names and photographs placed beside each door help residents locate their rooms.

Residents interact easily with the caring staff and enjoy regular physical and mental exercise. They also take part in supervised candle making. Cooking therapy is a favorite activity—several residents especially love preparing the side dishes and desserts for Thanksgiving. A paved courtyard lies at the heart of the facility. Black wrought iron chairs and a matching table furnish the inner patio. A walkway diverges in yet another secured courtyard; one path leads to a seating area, and the other leads to a pond surrounded by flowers and shrubs.

## AVALON—SPARROWS POINT A/D

5013 Sparrows Point
Plano, TX 75023

(214) 752-7050
(800) 696-6536
www.avalon-care.com

---

**GILBERT GUIDE OBSERVATIONS**

| Category | Rating | Category | Rating |
|---|---|---|---|
| Administration & Staff | g g g g g | Dietary & Food Selection | g g g g |
| Facility Aesthetics | g g g g | Activities | g g g |
| Facility Condition & Safety | g g g g g | Alzheimer's & Dementia Capabilities | g g g g |
| Residents | g g g g | | |

**DETAILS**

Year Built: 1977
Year Remodeled: 2002
Current Mgmt. Since: 2000
No. of Floors: 1
Resident Capacity: 16

**SPECIAL**

Alzheimer's/Dementia Only Facility
Diets Accommodated: Diabetic, Low-fat, Low-salt
Proximity to Emergency Svcs.: 16+ Miles
Nearby shopping and entertainment
No pets allowed

**STAFF**

Nurse/LVN/LPN: On-call 24/7
Caregiver Training: Dementia, Ethics, Family communication, Grief, Patient transfers, Stress management, Transition issues, Validation therapy
Criminal Background Check: Yes
Principal Staff Language(s): English

**FACILITY FEATURES**

Activities/Recreation
Beauty/Barber Shop
Chapel Services
Facility Parking
Guest Meals
Outside Patio/Gardens
Transportation
24-hour Security

**ROOM FEATURES**

Cable TV Ready ($)
Furnished
Private Bathrooms
Telephone Ready ($)

**COSTS**

PRICES MAY INCREASE. PLEASE CALL FOR MOST CURRENT INFORMATION.

| | |
|---|---|
| Alzheimer's Unit | $3,875–$4,275/month for private room |
| Costs of Care | $200/month for incontinence |
| Rate Increase | Annually; usually 2–3% |
| Reimbursement | Private pay |
| Security Deposit | $500 |

**PORTRAIT**

Avalon Sparrows Point is an upscale Alzheimer's facility that provides care for all stages of dementia. The staff works as a team to harbor a comforting environment. The large home sits on a calm tree-lined street in a safe neighborhood. The luxurious interior décor brings to mind a five-star hotel. The walls are painted in shades of mocha. Attractive artwork and contemporary furnishings add to the elegant ambience. Several residents were relaxing on the overstuffed sofas and chairs in the common areas when we visited. Although there was a large TV and entertainment center, we noticed that they were not being used, as residents preferred to socialize instead—a touching glimpse of the familial environment at Sparrow's Point.

The staff regularly performs room checks and are generally very attentive to residents. Residents are encouraged to decorate their own rooms, which are large and tidy, with plenty of space for personal items and lots of natural light. Multiple overhead fixtures throughout

AVALON—SPARROWS POINT (CONTINUED)

the facility produce bright lighting. There are no hallways; one spacious walkway leads to the rear of the facility.

Fruit, cookies, coffee and tea are daily snacks. A resident was helping prepare "Special Stew," a favorite meal at the facility, during our visit. Residents often relax on the patio, where they enjoy the trees, plants and flowers. There are weekly field trips to shopping malls, and daily activities may include game hour, exercise and cookie socials.

## Collin Oaks Assisted Living A/D

4045 West 15th Street
Plano, TX 75093

(972) 519-0480
www.emeritus.com

---

**GILBERT GUIDE OBSERVATIONS**

| | | | |
|---|---|---|---|
| Administration & Staff | g g g g | Dietary & Food Selection | g g g g |
| Facility Aesthetics | g g g g | Activities | g g g g g |
| Facility Condition & Safety | g g g | Alzheimer's & Dementia Capabilities | g g g g |
| Residents | g g g g | | |

### DETAILS

Year Built: 1995
Year Remodeled: 2005
Current Mgmt. Since: 2003
No. of Floors: 1
Resident Capacity: 74

### SPECIAL

Diets Accommodated: Diabetic, Low-fat, Low-salt
Proximity to Emergency Svcs.: Under 8 miles
Nearby shopping and entertainment
Some pets allowed

### STAFF

Nurse/LVN/LPN: 40 hours/week, On-call 24/7
Caregiver Training: Dementia, Ethics, Family communication, Grief, Patient transfers, Stress management, Transition issues, Validation therapy
Criminal Background Check: Yes
Principal Staff Language(s): English
Other Staff Language(s): Spanish

### FACILITY FEATURES

Activities/Recreation
Beauty/Barber Shop ($)
Chapel Services
Facility Parking
Guest Meals ($)
Outside Patio/Gardens
Pharmaceutical Service ($)
Private Dining Room

### ROOM FEATURES

Cable TV Ready
Emergency Call System
Furnished
Grab Bars
Kitchenette
Shared & Private Bathrooms
Telephone Ready ($)
Temperature Controls

FACILITY FEATURES (CONTINUED)

Room Service ($)
Separate Therapy Room
Transportation to MD Appointments, Scheduled Outings
24-hour Security

## COSTS

PRICES MAY INCREASE. PLEASE CALL FOR MOST CURRENT INFORMATION.

| | |
|---|---|
| Studio Apt. | \$2,250/month |
| One Bedroom Apt. | \$2,600–\$3,050/month<br>Double occupancy add \$1,750/month |
| Alzheimer's Unit | \$3,400–\$3,600/month for shared room |
| Costs of Care | Based on individual need |
| Rate Increase | Every 2–3 years; usually 2–3% |
| Reimbursement | LTCI, Private pay |
| Entrance Fee | \$1,000 |
| Pet Deposit | \$250 |

## PORTRAIT

Collin Oaks calls a busy portion of West 15th Street home. Lush greenery encircles a decorative water fountain in the park-like exterior and a bench provides an inviting place to sit. Shutters on the windows and a large wreath above the entrance add elements of charm. Inside, silk flower arrangements complement the hanging artwork that depicts butterflies and blossoms. Dark green carpet contrasts nicely with the elegant lavender window treatments. Ceiling fans generate a soft breeze in the common areas. The facility is brightened by a mixture of natural and fluorescent lighting. Handrails line the expansive hallways. Family members decorate residents' rooms with personal knickknacks to stimulate memory. Regular activities include afternoon strolls, exercises for cognitive stimulation, and listening to soothing music. Staff members possess intimate knowledge of residents' various stages of dementia, which allows them to prompt residents appropriately. A handful of residents chatted together cheerfully during our tour.

Residents enjoy low-sodium and low-sugar meals including grilled chicken sandwiches with vegetables. Alternate offerings such as salad are also available. Padded chairs surround cherrywood tables in the formal dining room. The floral wallpaper is striking against the room's mauve curtains and green upholstery. Diners have a view of the courtyard, located at the heart of the facility. Walkways lined with flowers meander across the lawn between oak trees.

## Colonial Lodge of Plano

5217 Village Creek Drive
Plano, TX 75093

(972) 735-0306
www.alcco.com

---

**GILBERT GUIDE OBSERVATIONS**

| | | | |
|---|---|---|---|
| Administration & Staff | g g g g | Residents | g g g g |
| Facility Aesthetics | g g g | Dietary & Food Selection | g g g |
| Facility Condition & Safety | g g g | Activities | g g g |

### DETAILS

Year Built: 1997
Current Mgmt. Since: 2001
No. of Floors: 1
Resident Capacity: 66

### SPECIAL

Mild dementia care provided
Diets Accommodated: Diabetic, Low-fat, Low-salt, Renal
Proximity to Emergency Svcs.: Under 8 miles
Nearby shopping and entertainment
Pet visits allowed

### STAFF

Nurse/LVN/LPN: 40 hours/week, On-call 24/7
Caregiver Training: Dementia, Ethics, Family communication, Grief, Transition issues
Criminal Background Check: Yes
Principal Staff Language(s): English
Other Staff Language(s): Spanish

### FACILITY FEATURES

Activities/Recreation
Beauty/Barber Shop ($)
Chapel Services
Facility Parking
Guest Meals ($)
Outside Patio/Gardens
Pharmaceutical Service
Private Dining Room
Separate Therapy Room
Transportation
24-hour Security

### ROOM FEATURES

Cable TV Ready ($)
Emergency Call System
Grab Bars
Kitchenette
Private Bathrooms
Telephone Ready ($)
Temperature Controls

### COSTS

PRICES MAY INCREASE. PLEASE CALL FOR MOST CURRENT INFORMATION.

| | |
|---|---|
| Studio Apt. | $81–$89/day |
| One Bedroom Apt. | $145/day |
| Costs of Care | $5–$57/day based on individual need |
| Rate Increase | Annually; usually 3–5% |
| Reimbursement | LTCI, Private pay |
| Entrance Fee | $1,250 |

## PORTRAIT

The veranda lined with stately white columns contrasts attractively with the brown brick exterior of Colonial Lodge of Plano, evoking a Southern mansion. Ivy thrives alongside the emerald lawn, while oak trees spread their branches over the parking lot. Sunny common rooms are located at the ends of the H-shaped building. Residents enjoy the facility's collection of comfortable furniture so much that it has become somewhat worn. Abundant sunlight has faded the pictures that adorn the walls. Handrails border the wide hallways. Residents paint and decorate their cozy rooms according to taste. The fluorescent lighting throughout the facility tends to be rather harsh in certain areas. Old favorites such as meatloaf, mashed potatoes, mixed vegetables and carrot cake are staples on the menu.

The director informed us that the outdoor areas had been recently replanted and we observed several residents there using the walkways and resting on wooden benches. Laughter rang throughout the facility on our visit. Residents chatted with one another and with staff members, who addressed each resident by name. The director praised the staff for their dedication to residents' comfort. Scheduled activities include exercise, bingo, movies, card games and religious services. Outings to retailers such as Wal-Mart encourage residents to get out and about.

Two residents who live across the hall from one another are in fierce competition to see whose bird feeder attracts the most birds. They are known to spend the better part of the day counting birds through their windows in an attempt to emerge victorious.

## COLONIAL RETIREMENT LODGE

2301 North Brook
McKinney, TX 75069

(972) 542-6006
www.assistedlivingconcepts.com

### GILBERT GUIDE OBSERVATIONS

| | | | |
|---|---|---|---|
| Administration & Staff | g g g g g | Residents | g g g g g |
| Facility Aesthetics | g g g g | Dietary & Food Selection | g g g |
| Facility Condition & Safety | g g g g | Activities | g g g g g |

### DETAILS

Year Built: 1993
Year Remodeled: 1996
Current Mgmt. Since: Unknown
No. of Floors: 1
Resident Capacity: 50

### SPECIAL

Mild dementia care provided
Diets Accommodated: Diabetic, Low-fat, Low-salt
Proximity to Emergency Svcs.: Under 8 miles
Nearby shopping and entertainment
Pets allowed

COLONIAL RETIREMENT LODGE (CONTINUED)

## STAFF

Nurse/LVN/LPN: 24 hours/week
Caregiver Training: Dementia, Ethics, Family communication, Grief
Criminal Background Check: Yes
Principal Staff Language(s): English
Other Staff Language(s): Spanish

## FACILITY FEATURES

Activities/Recreation
Beauty/Barber Shop ($)
Chapel Services
Facility Parking
Guest Meals ($)
Outside Patio/Gardens
Pharmaceutical Service
Private Dining Room
Separate Therapy Room
Transportation
24-hour Security

## ROOM FEATURES

Cable TV Ready ($)
Emergency Call System
Grab Bars
Kitchenette
Private Bathrooms
Telephone Ready ($)
Temperature Controls

## COSTS

PRICES MAY INCREASE. PLEASE CALL FOR MOST CURRENT INFORMATION.

| | |
|---|---|
| Studio Apt. | $61–$74/day |
| Costs of Care | $7–$14/day based on individual need |
| Rate Increase | Annually; usually 2% |
| Reimbursement | LTCI, Private pay, Veterans |
| Entrance Fee | $1,750 |
| Pet Deposit | $200 |

## PORTRAIT

Colonial Retirement Lodge enjoys peaceful seclusion on a quiet and safe street. The well-kept facility imparts Southern country charm. High ceilings, floral wallpaper and gold chandeliers add a warm ambience to the long entryway. Residents' rooms are spacious enough for personal furniture. Couples or friends often choose to share suites that feature living areas and updated kitchens. The rooms also have convenient walk-in showers and emergency call systems.

Residents played bingo, exercised and relaxed in the designated quiet area during our visit. The "Coca-Cola Corner" is a popular area, which has a soda fountain, old-fashioned seating with Coke decorations and a black-and-white checkered floor. For a moment, we felt transported back in time. Coffee is served all day, beginning at 4:30 am, with snacks served intermittently. There are two separate courtyards—one has umbrellas, large chairs, fountains and plants.

Bulletin boards hang from the softly lit hallways, noting cheerful announcements of congratulations on new grandchildren and great-grandchildren, as well as photographs depicting poker games, Red Hat Society celebrations, birthday parties and residents' family members. The staff appears to have a committed and loving relationship with the residents. The administrator is a registered dietician, who has worked at Colonial for twelve years.

## CORINTHIANS A/D

1029 West Seminole Trail
Carrollton, TX 75007

(972) 395-3553
www.corithiansalf.com

### GILBERT GUIDE OBSERVATIONS

| | | | |
|---|---|---|---|
| Administration & Staff | g g g g g | Dietary & Food Selection | g g g |
| Facility Aesthetics | g g g g g | Activities | g g g |
| Facility Condition & Safety | g g g g g | Alzheimer's & Dementia Capabilities | g g g g g |
| Residents | g g g g | | |

### DETAILS

Year Built: 1996
Current Mgmt. Since: 1996
No. of Floors: 1
Resident Capacity: 65

### SPECIAL

Diets Accommodated: Low-fat, Low-salt
Proximity to Emergency Svcs.: Under 8 miles
Nearby shopping and entertainment
Pets allowed

### STAFF

Nurse/LVN/LPN: 40 hours/week, On-call 24/7
Caregiver Training: Dementia, Ethics, Family communication, Grief, Patient transfers, Stress management, Transition issues, Validation therapy
Criminal Background Check: Yes
Principal Staff Language(s): English
Other Staff Language(s): Spanish

### FACILITY FEATURES

Activities/Recreation
Beauty/Barber Shop ($)
Chapel Services
Facility Parking
Guest Meals ($)
Outside Patio/Gardens
Overnight Guest Room ($)
Room Service
Separate Therapy Room
Transportation
24-hour Security

### ROOM FEATURES

Cable TV Ready ($)
Emergency Call System
Grab Bars
Kitchenette
Shared & Private Bathrooms
Temperature Controls

CORINTHIANS (CONTINUED)

## COSTS

PRICES MAY INCREASE. PLEASE CALL FOR MOST CURRENT INFORMATION.

| | |
|---|---|
| Studio Apt. | $2,200/month |
| One Bedroom Apt. | $2,395–$3,020/month<br>Double occupancy add $600/month |
| Alzheimer's Unit | $3,200–$3,350/month for shared room |
| Costs of Care | $300–$1,200/month based on individual need |
| Rate Increase | Annually; usually 1–2% |
| Reimbursement | LTCI, Private pay |
| Entrance Fee | $750 |
| Pet Deposit | $500 |

## PORTRAIT

A quaint scene greeted us at Corinthians—residents enjoying a cool evening on the porch, seated at a table topped with a vase of yellow tea roses. They looked past the circular driveway, between oak and fruit trees, at the comings and goings on tranquil West Seminole Trail. One resident played Chopin on the piano near the entrance.

A fireplace and comfortable couches, upholstered to complement the maroon, brown and white color scheme, furnish the homey foyer. Parakeets and finches chirp noisily from a white birdcage. Lithographs depicting scenes of milkmaids, shepherds and farmers, adorn the walls. Matching green wallpaper and carpet dominate the intimate dining area, which features an oak table dressed in white linen. The menu is comprised of American fare such as pot roast, mashed potatoes and vegetables. The dining area is also used for socials and board games. Some residents watch weekly football games on the big-screen TV in the comfortably furnished common area. Sunlight streams into the dining area, common areas and solarium. Dementia-appropriate lamps and fluorescent lighting illuminate the wide hallways, which are lined with oak handrails. Cushioned wooden chairs in the halls provide convenient resting spots. Cream-colored paint contrasts with dark wooden baseboards in residents' rooms. Each room features a closet with ample shelving and white window treatments.

A group of vivacious residents socialized with one another in the warm solarium when we visited. The solarium leads to a secured outer courtyard. Outings to shopping destinations such as Wal-Mart are popular among residents, who also take part in gospel singing, exercising, baking and gardening. Geraniums planted by residents bloom along the walkway in the courtyard.

## CREEKSIDE ALZHEIMER'S SPECIAL CARE CENTER A/D

2000 West Spring Creek Parkway
Plano, TX 75023

(972) 312-9993
www.jeaseniorliving.com

### GILBERT GUIDE OBSERVATIONS

| | | | |
|---|---|---|---|
| Administration & Staff | g g g g g | Dietary & Food Selection | g g g g |
| Facility Aesthetics | g g g g | Activities | g g g g g |
| Facility Condition & Safety | g g g g g | Alzheimer's & Dementia Capabilities | g g g g |
| Residents | g g g g | | |

### DETAILS

Year Built: 1999
Current Mgmt. Since: 1999
No. of Floors: 1
Resident Capacity: 56

### SPECIAL

Alzheimer's/Dementia Only Facility
Diets Accommodated: Diabetic, Low-fat, Low-salt, Renal
Proximity to Emergency Svcs.: Under 8 miles
Nearby shopping and entertainment
Pet visits allowed

### STAFF

Nurse/LVN/LPN: Onsite 24/7
Caregiver Training: Dementia, Ethics, Family communication, Grief, Patient transfers, Stress management, Transition issues, Validation therapy
Criminal Background Check: Yes
Principal Staff Language(s): English
Other Staff Language(s): Spanish

### FACILITY FEATURES

Activities/Recreation
Beauty/Barber Shop ($)
Chapel Services
Guest Meals ($)
Outside Patio/Gardens
Pharmaceutical Service
Private Dining Room
Room Service ($)
Transportation to MD Appointments ($), Personal Outings ($)
24-hour Security

### ROOM FEATURES

Cable TV Ready ($)
Furnished
Grab Bars
Shared & Private Bathrooms
Telephone Ready ($)
Temperature Controls

### COSTS

PRICES MAY INCREASE. PLEASE CALL FOR MOST CURRENT INFORMATION.

| | |
|---|---|
| Alzheimer's Unit | $3,450–$4,510/month for shared room |
| Respite Stays | $125/day for shared room |
| Costs of Care | Included in monthly rate |
| Rate Increase | Annually; usually 1.5% |
| Reimbursement | LTCI, Private pay |
| Application Fee | $650 |

CREEKSIDE ALZHEIMER'S SPECIAL CARE CENTER (CONTINUED)

### PORTRAIT

Creekside is situated on lively West Spring Creek Parkway. The trimmed front lawn is peppered with shapely hedges and shrubs. The gold and green interior color scheme is illuminated by plentiful natural light. The lobby is comfortably furnished with sofas and chairs, beckoning residents to relax in front of the stone fireplace.

Residents' rooms are moderately sized with large windows. Residents decorate and furnish to suit their tastes. The dining room is a lovely setting of whitewashed wood tables and chairs upholstered in floral fabrics. The soft lighting in this room gives it a cozy feel. Staff encourages the residents to dine together. The kitchen staff prepares favorites such as meatloaf with mixed vegetables. We observed one delighted resident in the middle of her apple pie. Residents gather in the living room and enjoy the warmth of a second fireplace. The secured outdoor patio is furnished. The stone planter is the garden centerpiece among young trees, walkways and freshly cut grass. The interior is brightened by an abundance of windows and recessed lighting. Elegant glass and brass sconces add a decorative touch. The hallways are spacious and features handrails; rest areas are furnished intermittently.

The staff facilitates an active community. Residents enjoy an array of activities, including arts and crafts, sing-alongs, morning exercise and movie nights. The environment is a positive one. It was plain to see the mutual respect between residents and caregivers.

## DAY SPRING ASSISTED LIVING

6400 Cheyenne Trail
Plano, TX 75023

(972) 769-1109
www.seniorhousing.net

---

### GILBERT GUIDE OBSERVATIONS

| | | | |
|---|---|---|---|
| Administration & Staff | g g g g | Residents | g g g g g |
| Facility Aesthetics | g g g g | Dietary & Food Selection | g g g g g |
| Facility Condition & Safety | g g g g | Activities | g g g g g |

### DETAILS

Year Built: 1998
Year Remodeled: 2003
Current Mgmt. Since: 1998
No. of Floors: 1
Resident Capacity: 70

### SPECIAL

Mild dementia care provided
Diets Accommodated: Diabetic, Low-fat, Low-salt
Proximity to Emergency Svcs.: Under 8 miles
Nearby shopping and entertainment
Some pets allowed

## STAFF

Nurse/LVN/LPN: None on staff
Caregiver Training: Dementia, Ethics, Family communication, Grief, Patient transfers, Stress management, Transition issues, Validation therapy
Criminal Background Check: Yes
Principal Staff Language(s): English
Other Staff Language(s): Spanish

## FACILITY FEATURES

Activities/Recreation
Beauty/Barber Shop ($)
Chapel Services
Computer/Internet Access
Facility Parking ($)
Guest Meals ($)
Outside Patio/Gardens
Pharmaceutical Service
Private Dining Room
Room Service ($)
Transportation

## ROOM FEATURES

Cable TV Ready
Emergency Call System
Grab Bars
Kitchenette
Private Bathrooms
Telephone Ready ($)
Temperature Controls

## COSTS

PRICES MAY INCREASE. PLEASE CALL FOR MOST CURRENT INFORMATION.

| | |
|---|---|
| Studio Apt. | $2,390–$2,960/month |
| Costs of Care | $300–$900/month based on individual need |
| Rate Increase | Annually; usually 1–6% |
| Reimbursement | LTCI, Private pay |
| Security Deposit | $500 |
| Pet Deposit | $500 (refundable) |

## PORTRAIT

Visitors to Day Spring Assisted Living follow a covered walkway to a large door with a decorative wreath. Located in a peaceful residential neighborhood, the facility is close to a church. A heavily attended bingo game was taking place during our visit. The hall rang with laughter—evidence of the camaraderie between residents and staff. The long list of activities includes painting classes, group crossword puzzles, Bible study, yarn club, musical entertainment, variety shows, and movies on the big-screen TV.

The interior décor consists of well-coordinated furnishings. Fluorescent lighting illuminates the wide hallways. Each hall is equipped with handrails and leads to a private seating area. The dining and common areas feature more subdued lighting. Cherrywood furniture creates a homey ambiance in the dining area, where a variety of homestyle meals are served. A small resident-tended flower garden rounds out the limited areas for socializing. Residents decorate and furnish their small rooms to suit their tastes.

## Edenbrook of Plano Assisted Living & Alzheimer's Unit A/D

3000 Midway Drive
Plano, TX 75093

(972) 473-7400
www.sunriseseniorliving.com

---

**GILBERT GUIDE OBSERVATIONS**

| | | | |
|---|---|---|---|
| Administration & Staff | g g g | Dietary & Food Selection | g g g g g |
| Facility Aesthetics | g g g g g | Activities | g g g |
| Facility Condition & Safety | g g g g g | Alzheimer's & Dementia Capabilities | g g g g |
| Residents | g g g | | |

### DETAILS

Year Built: 1999
Current Mgmt. Since: 2003
No. of Floors: 2
Resident Capacity: 85 (AL), 20 (ALZ)

### SPECIAL

Diets Accommodated: Diabetic, Low-fat, Low-salt
Proximity to Emergency Svcs.: 16+ miles
Pets allowed

### STAFF

Nurse/LVN/LPN: Onsite 24/7
Caregiver Training: Dementia, Ethics, Family communication, Grief, Patient transfers, Stress management, Transition issues, Validation therapy
Criminal Background Check: Yes
Principal Staff Language(s): English

### FACILITY FEATURES

Activities/Recreation
Beauty/Barber Shop
Chapel Services
Computer/Internet Access
Fitness Room/Gym
Guest Meals
Outside Patio/Gardens
Overnight Guest Room
Pharmaceutical Service
Private Dining Room
Room Service
Separate Therapy Room
Transportation
24-hour Security

### ROOM FEATURES

Cable TV Ready ($)
Emergency Call System
Furnished
Grab Bars
Private Bathrooms
Telephone Ready ($)
Temperature Controls

### COSTS

PRICES MAY INCREASE. PLEASE CALL FOR MOST CURRENT INFORMATION.

| | |
|---|---|
| Studio Apt. | $2,950/month |
| One Bedroom Apt. | $4,600/month<br>Double occupancy add $900/month |
| Costs of Care | $22–$52/day based on individual need |

| | |
|---|---|
| Rate Increase | Annually; usually 5% |
| Reimbursement | Private pay, Veterans |
| Application Fee | $2,500 |
| Pet Deposit | $500 |

**PORTRAIT**

A luxurious atmosphere pervades Edenbrook of Plano Assisted Living and its sister Alzheimer's unit. Expansive landscaping with hedges, trees and a manicured lawn leads to beautiful French doors. A gorgeous stone fountain welcomes visitors to the facility. The warm coffee-and-cream colored interior has marble flooring and a contemporary reception area with fresh flowers. The facility implements a strict no-fluorescent-lighting policy; a combination of soft recessed lighting, dome-style fixtures and natural lighting is used instead.

The residents' furnished rooms all have large windows. The formal dining room features linen tablecloths, china and fine silver. The restaurant-style menu provides several options. A sample lunch menu lists prime rib with au jus, baked potatoes and broccoli. The numerous common rooms are comfortably and strategically furnished to promote socialization between residents. The hallways are equipped with handrails and are wide enough to accommodate wheelchairs and foot traffic. Tall trees shade the outdoor area, where residents often relax on the porch swing or patio furniture.

Five activities are offered each day, including outside entertainment, cookie socials, exercise and birthday parties. During our visit, a group of residents were enjoying a card game. A social atmosphere filled the home and residents chatted in small groups. Familiar activities form the basis of the Alzheimer's program, which is tailored to the interests, preferences and life skills of the residents. The activities, which include exercise and Name That Tune, are designed to enhance physical and mental wellness. We noted that the staff was extremely comforting to these residents, who were somewhat quiet and reserved. The staff was pleasant and wore immaculate uniforms, in keeping with the upscale feeling of the community.

## THE GARDENS OF RICHARDSON

1111 West Shore Drive (972) 783-8000
Richardson, TX 75080

---

**GILBERT GUIDE OBSERVATIONS**

| | | | |
|---|---|---|---|
| Administration & Staff | g g g g | Residents | g g g |
| Facility Aesthetics | g g g | Dietary & Food Selection | g g g |
| Facility Condition & Safety | g g g | Activities | g g g |

THE GARDENS OF RICHARDSON (CONTINUED)

## DETAILS

Year Built: 1988
Year Remodeled: 2002
Current Mgmt. Since: 2000
No. of Floors: 1
Resident Capacity: 86

## SPECIAL

Mild dementia care provided
Diets Accommodated: Diabetic, Low-fat, Low-salt
Proximity to Emergency Svcs.: Under 8 miles
Pets allowed

## STAFF

Nurse/LVN/LPN: 40 hours/week, On-call 24/7
Caregiver Training: Dementia, Patient transfers, Validation therapy
Criminal Background Check: Yes
Principal Staff Language(s): English

## FACILITY FEATURES

Activities/Recreation
Facility Parking
Guest Meals
Outside Patio/Gardens
Transportation
24-hour Security

## ROOM FEATURES

Cable TV Ready ($)
Emergency Call System
Furnished
Grab Bars
Kitchenette
Private Bathrooms
Telephone Ready ($)
Temperature Controls

## COSTS

PRICES MAY INCREASE. PLEASE CALL FOR MOST CURRENT INFORMATION.

| | |
|---|---|
| One Bedroom Apt. | $2,165/month |
| Two Bedroom Apt. | $2,815–$2,975/month |
| Costs of Care | Included in monthly rate |
| Rate Increase | Annually; usually 2–5% |
| Reimbursement | Private pay |
| Security Deposit | $500 |

## PORTRAIT

The Gardens of Richardson is located in the peaceful, residential heart of North Dallas, next to Richardson Senior Center, which offers numerous activities. The brown brick facility has a covered entry that shelters wooden benches and colorful potted flowers. The foyer is decorated with wing chairs and Queen Anne tables. Mirrors and painted portraits line the dark blue walls. A chandelier provides an elegant focal point and highlights bright silk flower arrangements. The receptionist warmly greets visitors.

Expansive windows flood residents' spacious rooms with cheery sunlight. The walls are painted in a neutral color—a blank canvas that residents are encouraged to adorn. The common rooms are brightened with natural light; fluorescent lighting dominates the hallways. Seating areas are located throughout the wide hallways.

Residents are served by a waitstaff in the formal dining area. The mouthwatering smell of oven roasted turkey, served on the day of our visit, reminded us of Thanksgiving. The dining room is also used for socializing. There is also a private dining room with cherrywood furniture, including a hutch displaying decorative dishes. A bright chandelier hangs over the dining table. The entertainment room features card tables and a grand piano often used for sing-alongs. Two sunrooms open onto courtyards with lighted walkways. Many activities are offered, including morning coffee socials, card games, exercise, Bible study and scenic drives. A number of energetic residents socialized with one another when we visited.

## Hearthstone at Vista Ridge

400 Highland Drive
Lewisville, TX 75067

(972) 315-1532
(214) 533-5743
www.hearthstoneassisted.com

---

### GILBERT GUIDE OBSERVATIONS

| | | | |
|---|---|---|---|
| Administration & Staff | g g g g | Residents | g g g |
| Facility Aesthetics | g g g | Dietary & Food Selection | g g g |
| Facility Condition & Safety | g g g | Activities | g g g |

### DETAILS

Year Built: 1998
Current Mgmt. Since: 1998
No. of Floors: 1
Resident Capacity: 118

### SPECIAL

Mild dementia care provided
Diets Accommodated: Low-fat
Proximity to Emergency Svcs.: Under 8 miles
Nearby shopping and entertainment
Pets allowed

### STAFF

Nurse/LVN/LPN: On-call 24/7
Caregiver Training: Ethics, Grief, Stress management
Criminal Background Check: Yes
Principal Staff Language(s): English
Other Staff Language(s): Spanish

### FACILITY FEATURES

Activities/Recreation
Beauty/Barber Shop ($)
Facility Parking
Guest Meals ($)
Outside Patio/Gardens
Pharmaceutical Service ($)
Transportation
24-hour Security

### ROOM FEATURES

Cable TV Ready ($)
Emergency Call System
Grab Bars
Kitchenette
Private Bathrooms
Telephone Ready ($)
Temperature Controls

HEARTHSTONE AT VISTA RIDGE (CONTINUED)

## COSTS

PRICES MAY INCREASE. PLEASE CALL FOR MOST CURRENT INFORMATION.

| | |
|---|---|
| Studio Apt. | $3,295/month |
| One Bedroom Apt. | $3,495/month |
| Two Bedroom Apt. | $3,895/month |
| Costs of Care | $175–$1,925/month based on individual need |
| Rate Increase | Annually; usually 1–3% |
| Reimbursement | LTCI, Private pay, Veterans |
| Entrance Fee | $1,500 |
| Pet Deposit | $250 |

## PORTRAIT

Residents of Hearthstone at Vista Ridge enjoy attractive views of their Louisville neighborhood from comfortable rocking chairs on the home's porch. Black shutters, white trim and cupolas add distinctive elements to the red brick building. The receptionist cheerfully greeted us and immediately located our tour guide. A stone fireplace dominates the white-walled entry room known as the "great room." Rich earth-toned upholstery accents the dark wooden furnishings. An adjacent activity room doubles as a library.

Several residents talked and laughed in the great room. We overhead one resident ask the activity director, "Where's the action going to be?" A fresh round of smiles and laughter greeted his question. The popular activity director incorporates walking, religious services, guest musical performances, educational seminars and current events discussions in the full roster of activities. The polite staff members know each resident by name. Residents' rooms come in three floor plans, each of which is moderately sized. Closets and cabinets provide additional storage space. Residents are free to express themselves in their choice of wall paint.

Residents attend socials in the dining room, which is furnished with dark wooden tables and chairs. Striped upholstery adds a bright shot of color. The dinner menu listed an appetizing meal of tomato salad, sautéed beef with mushrooms, brussels sprouts and banana pudding on the day of our visit. Fluorescent lighting supplemented with brass and glass sconces brighten the home. Floral borders accent the green wallpaper and carpets in the wide, handrail-lined hallways. The sunroom opens to the courtyard, where blooming magnolia trees entice residents to walk along the pathway. White wicker furniture provides comfortable places for residents to sit as they barbecue outdoors.

## Lewisville Estates

800 College Parkway
Lewisville, TX 75077

(972) 434-1727
www.wellstoneretirement.com

### GILBERT GUIDE OBSERVATIONS

| | | | |
|---|---|---|---|
| Administration & Staff | g g g | Residents | g g g |
| Facility Aesthetics | g g g | Dietary & Food Selection | g g g |
| Facility Condition & Safety | g g g | Activities | g g g |

### DETAILS

Year Built: 1999
Current Mgmt. Since: 2002
No. of Floors: 1
Resident Capacity: 56

### SPECIAL

Mild dementia care provided
Diets Accommodated: Diabetic, Low-fat, Low-salt
Proximity to Emergency Svcs.: Under 8 miles
Nearby shopping and entertainment
Pets allowed

### STAFF

Nurse/LVN/LPN: Onsite 24/7
Caregiver Training: Dementia, Ethics, Family communication, Grief, Stress management, Transition issues, Validation therapy
Criminal Background Check: Yes
Principal Staff Language(s): English
Other Staff Language(s): Spanish

### FACILITY FEATURES

Activities/Recreation
Beauty/Barber Shop
Chapel Services
Computer/Internet Access
Facility Parking
Fitness Room/Gym
Guest Meals
Outside Patio/Gardens
Overnight Guest Room
Pharmaceutical Service
Private Dining Room
Separate Therapy Room
Transportation

### ROOM FEATURES

Cable TV Ready ($)
Emergency Call System
Furnished
Grab Bars
Private Bathrooms
Telephone Ready ($)
Temperature Controls

### COSTS

PRICES MAY INCREASE. PLEASE CALL FOR MOST CURRENT INFORMATION.

| | |
|---|---|
| Studio Apt. | $2,495/month |
| One Bedroom Apt. | Call for rates |
| Two Bedroom Apt. | Call for rates |
| Costs of Care | $200–$1,000/month |
| Rate Increase | Annually |

LEWISVILLE ESTATES (CONTINUED)

| | |
|---|---|
| Reimbursement | Private pay |
| Entrance Fee | $500 |
| Pet Deposit | $250 |

### PORTRAIT

Located in a residential neighborhood two blocks from Interstate 35, Lewisville Estates is easily accessible and provides all the comforts of home. Oak trees, boxwood shrubs and various flowering plants grace the entrance to this stately facility. A combination of neutral-colored walls strewn with serene landscape paintings and plush furniture create a restful atmosphere. The residents have spacious rooms and are encouraged to decorate to suit their tastes. Lewisville Estates keeps guest suites to accommodate overnight visitors.

The spacious common areas are beautifully arranged with rich wood furniture. A variety of snacks supplement the extensive menu. Residents may reserve the private dining room for intimate parties. Subtle crisscross patterns in the dark carpeting that lines the hallways are curiously charming. The hallways are equipped with adequate support systems. Soft lighting radiates from elegant glass lamps and brass fixtures. The outdoor patio area is expansive and well kept. Padded chairs, shaded tables and chaise lounges allow residents to relax in this natural setting. In the background, soothing aquatic sounds from the water fountain trickle into a nearby pond.

The activities calendar lists resident favorites including bingo and card games. Staff and residents interacted pleasantly with one another during our visit.

## MERCER HOUSE

5701 Dexham Road
Rowlett, TX 75088

(972) 463-1646
www.alcco.com

### GILBERT GUIDE OBSERVATIONS

| | | | |
|---|---|---|---|
| Administration & Staff | g g g g g | Residents | g g g g g |
| Facility Aesthetics | g g g g g | Dietary & Food Selection | g g g |
| Facility Condition & Safety | g g g g g | Activities | g g g g |

### DETAILS

Year Built: 1996
Current Mgmt. Since: 1996
No. of Floors: 1
Resident Capacity: 34

### SPECIAL

Diets Accommodated: Low-salt
Proximity to Emergency Svcs.: Under 8 miles
Nearby shopping and entertainment
Pets allowed

## STAFF

Nurse/LVN/LPN: On-call 24/7
Caregiver Training: Ethics, Family communication, Grief, Patient transfers, Stress management, Transition issues, Validation therapy
Criminal Background Check: Yes
Principal Staff Language(s): English

## FACILITY FEATURES

Activities/Recreation
Beauty/Barber Shop ($)
Chapel Services
Guest Meals ($)
Outside Patio/Gardens
Room Service
Transportation

## ROOM FEATURES

Cable TV Ready ($)
Emergency Call System
Grab Bars
Kitchenette
Private Bathrooms
Telephone Ready
Temperature Controls

## COSTS

PRICES MAY INCREASE. PLEASE CALL FOR MOST CURRENT INFORMATION.

| | |
|---|---|
| Studio Apt. | $64.86/day |
| One Bedroom Apt. | $76.19/day<br>Double occupancy add $27.37/day |
| Respite Stays | $100/day for private room |
| Costs of Care | $11.55–$70/day based on individual need |
| Rate Increase | Annually; usually 1% |
| Reimbursement | Private pay |
| Entrance Fee | $1,250 |
| Pet Deposit | $300 |

## PORTRAIT

Mercer House is located on a quiet street near Highway 66. The downhill slope of the facility gives passersby a magnificent view of the red brick building with white shutters. The entrance is electronically secured.

The interior color scheme is white, green and maroon. Decorative prints of country landscapes and opulent urns adorn the walls. The comfortable furniture in the living room is both inviting and spaced appropriately, to accommodate residents who use wheelchairs and walkers. Residents regularly gather around the piano in the dining room for sing-alongs. The common areas are a homey setting for residents to watch TV, catch up on reading or visit with one another. The building is brightened by a combination of natural and fluorescent lighting. The carpeted hallways are equipped with handrails and are furnished with chairs and tables. Residents furnish their rooms, which are moderately sized. All have windows with decorative treatments. The kitchen staff uses fresh produce and specializes in home-style and Mexican cooking.

Mercer House has three separate outdoor areas—a front porch, central courtyard and back deck. Residents enjoy the cheerful atmosphere in the courtyard, with its hanging birdfeeders

MERCER HOUSE (CONTINUED)

and colorful poppies and begonias. The courtyard is also a summer hot spot for barbeques and socials. Residents are very active. Regular activities include church services, bingo, board games and shopping trips. During our visit, all thirty-four residents were gathered in the dining room for lunch. The room was filled with conversation and laughter.

## Morrison Residence at Denton Good Samaritan Village

2500 Hinkle Drive
Denton, TX 76201

(940) 383-6352
www.good-sam.com

### GILBERT GUIDE OBSERVATIONS

| | | | |
|---|---|---|---|
| Administration & Staff | g g g g g | Residents | g g g g |
| Facility Aesthetics | g g g | Dietary & Food Selection | g g g |
| Facility Condition & Safety | g g g g g | Activities | g g g g g |

### DETAILS

Year Built: 2004
Current Mgmt. Since: 2004
No. of Floors: 1
Resident Capacity: 14–16

### SPECIAL

Mild dementia care provided
Diets Accommodated: Low-fat, Low-salt
Proximity to Emergency Svcs.: Under 8 miles
Nearby shopping and entertainment
No pets allowed

### STAFF

Nurse/LVN/LPN: 20 hours/week, On-call 24/7
Caregiver Training: Dementia, Ethics, Family communication, Grief, Stress management, Transition issues
Criminal Background Check: Yes
Principal Staff Language(s): English

### FACILITY FEATURES

Activities/Recreation
Beauty/Barber Shop ($)
Chapel Services
Facility Parking
Guest Meals ($)
Overnight Guest Room ($)
Pharmaceutical Service
Private Dining Room
Room Service
Separate Therapy Room
Transportation to MD Appointments ($), Personal Outings ($), Scheduled Outings
24-hour Security

### ROOM FEATURES

Cable TV Ready
Emergency Call System
Grab Bars
Kitchenette
Private Bathrooms
Telephone Ready
Temperature Controls

## COSTS

PRICES MAY INCREASE. PLEASE CALL FOR MOST CURRENT INFORMATION.

| | |
|---|---|
| Studio Apt. | \$2,250–\$2,550/month |
| Respite Stays | \$2,250–\$2,550/month for private room |
| Costs of Care | \$200–\$500/month based on individual need |
| Rate Increase | Annually |
| Reimbursement | LTCI, Private pay |
| Application Fee | \$500 (refundable) |

## PORTRAIT

Morrison Residence was created to bridge the gap between independent and skilled nursing care at a local retirement community, Denton Good Samaritan Village. Residents who joined the community at the independent living level are given priority for entering the assisted living unit. The front door, which remains locked at all times, opens to an immaculate entry and living room. Numerous photographs of residents engaged in activities are prominently displayed on a bulletin board next to framed prints. Comfortable seating faces a TV and VCR. A grand piano and a record player (along with a collection of records) provide options for residents' listening pleasure. The broad hallways are short and sunny. Knockers on residents' doors allow visitors to formally announce themselves. Four of the fourteen suites are wheelchair-accessible; all are furnished by residents. A door at the end of the main hall connects the assisted living and independent living areas. All residents share a library.

Placemats and tablecloths dress the tables in the dining and activity area, where residents often opt for a light dinner of soup and sandwiches. Residents enjoy snacks such as cookies, yogurt and lemonade daily. The space also houses an oven, refrigerator, microwave and sink, which are utilized for cooking activities. The assisted living unit shares an attractively appointed private dining room, accessed through French doors, with independent living. Thanks to the facility's small size, residents have a big say in their activities. They keep an artificial Christmas tree up year-round and adorn it with seasonal decorations; we admired the charming ceramic hearts that they had crafted and hung on the tree for Valentine's Day. Our guide told us about the "Name the Betta" contest that residents held to christen their betta fish. Residents hold birthday celebrations individually, so there is nearly always a party on the horizon! The facility also hosts music recitals for local children, which are much-anticipated events.

## Provident Living Centers A/D

1601 West El Dorado Parkway (972) 569-8660
McKinney, TX 75069

---

**GILBERT GUIDE OBSERVATIONS**

| | | | |
|---|---|---|---|
| Administration & Staff | g g g | Dietary & Food Selection | g g g g |
| Facility Aesthetics | g g g g | Activities | g g g g g |
| Facility Condition & Safety | g g g g g | Alzheimer's & Dementia Capabilities | g g g g g |
| Residents | g g g g | | |

### DETAILS

Year Built: 1999
Year Remodeled: 1999
Current Mgmt. Since: 1999
No. of Floors: 1
Resident Capacity: 72

### SPECIAL

Alzheimer's/Dementia Only Facility
Diets Accommodated: Diabetic, Low-fat, Low-salt
Proximity to Emergency Svcs.: Under 8 miles
Nearby shopping and entertainment
Pets allowed

### STAFF

Nurse/LVN/LPN: Onsite 24/7
Caregiver Training: Dementia, Ethics, Family communication, Stress management, Transition issues
Criminal Background Check: Yes
Principal Staff Language(s): English
Other Staff Language(s): Spanish

### FACILITY FEATURES

Activities/Recreation
Beauty/Barber Shop ($)
Chapel Services
Facility Parking
Guest Meals
Outside Patio/Gardens
Private Dining Room
Room Service
24-hour Security

### ROOM FEATURES

Emergency Call System
Grab Bars
Shared & Private Bathrooms
Telephone Ready
Temperature Controls

### COSTS

PRICES MAY INCREASE. PLEASE CALL FOR MOST CURRENT INFORMATION.

| | |
|---|---|
| Alzheimer's Unit | $3,100/month for shared room<br>$3,700/month for private room |
| Respite Stays | $140/day for private room |
| Costs of Care | $120/month for incontinence supplies |
| Rate Increase | Periodically |
| Reimbursement | LTCI, Private pay |
| Application Fee | $500 (refundable) |

## PORTRAIT

Provident Living Centers is situated in a thriving neighborhood of McKinney. Only a few minutes east of Central Expressway, the facility is close to lots of local stores. The receptionist greets visitors in the lobby, which also houses the administrator's office. Inside, the brightly colored hallways are spacious and neat. The cheerful color scheme helps residents navigate through the facility with ease and familiarity. Built-in hallway benches are comfortable rest stops; handrails provide adequate support. Pretty hanging fixtures bathe the facility in soft artificial light. The nurses have a clear vantage point of each hallway from their corner desks.

Outside the main activity area, an oversized bulletin board lists upcoming activities. The activity director organizes a variety of fun and stimulating activities, including map games, spelling bees, storytelling and poem reading, chatting on the porch, "Fill in the Blank" and "Words Ending in 'A'" (both mind-stimulating games), rhythm band, charades and flower arranging. A volunteer leads weekly dominoes and card games. We observed the activity director guiding an enthusiastic exercise class; the residents were clearly energized by the high-spirited sounds of a marching band playing in the background! Activities are an integral part of the Provident Living program. In fact, residents' rooms remained locked during daytime hours to encourage their participation in the numerous activities, which are scheduled until eight each evening. In the activity area, a "career wall" strewn with framed photos captures highlights of the residents' careers. The dining area is an elegant setting with vaulted ceilings and grand windows, where residents are served by a waitstaff. Several snacks are served throughout the day.

Most of residents' rooms are private; all are generously sized. The brightly painted décor makes each room recognizable to its tenant. Each is equipped with built-in dressers, closet space and an oversized window. Participants of the affiliated day care and respite programs gather in comfortably furnished seating areas throughout the facility. For outdoor leisure, residents often take to the furnished patio, which features waist-high planters for easy gardening!

Despite the majority of the staff having minimal training in dementia, the Provident Living program is an excellent one, with many thoughtful provisions. The current administrator has a long history with the facility, dating back to her days as the owner's administrative secretary. During our tour, we were pleased by her friendly rapport with the residents; she demonstrated familiarity with several of their personal histories, in addition to greeting resident by name as we passed.

## Redbud House

101 West Wilson Creek Parkway
McKinney, TX 75069

(972) 562-9698
www.assistedlivingconcepts.com

### GILBERT GUIDE OBSERVATIONS

| | | | |
|---|---|---|---|
| Administration & Staff | g g g g | Residents | g g g |
| Facility Aesthetics | g g g | Dietary & Food Selection | g g g |
| Facility Condition & Safety | g g g g | Activities | g g g g |

### DETAILS

Year Built: 1996
Year Remodeled: Ongoing
Current Mgmt. Since: 1996
No. of Floors: 1
Resident Capacity: 48

### SPECIAL

Mild dementia care provided
Diets Accommodated: Diabetic, Low-fat, Low-salt
Proximity to Emergency Svcs.: Under 8 miles
Nearby shopping and entertainment
Pets allowed

### STAFF

Nurse/LVN/LPN: 24 hours/week
Caregiver Training: Family communication, Stress management
Criminal Background Check: Yes
Principal Staff Language(s): English
Other Staff Language(s): Spanish

### FACILITY FEATURES

Activities/Recreation
Beauty/Barber Shop ($)
Chapel Services
Computer/Internet Access
Facility Parking
Guest Meals ($)
Outside Patio/Gardens
Pharmaceutical Service
Private Dining Room ($)
Room Service ($)
Transportation
24-hour Security

### ROOM FEATURES

Cable TV Ready ($)
Emergency Call System
Grab Bars
Kitchenette
Private Bathrooms
Telephone Ready ($)
Temperature Controls

### COSTS

PRICES MAY INCREASE. PLEASE CALL FOR MOST CURRENT INFORMATION.

| | |
|---|---|
| Studio Apt. | $58.52/day |
| One Bedroom Apt. | $74.13/day |
| Respite Stays | $68.50/day for private room |
| Costs of Care | $11.75–$70/day based on individual need |
| Rate Increase | Periodically |
| Reimbursement | LTCI, Private pay, Veterans |

| | |
|---|---|
| Entrance Fee | $1,750 |
| Pet Deposit | $500 (refundable) |

**PORTRAIT**

There is an unmistakable country charm about Redbud House. Although the facility neighbors a residential area, its surrounding landscape imparts a feeling of a secluded refuge. Skirting the building's entrance, a large wooden porch furnished with several rockers invites residents to bask outdoors.

Residents' bright, spacious rooms all feature extra storage space. Furnished respite rooms are available as well. In the hallways, freshly painted walls and updated light fixtures are telltale signs of management's ongoing remodeling project. We observed residents visiting in the comfortable seating areas found here. Soft artificial lighting, along with natural light, provides a warm glow.

Residents enjoy the simple and cozy layout of the L-shaped building; it promotes frequent interaction between residents and staff. In one area, we noted residents participating in their daily exercise routine with a fitness instructor. Another common area featured a library, where many residents were checking out books. The energetic residents at Redbud House seem comfortable in their quaint environment.

## Signature Pointe on the Lake A/D

14655 Preston Road
Dallas, TX 75254

(972) 726-7575
www.seniorhousingnet.com

**GILBERT GUIDE OBSERVATIONS**

| | | | |
|---|---|---|---|
| Administration & Staff | g g g g g | Dietary & Food Selection | g g g g g |
| Facility Aesthetics | g g g g g | Activities | g g g g g |
| Facility Condition & Safety | g g g g g | Alzheimer's & Dementia Capabilities | g g g g g |
| Residents | g g g g g | | |

**DETAILS**

Year Built: 1997
Current Mgmt. Since: 1997
No. of Floors: 4
Resident Capacity: 76

**SPECIAL**

Diets Accommodated: Diabetic, Low-fat, Low-salt, Renal
Proximity to Emergency Svcs.: Under 8 miles
Nearby shopping and entertainment
No pets allowed

**STAFF**

Nurse/LVN/LPN: Onsite 24/7
Caregiver Training: Dementia, Family communication, Grief, Transition issues
Criminal Background Check: Yes

SIGNATURE POINTE ON THE LAKE (CONTINUED)

Principal Staff Language(s): English
Other Staff Language(s): Spanish

### FACILITY FEATURES

Activities/Recreation
Beauty/Barber Shop ($)
Chapel Services
Facility Parking
Fitness Room/Gym
Guest Meals ($)
Outside Patio/Gardens
Pharmaceutical Service ($)
Private Dining Room
Room Service ($)
Separate Therapy Room
Transportation
24-hour Security

### ROOM FEATURES

Cable TV Ready ($)
Emergency Call System
Grab Bars
Kitchenette
Private Bathrooms
Telephone Ready ($)
Temperature Controls

### COSTS

PRICES MAY INCREASE. PLEASE CALL FOR MOST CURRENT INFORMATION.

| | |
|---|---|
| Studio Apt. | $2,465–$3,645/month |
| One Bedroom Apt. | $3,830–$3,965/month<br>Double occupancy add $600/month |
| Alzheimer's Unit | $131–$133/day for shared room, $152-$235/day for private room |
| Costs of Care | Included in monthly and daily rates |
| Rate Increase | Annually; usually 2–3% |
| Reimbursement | LTCI, Private pay |
| Security Deposit | $500 (refundable) |

### PORTRAIT

A posh Dallas community is home to Signature Pointe on the Lake, which sits on lively Preston Road. Shade trees abound in the pastoral setting surrounding the red brick building. Ducks paddle in the fountain at the center of the facility's man-made lake. A quaint seating area is located onshore. Breathtaking chandeliers hang from the vaulted ceiling in the foyer. The upscale furnishings include wooden tables and hutches. Green and gold carpeting extends from wall to wall. A cheerful group of residents waited for their families to pick them up for holiday activities as we began our tour. Light from large windows and elegant fixtures brighten the facility. Beautiful flower arrangements and comfortable chairs fill the expansive hallways. Crown moldings accent the earth-toned walls in residents' rooms. Some rooms boast private patios; all enjoy lovely views of the landscaped grounds.

The waitstaff make a formal appearance in jackets and ties in the elegant dining room, where they serve meals. Our mouths watered as we read the menu, which listed turkey, mashed potatoes and pumpkin pie. The staff frequently holds socials and happy hours for the residents. Other activities include exercise, games, arts and crafts, and outings to movie theaters and shopping destinations. Guest musicians entertain the residents on the facility's grand piano.

Signature Pointe offers Alzheimer's and skilled nursing care in addition to assisted living. The secured Alzheimer's unit is divided between residents in the early stages of the disease and those in the more advanced stages. Therapeutic activities for Alzheimer's residents often involve pets and music. It is plain to see that the staff genuinely cares about the residents. One example of supportive behavior includes validating action, such as helping residents who believe they must prepare for a job or other activity they performed in the past.

## SILVERADO SENIOR LIVING A/D

5521 Village Creek Drive
Plano, TX 75093

(972) 447-0038
www.silveradosenior.com

### GILBERT GUIDE OBSERVATIONS

| | | | |
|---|---|---|---|
| Administration & Staff | g g g g | Dietary & Food Selection | g g g g g |
| Facility Aesthetics | g g g g | Activities | g g g g |
| Facility Condition & Safety | g g g | Alzheimer's & Dementia Capabilities | g g g g g |
| Residents | g g g g g | | |

### DETAILS

Year Built: 1998
Year Remodeled: 2006
Current Mgmt. Since: 2005
No. of Floors: 1
Resident Capacity: 56

### SPECIAL

Alzheimer's/Dementia Only Facility
Diets Accommodated: Diabetic, Low-fat, Low-salt
Proximity to Emergency Svcs.: Under 8 miles
Nearby shopping and entertainment
Pets allowed

### STAFF

Nurse/LVN/LPN: 40 hours/week, On-call 24/7
Caregiver Training: Dementia, Ethics, Family communication, Grief, Patient transfers, Transition issues
Criminal Background Check: Yes
Principal Staff Language(s): English
Other Staff Language(s): Spanish

### FACILITY FEATURES

Activities/Recreation
Beauty/Barber Shop ($)
Chapel Services
Facility Parking
Guest Meals
Outside Patio/Gardens
Private Dining Room

### ROOM FEATURES

Cable TV Ready
Emergency Call System
Grab Bars
Kitchenette
Shared & Private Bathrooms
Telephone Ready
Temperature Controls

SILVERADO SENIOR LIVING (CONTINUED)

**FACILITY FEATURES (CONTINUED)**

Room Service
Transportation to MD Appointments ($), Personal Outings ($), Scheduled Outings
24-hour Security

## COSTS

PRICES MAY INCREASE. PLEASE CALL FOR MOST CURRENT INFORMATION.

| | |
|---|---|
| Alzheimer's Unit | $150–$170/day for shared room<br>$200–$250/day for private room |
| Respite Stays | $155/day for shared room |
| Costs of Care | $375/month for incontinence care |
| Rate Increase | Annually; usually 3–6% |
| Reimbursement | LTCI, Private pay |
| Security Deposit | $2,500 (refundable) |
| Pet Deposit | $35–$65/month for supplies and care |

## PORTRAIT

Silverado Senior Living was undergoing extensive renovations at the time of our visit. The boisterous laughter of children reached our ears from the day care next door. Staff members' children romp on the colorful playground equipment in the front yard when their parents bring them to work. We learned from the staff that the new owners intend to create large, open areas that encourage residents to move freely in and out of the home.

After renovations are complete, the home will offer eight floor plans, including private rooms as well as suites that share a living area and bathroom. Memory boxes filled with photographs and knickknacks hang beside the doors to residents' rooms. Birds sing in a cage in the homey dining area, which features a refrigerator stocked with snacks. A fireplace and comfortable rocking chairs make the activity area feel like one's own living room. We observed residents participating in a current events discussion, in which a staff member would read a portion of an article and then ask questions. Two residents pored over an album with photographs of 1940s movie stars, which prompted them to share their memories. Many of the residents have scrapbooks that document their activities with photographs. The staff informed us that future activities will be geared toward building self-esteem and stimulating residents' senses.

Two cats share the home, which accommodates dementia residents with behavioral issues. The nursing director possesses two decades of dementia-related experience, and the staff has been specially trained to deal with angry outbursts and other difficult behavior.

## VILLAGE OAKS AT FARMERS BRANCH A/D

13505 Webb Chapel Road
Farmers Branch, TX 75234
(972) 241-3955
www.emeritus.com

### GILBERT GUIDE OBSERVATIONS

| | |
|---|---|
| Administration & Staff | g g g g g |
| Facility Aesthetics | g g g g |
| Facility Condition & Safety | g g g g g |
| Residents | g g g g g |
| Dietary & Food Selection | g g g |
| Activities | g g g |
| Alzheimer's & Dementia Capabilities | g g g g g |

### DETAILS

Year Built: 1997
Year Remodeled: 2002
Current Mgmt. Since: 2002
No. of Floors: 1
Resident Capacity: 65 (AL), 20 (ALZ)

### SPECIAL

Diets Accommodated: Diabetic, Low-fat, Low-salt
Proximity to Emergency Svcs.: Under 8 miles
Nearby shopping and entertainment
Pet visits allowed

### STAFF

Nurse/LVN/LPN: Onsite 24/7
Caregiver Training: Dementia, Ethics, Family communication, Grief, Patient transfers, Stress management, Transition issues, Validation therapy
Criminal Background Check: Yes
Principal Staff Language(s): English
Other Staff Language(s): Spanish

### FACILITY FEATURES

Activities/Recreation
Beauty/Barber Shop ($)
Chapel Services
Facility Parking
Fitness Room/Gym
Guest Meals ($)
Outside Patio/Gardens
Pharmaceutical Service
Private Dining Room
Room Service ($)
Separate Therapy Room
Transportation
24-hour Security

### ROOM FEATURES

Cable TV Ready
Emergency Call System
Grab Bars
Kitchenette
Private Bathrooms
Telephone Ready ($)
Temperature Controls

### COSTS

PRICES MAY INCREASE. PLEASE CALL FOR MOST CURRENT INFORMATION.

| | |
|---|---|
| Studio Apt. | $2,100/month |
| One Bedroom Apt. | $2,300–$2,600/month |
| Alzheimer's Unit | $2,500–$2,700/month for private room |
| Respite Stays | $125/day for private room |

VILLAGE OAKS AT FARMERS BRANCH (CONTINUED)

| | |
|---|---|
| Costs of Care | \$200–\$1,000/month based on individual need |
| Rate Increase | Annually; usually 5% |
| Reimbursement | LTCI, Private pay, SSI, Veterans |
| Entrance Fee | \$1,000 |

**PORTRAIT**

Village Oaks is located in a residential neighborhood of Farmers Branch, just four blocks north of Interstate 635. Tall maples and oaks shade much of the street. The facility is housed in a brown brick building with a white portico. A Protestant church holds services next door. Several outdoor common areas include a garden patio with a gazebo, an extensive porch furnished with iron tables and chairs, and concrete walkways that feature perennial plants. Double doors at the facility's entrance lead to a small atrium. Vividly colored tropical fish swim in a 175-gallon aquarium across from the reception desk.

Friendly peals of laughter between the animated residents and the attentive staff were noted frequently during our visit. Meals are served cafeteria-style in the spacious dining hall. A salad bar adds variety to the menu, which features traditional staples like meatloaf. A soft serve ice cream machine supplements dessert offerings.

The living room is furnished with numerous sofas and a big-screen TV. A common area serves as the library, private dining room and conference space. The secured Alzheimer's area has a nautical theme with soothing colors. A mixture of fluorescent and natural lighting brightens the facility. The hallways are wide and equipped with handrails. Residents' rooms are moderately sized; all have closets, windows and built-in bookshelves. Baking and cooking class participants use the oven in the activity room, where dancing and a variety of games also take place. Weekly restaurant outings are another popular activity.

## THE WATERFORD AT PLANO

3401 Premier Drive
Plano, TX 75075

(972) 423-7400
www.capitalsenior.com

---

**GILBERT GUIDE OBSERVATIONS**

| | | | |
|---|---|---|---|
| Administration & Staff | g g g g g | Residents | g g g g |
| Facility Aesthetics | g g g g | Dietary & Food Selection | g g g g g |
| Facility Condition & Safety | g g g g | Activities | g g g g |

**DETAILS**

Year Built: 2000
Current Mgmt. Since: 2000
No. of Floors: 1

**SPECIAL**

Mild dementia care provided
Diets Accommodated: Diabetic, Low-fat, Low-salt, Renal

DETAILS (CONTINUED)
Resident Capacity: 42
Nearby shopping and entertainment
Pets allowed

SPECIAL (CONTINUED)
Proximity to Emergency Svcs.: Under 8 miles

## STAFF

Nurse/LVN/LPN: On-call 24/7
Caregiver Training: Dementia, Ethics, Family communication, Patient transfers, Stress management, Transition issues
Criminal Background Check: Yes
Principal Staff Language(s): English
Other Staff Language(s): Spanish

## FACILITY FEATURES

Activities/Recreation
Beauty/Barber Shop ($)
Chapel Services
Computer/Internet Access
Facility Parking
Guest Meals ($)
Outside Patio/Gardens
Pharmaceutical Service
Private Dining Room
Room Service ($)
Transportation
24-hour Security

## ROOM FEATURES

Cable TV Ready
Emergency Call System
Grab Bars
Kitchenette
Private Bathrooms
Telephone Ready ($)
Temperature Controls

## COSTS

PRICES MAY INCREASE. PLEASE CALL FOR MOST CURRENT INFORMATION.

| | |
|---|---|
| Studio Apt. | $2,080–$2,625/month |
| One Bedroom Apt. | $2,850–$3,150/month<br>Double occupancy add $600/month |
| Costs of Care | Included in monthly rate |
| Rate Increase | Annually; usually 4% |
| Reimbursement | Private pay |
| Security Deposit | $500 |
| Pet Deposit | $500 |

## PORTRAIT

The immaculate brick building that houses Waterford at Plano is set well back from Premier Drive, although restaurants and shops are still within sight. Saplings flank the circular driveway leading to the portico. The interior exudes elegance. Custom drapes on the floor-to-ceiling windows coordinate with the burgundy, green and yellow carpet. A crystal chandelier hangs in the foyer. Mahogany tables, plush seating and a fireplace continue the upscale theme.

Residents enjoy two snacks a day. The menu lists meals such as meatloaf with mashed potatoes and green beans and apple pie. High ceilings crisscrossed with support beams soar

THE WATERFORD AT PLANO (CONTINUED)

above the dining and common areas. Brass chandeliers shed mellow light over cherrywood furniture and comfortable chairs. Recessed fixtures supplement the abundant natural lighting. Handrails line the wide hallways. Each resident's apartment features an amply sized living area as well as a spacious bedroom. Residents furnish their rooms to suit their tastes.

Tall trees shade the two courtyards, where a fountain shoots water into the air. Residents take part in frequent outings, including shopping and dining. They also attend church services and Bible study. Happy hour, teatime and exercise are other popular activities. Residents and staff smiled frequently during our tour while they conversed warmly with one another.

## The Wellington at Arapaho

600 West Arapaho Road
Richardson, TX 75080

(469) 330-2800
www.capitalsenior.com

---

**GILBERT GUIDE OBSERVATIONS**

| | | | |
|---|---|---|---|
| Administration & Staff | g g g | Residents | g g g g g |
| Facility Aesthetics | g g g g | Dietary & Food Selection | g g g g g |
| Facility Condition & Safety | g g g g | Activities | g g g g g |

### DETAILS

Year Built: 2002
Current Mgmt. Since: 2002
No. of Floors: 1
Resident Capacity: 86

### SPECIAL

Mild dementia care provided
Diets Accommodated: Diabetic, Low-salt
Proximity to Emergency Svcs.: Under 8 miles
Nearby shopping and entertainment
Some pets allowed

### STAFF

Nurse/LVN/LPN: 40 hours/week, On-call 24/7
Caregiver Training: Dementia, Ethics, Family communication, Grief, Patient transfers, Stress management, Transition issues, Validation therapy
Criminal Background Check: Yes
Principal Staff Language(s): English
Other Staff Language(s): Spanish

### FACILITY FEATURES

Activities/Recreation
Beauty/Barber Shop ($)
Chapel Services
Computer/Internet Access
Facility Parking
Fitness Room/Gym ($)
Guest Meals ($)

### ROOM FEATURES

Cable TV Ready
Emergency Call System
Grab Bars
Kitchenette
Private Bathrooms
Telephone Ready ($)
Temperature Controls

FACILITY FEATURES (continued)
Overnight Guest Room ($)
Pharmaceutical Service
Private Dining Room
Room Service ($)
Transportation to MD Appointments, Scheduled Outings

## COSTS

PRICES MAY INCREASE. PLEASE CALL FOR MOST CURRENT INFORMATION.

| | |
|---|---|
| Studio Apt. | $2,345–$4,600/month |
| One Bedroom Apt. | $3,290/month<br>Double occupancy add $600/month |
| Two Bedroom Apt. | Up to $4,600/month |
| Respite Stays | $85/day for private room |
| Costs of Care | Included in monthly rate |
| Rate Increase | Annually; usually 4% |
| Reimbursement | LTCI, Private pay |
| Security Deposit | $500 (refundable) |
| Pet Deposit | $1,000 (refundable) |

## PORTRAIT

Wood trim accentuates the red brick building that houses The Wellington at Arapaho. The tidy exterior features a covered driveway and potted plants. Comfortable furnishings and pale green carpet with a border of triangles lend an inviting air to the entrance. The facility features arched doorways throughout. Books line shelves in the library, where residents enjoy web access. Natural lighting supplements the chandeliers and recessed fixtures. Along with high ceilings, the lighting creates an open, welcoming atmosphere in the common rooms. Handrails line the spacious hallways.

White crown moldings accent the dining area's pale walls. Support beams are visible beneath the high ceiling. Padded chairs surround the linen-covered tables. Chandeliers and custom window treatments add to the facility's upscale quality. The menu features hearty meals such as chicken fried steak or grilled chicken with mashed potatoes, country vegetables and pie. Alternate choices are also available.

Resident furnish their own rooms, which range in size from small to large, and include either one or two windows. Several friendly residents wished us a good morning. Staff members address residents by their first names. Residents enjoy guest musicians and speakers, as well as aquatic exercise and variety of crafts, including crocheting and knitting. Religious services are also popular. The Wellington features abundant landscaped outdoor areas shaded by trees, where residents tend a vegetable and herb garden.

SKILLED NURSING FACILITIES

## Heritage Manor Healthcare Center

1621 Coit Road
Plano, TX 75075
(972) 596-7930

**TOTAL GOVERNMENT DEFICIENCIES: 6** — Reviewed on: August 18, 2005

| Environmental | Nutrition and Dietary | Pharmacy Service |
|---|---|---|
| 1 | 1 | 2 |
| **Quality Care** | **Resident Rights** | |
| 1 | 1 | |

* IMPORTANT: REVIEW DETAILS OF EACH DEFICIENCY AT WWW.MEDICARE.GOV

**GILBERT GUIDE OBSERVATIONS**

| Category | Rating | Category | Rating |
|---|---|---|---|
| Administration & Staff | g g g | Dietary & Food Selection | g g g |
| Facility Aesthetics | g g g | Activities | g g |
| Facility Condition & Safety | g g g | Access to Medical Care | g g g g |
| Residents | g g g g | | |

### DETAILS

Year Built: 1976
Year Remodeled: 1990
Current Mgmt. Since: 2003
No. of Floors: 1
Resident Capacity: 160
Facility Type: Long-term care, Short-term rehab

### SPECIAL

Special diets accommodated
Proximity to Emergency Svcs.: Under 8 miles

### STAFF

Caregiver Training: Dementia, Ethics, Family communication, Grief, Pain management, Patient transfers, Stress management, Transition issues, Universal precautions, Validation therapy, Wound care
Criminal Background Check: Yes
Principal Staff Language(s): English
Other Staff Language(s): Cantonese, German, Italian, Mandarin, Spanish, Vietnamese

### FACILITY FEATURES

Activities/Recreation
Beauty/Barber Shop ($)
Chapel Services
Guest Meals ($)
Outside Patio/Gardens
Private Dining Room
Separate Therapy Room
Wanderguard
Whirlpool Baths

### ROOM FEATURES

Cable TV Ready
Space for personal items
Shared & Private Bathrooms
Telephone Ready

### COSTS

PRICES MAY INCREASE. PLEASE CALL FOR MOST CURRENT INFORMATION.

| | |
|---|---|
| Shared Room | $132/day |
| Private Room | $153–$234/day |
| Respite Stays | $132/day for shared room |
| Rate Increase | Annually; usually 4–6% |
| Reimbursement | Medicare, Medicaid, LTCI, Private pay |

### PORTRAIT

The enclosed porch outfitted with benches and glass double doors creates a welcoming entrance to Heritage Manor. A majestic chandelier brightens the lobby. Comfortable seating in the living room allows residents and guests to enjoy the crackling fireplace and tinkling of the grand piano. A podium commands attention in a nearby activity area. Floor-to-ceiling bookcases dominate a second activity space, where residents enjoy watching old movies on the big-screen TV. Leather chairs and matching sofas provide plush seating.

Wooden panels, knockers and doorbells add luxury to the outside of residents' sunny rooms—all of which are certified by Medicare. Most rooms feature unique floor plans (very few are square or rectangle) and all are generously sized. Some rooms feature carpeting and full baths. The facility supplies each resident with a hospital bed, an armoire, a table and a chair. Ample closets fitted with large mirrors offer additional storage.

Sturdy handrails and wainscoting border the hallways, where recessed lighting illuminates photographs of residents and trivia posted by the activity director. A sea of tables and chairs surrounds a piano in the main dining area. The ice cream parlor in the corner hosts ice cream socials and other activities. An elegant wrought iron fence secures the paved patio area, which is furnished with weatherproof tables and chairs.

Heritage Manor staff struck us as a strong team. The current administrator has worked at the facility for twenty-seven years, under multiple owners. The facility also boasts three staff social workers! Prior to our tour, we received a packet of information in which we were delighted to find touching personal stories authored by residents, their families and the administrator.

## Lake Village Nursing & Rehabilitation Center

169 Lake Park Road
Lewisville, TX 75057
(972) 436-7571

**TOTAL GOVERNMENT DEFICIENCIES: 2** Reviewed on: March 10, 2005

| Environmental | Nutrition and Dietary |
|---|---|
| 1 | 1 |

* IMPORTANT: REVIEW DETAILS OF EACH DEFICIENCY AT WWW.MEDICARE.GOV

**GILBERT GUIDE OBSERVATIONS**

| | | | |
|---|---|---|---|
| Administration & Staff | g g g g | Dietary & Food Selection | g g g |
| Facility Aesthetics | g g g | Activities | g g g |
| Facility Condition & Safety | g g g | Access to Medical Care | g g g |
| Residents | g g g | | |

### DETAILS

Year Built: 1980
Year Remodeled: Ongoing
Current Mgmt. Since: 1993
No. of Floors: 1
Resident Capacity: 114
Facility Type: Long-term care, Short-term rehab

### SPECIAL

Special diets accommodated
Proximity to Emergency Svcs.: Under 8 miles

### STAFF

Caregiver Training: Ethics, Pain management, Stress management, Wound care
Criminal Background Check: Yes
Principal Staff Language(s): English
Other Staff Language(s): Spanish

### FACILITY FEATURES

Activities/Recreation
Beauty/Barber Shop ($)
Separate Therapy Room
24-hour Security
Wanderguard

### ROOM FEATURES

Cable TV Ready ($)
Space for personal items
Shared & Private Bathrooms
Telephone Ready ($)

### COSTS

PRICES MAY INCREASE. PLEASE CALL FOR MOST CURRENT INFORMATION.

| | |
|---|---|
| Shared Room | $125/day |
| Private Room | $165/day |
| Rate Increase | Annually; usually 1–3% |
| Reimbursement | Medicare, Medicaid, LTCI, Private pay |

## PORTRAIT

Lake Village Nursing and Rehabilitation Center neighbors the expansive park and recreation grounds of Lewisville Lake; it is also adjacent to Lake Park Golf Course. The building is well-maintained. Star-shaped moldings embedded in the stone brick frame add delightful character to the exterior. The entrance opens up to a furnished common area. Residents gathered in front of the big-screen TV to watch their favorite soap opera during our visit.

Residents' rooms are small, but each has a window. All of the rooms are equipped with hospital beds. The dining area is adequately sized to accommodate all of the residents at one time. Although furniture and decorative ornaments are sparse, the area is perfectly functional. The nursing station is positioned at the center of the building, providing a clear vantage point to the six outlying wings. Each hall is named after one of the six flags that has waved over Texas in the course of its history—the Spanish, French, Mexican, Confederate, and American flags—and, of course, the Texas state flag. Recessed and fluorescent lighting maintain a bright environment. The outdoor area features lovely wrought iron patio furniture. Residents voiced their enjoyment of the surrounding landscape of towering trees and various shrubs.

Lake Village's owner is incredibly caring and dedicated to the residents, and is very involved with the daily operations of the facility.

# LINDAN PARK CARE CENTER LP

1510 North Plano Road
Richardson, TX 75081

(972) 234-4786

---

**TOTAL GOVERNMENT DEFICIENCIES: 1** — Reviewed on: April 28, 2005

Nutrition and Dietary

1

* IMPORTANT: REVIEW DETAILS OF EACH DEFICIENCY AT WWW.MEDICARE.GOV

**GILBERT GUIDE OBSERVATIONS**

| Category | Rating | Category | Rating |
|---|---|---|---|
| Administration & Staff | g g g g g | Dietary & Food Selection | g g g |
| Facility Aesthetics | g g g | Activities | g g g g g |
| Facility Condition & Safety | g g g | Access to Medical Care | g g g |
| Residents | g g g g | | |

## DETAILS

Year Built: 1965
Year Remodeled: 2005
Current Mgmt. Since: 5
No. of Floors: 1

## SPECIAL

Special diets accommodated
Proximity to Emergency Svcs.: 16+ Miles

LINDAN PARK CARE CENTER LP (CONTINUED)

**DETAILS (CONTINUED)**

Resident Capacity: 126
Facility Type: Long-term care

## STAFF

Caregiver Training: Dementia, Ethics, Family communication, Grief, Pain management, Patient transfers, Stress management, Transition issues, Universal precautions, Validation therapy, Wound care
Criminal Background Check: Yes
Principal Staff Language(s): English
Other Staff Language(s): Farsi, Spanish

## FACILITY FEATURES

Activities/Recreation
Beauty/Barber Shop
Chapel Services
Facility Parking
Guest Meals ($)
Outside Patio/Gardens
Private Dining Room
Separate Therapy Room
Wanderguard

## ROOM FEATURES

Cable TV Ready ($)
Space for personal items
Shared & Private Bathrooms
Telephone Ready ($)

## COSTS

PRICES MAY INCREASE. PLEASE CALL FOR MOST CURRENT INFORMATION.

| | |
|---|---|
| Shared Room | $100/day |
| Private Room | $150/day |
| Rate Increase | Periodically |
| Reimbursement | Medicare, Medicaid, LTCI, Private pay |

## PORTRAIT

A sheltered walkway leads visitors to Lindan Park Care Center wjere the front porch features benches and overhead fans. Fluorescent lighting brightens the home's interior. A grand piano adds an upscale quality to a seating area decorated in earthy tones. The spacious hallways are lined with handrails. Residents' rooms feature charming wooden shutters. A tall fence, cheerfully painted with nature scenes, encircles the designated smoking area. Colorful crepe myrtles grow in the landscaped outdoor area. At the time of our visit, the facility was constructing another landscaped area with a gazebo.

Lindan Park's common areas double as activity spaces. Activities include exercise, coffee socials, book clubs, Red Hat Society functions, sing-alongs, and performances by local entertainers. Residents also attend church services and visit shopping areas.

Most residents on our visit were smiling and socializing—some even held hands. One resident, who was clearly distressed and confused, was being soothed by several concerned residents and staff members.

## ROWLETT HEALTH AND REHABILITATION CENTER

9300 Lakeview Parkway
Rowlett, TX 75088

(972) 475-4700
(469) 853-5944
www.scc-texas.com

---

**TOTAL GOVERNMENT DEFICIENCIES: 6** Reviewed on: April 15, 2005

| Administration | Nutrition and Dietary | Pharmacy Service | Quality Care |
|---|---|---|---|
| 1 | 3 | 1 | 1 |

* IMPORTANT: REVIEW DETAILS OF EACH DEFICIENCY AT WWW.MEDICARE.GOV

**GILBERT GUIDE OBSERVATIONS**

| | | | |
|---|---|---|---|
| Administration & Staff | g g g | Dietary & Food Selection | g g g |
| Facility Aesthetics | g g g | Activities | g g g |
| Facility Condition & Safety | g g g | Access to Medical Care | g g g |
| Residents | g g g | | |

### DETAILS

Year Built: 1990
Year Remodeled: 1997
Current Mgmt. Since: 1990
No. of Floors: 1
Resident Capacity: 169
Facility Type: Long-term care, Short-term rehab

### SPECIAL

Special diets accommodated
Proximity to Emergency Svcs.: Under 8 miles

### STAFF

Caregiver Training: Dementia, Ethics, Family communication, Grief, Pain management, Patient transfers, Stress management, Transition issues, Universal precautions, Validation therapy, Wound care
Criminal Background Check: Yes
Principal Staff Language(s): English

### FACILITY FEATURES

Activities/Recreation
Beauty/Barber Shop
Chapel Services
Outside Patio/Gardens
Separate Therapy Room
24-hour Security

### ROOM FEATURES

Cable TV Ready
Space for personal items
Shared Bathrooms
Telephone Ready

### COSTS

PRICES MAY INCREASE. PLEASE CALL FOR MOST CURRENT INFORMATION.

| | |
|---|---|
| Shared Room | $118–$125/day |
| Respite Stays | $118–$125/day for shared room |

ROWLETT HEALTH AND REHABILITATION CENTER (CONTINUED)

| | |
|---|---|
| Rate Increase | Annually; usually 1% |
| Reimbursement | Medicare, Medicaid, Private pay |

**PORTRAIT**

Rowlett Health is located three miles north of Interstate 30 on Highway 66. Adjacent to a local pottery shop, the white brick facility is nestled in a hilly residential area. Management expanded the facility—and clientele—in 1997, adding a new wing for short-term rehabilitation patients.

The somewhat outdated interior is decorated in blue, white and maroon. Painted landscapes and wallpaper with a fern motif adorn the cream-colored walls. The common areas are furnished with dark wooden pieces upholstered in a blue-and-white flowered pattern. We witnessed a group of residents chatting in unison with the animated twittering of canaries and finches. Blue tabletops against white linoleum floors set the stage in the dining room. The large windows in the common areas usher natural light into the facility and supplement the overhead fluorescent lighting. The hallways are neat and wide. White painted handrails trace the halls throughout.

Residents' rooms are large enough to accommodate two people and are furnished with a bed, armoire and nightstand. The cherrywood furniture looks especially rich against the subdued wallpaper. Residents regularly gather on the outdoor patio, a comfortable shaded spot with white wooden furniture. Some enjoy socializing near the hanging bird feeders; others prefer the large grassy area colored by bright yellow and purple pansies. During our visit, the staff seemed focused on working efficiently, while residents were content socializing amongst themselves.

## SIGNATURE POINTE ON THE LAKE

14655 Preston Road  
Dallas, TX 75254

(972) 726-7575  
www.signaturepointe.com

**TOTAL GOVERNMENT DEFICIENCIES: 12** — Reviewed on: July 13, 2005

| Quality Care | Residential Assessment | Nutrition and Dietary | Pharmacy Service |
|---|---|---|---|
| 1 | 3 | 2 | 3 |
| **Environmental** | **Administration** | | |
| 1 | 2 | | |

* IMPORTANT: REVIEW DETAILS OF EACH DEFICIENCY AT WWW.MEDICARE.GOV

**GILBERT GUIDE OBSERVATIONS**

| | | | |
|---|---|---|---|
| Administration & Staff | g g g g g | Dietary & Food Selection | g g g g g |
| Facility Aesthetics | g g g g g | Activities | g g g g g |
| Facility Condition & Safety | g g g g | Access to Medical Care | g g g g g |
| Residents | g g g g g | | |

## DETAILS

Year Built: 1997
Current Mgmt. Since: 1997
No. of Floors: 4
Resident Capacity: 195
Facility Type: Long-term care, Short-term rehab

## SPECIAL

Special diets accommodated
Proximity to Emergency Svcs.: Under 8 miles

## STAFF

Caregiver Training: Ethics, Family communication, Grief, Pain management, Patient transfers, Transition issues, Wound care
Criminal Background Check: Yes
Principal Staff Language(s): English
Other Staff Language(s): Spanish

## FACILITY FEATURES

Activities/Recreation
Beauty/Barber Shop ($)
Chapel Services
Guest Meals ($)
Outside Patio/Gardens
Private Dining Room
Separate Therapy Room
24-hour Security
Wanderguard

## ROOM FEATURES

Cable TV Ready ($)
Space for personal items
Shared & Private Bathrooms
Telephone Ready ($)

## COSTS

PRICES MAY INCREASE. PLEASE CALL FOR MOST CURRENT INFORMATION.

| | |
|---|---|
| Shared Room | $119/day |
| Private Room | $170–$221/day |
| Rate Increase | Annually; usually 2–3% |
| Reimbursement | Medicare, LTCI, Private pay |

## PORTRAIT

A stately red brick building houses Signature Pointe on the Lake's skilled nursing, assisted living and Alzheimer's units. Beautiful landscaped grounds surround the facility, which features a portico to ease entering and exiting vehicles in inclement weather. The man-made lake that sits on the wooded property is home to a number of ducks.

SIGNATURE POINTE ON THE LAKE (CONTINUED)

Chandeliers hang from the vaulted ceiling in the foyer, casting soft light over green-and-gold patterned carpet. Comfortable chairs and wooden tables are just some of the elegant furnishings in the common areas. Light from tasteful fixtures and expansive windows illuminate the home. The wide hallways easily accommodate multiple wheelchair and walker users. Residents' upscale rooms are sunny and have ample space for personal belongings.

Residents enjoy restaurant-style service in the dining room. During the tour, our guide smiled at each resident we came across—we noted several small groups socializing in the common areas. The guide informed us that the staff makes a special effort to introduce new residents to everyone to help them begin forming relationships. The residents at Signature Pointe on the Lake seem very much at home.

## THE VILLAGE AT RICHARDSON

1111 Rockingham Lane
Richardson, TX 75080

(972) 231-8833
www.thicare.com

**TOTAL GOVERNMENT DEFICIENCIES: 11** Reviewed on: September 16, 2005

| Environmental | Nutrition and Dietary | Pharmacy Service |
|---|---|---|
| 3 | 1 | 4 |
| **Quality Care** | **Resident Rights** | |
| 2 | 1 | |

* IMPORTANT: REVIEW DETAILS OF EACH DEFICIENCY AT WWW.MEDICARE.GOV

**GILBERT GUIDE OBSERVATIONS**

| | | | |
|---|---|---|---|
| Administration & Staff | g g g | Dietary & Food Selection | g g g |
| Facility Aesthetics | g g g | Activities | g g g |
| Facility Condition & Safety | g g g | Access to Medical Care | g g g g |
| Residents | g g g | | |

### DETAILS

Year Built: 1970
Year Remodeled: Ongoing
Current Mgmt. Since: 2000
No. of Floors: 1
Resident Capacity: 273
Facility Type: Long-term care, Short-term rehab

### SPECIAL

Special diets accommodated
Proximity to Emergency Svcs.: Under 8 miles

## STAFF

Caregiver Training: Dementia, Ethics, Family communication, Grief, Pain management, Patient transfers, Stress management, Transition issues, Universal precautions, Validation therapy, Wound care
Criminal Background Check: Yes
Principal Staff Language(s): English
Other Staff Language(s): Russian, Spanish

## FACILITY FEATURES

Activities/Recreation
Beauty/Barber Shop ($)
Chapel Services
Guest Meals ($)
Outside Patio/Gardens
Private Dining Room ($)
Private Visiting Room
Separate Therapy Room ($)
Whirlpool Baths

## ROOM FEATURES

Space for personal items
Shared Bathrooms
Telephone Ready ($)

## COSTS

PRICES MAY INCREASE. PLEASE CALL FOR MOST CURRENT INFORMATION.

| | |
|---|---|
| Shared Room | $3,600/monthly |
| Respite Stays | $112/day for shared room |
| Rate Increase | Every 2–3 years; usually 1–5% |
| Reimbursement | Medicare, Medicaid, LTCI, Private pay |

## PORTRAIT

A peaceful residential area harbors The Village at Richardson. The covered driveway facilitates entering and exiting comfortably in inclement weather. Colorful furniture with brass accents decorates the lobby. Residents relaxed and socialized in the comfortable seating areas when we visited. Handrails line the wide hallways. Chandeliers and sconces illuminate the facility. Lamps provide soft lighting in residents' rooms, which are set up so that wheelchair users may maneuver easily.

Tai chi, movies, religious services and shopping excursions are all popular activities among residents. Residents also enjoy the use of a whirlpool and spa. Assorted games and arts and crafts take place in the spacious and well-lit dining area, where a grand piano takes center stage. Here, yellow tablecloths add cheery elements. The facility boasts several patio areas, two of which open off of the dining room. One area is designated for smoking. The patio furniture appeared well worn and the landscaping was somewhat neglected. Residents who left a pet behind at their original homes are allowed pet visitation, as management recognizes the importance of this special bond.

## VISTA RIDGE NURSING AND REHABILITATION

700 East Vista Ridge Mall Drive
Lewisville, TX 75067

(972) 906-9789
www.vrsnf.com

**TOTAL GOVERNMENT DEFICIENCIES: 11** Reviewed on: October 13, 2005

| Administration | Environmental | Mistreatment | Nutrition and Dietary |
|---|---|---|---|
| 2 | 2 | 1 | 4 |
| **Pharmacy Service** | **Quality Care** | | |
| 1 | 1 | | |

* IMPORTANT: REVIEW DETAILS OF EACH DEFICIENCY AT WWW.MEDICARE.GOV

**GILBERT GUIDE OBSERVATIONS**

| | | | |
|---|---|---|---|
| Administration & Staff | g g g g | Dietary & Food Selection | g g g g g |
| Facility Aesthetics | g g g g | Activities | g g g |
| Facility Condition & Safety | g g g g | Access to Medical Care | g g g g g |
| Residents | g g g | | |

### DETAILS

Year Built: 2004
Current Mgmt. Since: 2004
No. of Floors: 1
Resident Capacity: 132
Facility Type: Long-term care, Short-term rehab

### SPECIAL

Special diets accommodated
Proximity to Emergency Svcs.: Under 8 miles

### STAFF

Caregiver Training: Dementia, Ethics, Family communication, Grief, Pain management, Patient transfers, Stress management, Transition issues, Universal precautions, Validation therapy, Wound care
Criminal Background Check: Yes
Principal Staff Language(s): English
Other Staff Language(s): Spanish

### FACILITY FEATURES

Activities/Recreation
Beauty/Barber Shop ($)
Chapel Services
Facility Parking
Guest Meals
Outside Patio/Gardens
Private Dining Room
Private Visiting Room
Separate Therapy Room
Whirlpool Baths

### ROOM FEATURES

Cable TV Ready
Space for personal items
Shared & Private Bathrooms
Telephone Ready ($)

## COSTS

PRICES MAY INCREASE. PLEASE CALL FOR MOST CURRENT INFORMATION.

| | |
|---|---|
| Shared Room | $3,875–$4,185/month |
| Private Room | $6,510–$6,820/month |
| Respite Stays | Call for shared room rates |
| Rate Increase | Annually |
| Reimbursement | Medicare, Medicaid, LTCI, HMO, Private pay, SSI |

## PORTRAIT

Vista Ridge Nursing and Rehab is located in peaceful Lewisville, north of Dallas. The sheltered entrance dominates the red brick exterior. Flowers and trees grace the front lawn surrounding the parking lot. The facility has a convenient location near Vista Ridge Regional Mall and numerous restaurants, yet it is distant enough from major roads to retain its serene atmosphere.

The brightly lit entryway features seating areas and distinctive white columns. The large nurses' station at the front provides an excellent vantage point of each hallway. The hallways are wide and equipped with safety rails. Lighting throughout the facility is soft and natural. The residents who were socializing in the common areas seemed to be well acquainted; two of them were in the midst of a spirited conversation over seating arrangements. The entertainment areas feature comfortable Queen Anne furnishings and red and brown patterned carpet. Paintings of Grecian vases adorn the walls. The modern dining area is somewhat institutional. There are two sunny patio areas that feature plentiful seating.

Natural light fills the residents' small rooms. In addition to a hospital bed, which is attractively designed with a wooden headboard, each room also features built-in drawers and a cable outlet. During the tour, our guide stepped away to help a resident who was having difficulty walking. Gold stars mark the doors of residents who are prone to falls; this "falling star" system provides a reminder to staff to check on those residents frequently. To further facilitate safety, the staff is also mindful of keeping residents' rooms free of potential tripping hazards.

IN-HOME CARE PROVIDERS

## Anchor Home Health Services

310 Crooked Creek (972) 279-1846
Garland, TX 75043

SEE CHAPTER 1 FOR A DESCRIPTION OF IN-HOME CARE SERVICES.

### DETAILS

Years in Business: 6 months
Home Health Services Provided: Yes
Care Visits Provided Within a Facility: No
Dementia Care Provided: No
Will Replace Caregiver Within 48 Hours Upon Request: Yes

### CAREGIVERS

RN on Staff: Yes
Hiring Qualifications: 2 years of experience, DMV check, TB test, Criminal background check, CNA certification, 3 references required
Caregiver Training: Dementia, Ethics, Family communication, Grief, Patient transfers, Stress management
Frequency of Caregiver Training: Initial formal training program, Semiannual
Language(s) Spoken: English, Spanish

### AVAILABILITY

Service Availability: 24/7
On-call Supervisor Availability: 24/7

### COSTS

PRICES MAY INCREASE. PLEASE CALL FOR MOST CURRENT INFORMATION.

Rate: Call for rates
Minimum Hours per Day: None
Minimum Days per Week: None
Sliding Fee Schedule Available: Yes

### UNIQUE QUALITIES

Anchor Home Health Services takes great pride in the care they offer; they put clients' needs ahead of all else. They believe in establishing close relationships with clients and their families. Anchor Home is certified by Medicare and Medicaid.

## At Home Companions

1500 South Central Expressway
McKinney, TX 75070

(214) 726-1591
www.athomecompanions.net

SEE CHAPTER 1 FOR A DESCRIPTION OF IN-HOME CARE SERVICES.

### DETAILS

Years in Business: 1
Home Health Services Provided: No
Care Visits Provided Within a Facility: Yes
Dementia Care Provided: Yes
Will Replace Caregiver Within 48 Hours Upon Request: Yes

### CAREGIVERS

RN on Staff: Yes
Hiring Qualifications: DMV check, Criminal background check, 3 references required
Caregiver Training: Dementia, Ethics, Family communication, Grief, Patient transfers, Stress management
Frequency of Caregiver Training: Initial formal training program, Monthly
Language(s) Spoken: English, Spanish

### AVAILABILITY

Service Availability: 24/7
On-call Supervisor Availability: 24/7

### COSTS

PRICES MAY INCREASE. PLEASE CALL FOR MOST CURRENT INFORMATION.

Rate: $17/hour
Live-In: $250/day
Minimum Hours per Day: 3
Minimum Days per Week: None
Sliding Fee Schedule Available: No

### UNIQUE QUALITIES

At Home Companions tries to maintain its clients' independence and dignity for as long possible. The agency promotes a relationship based on trust between caregivers, clients and their families.

## Aunt Mae's Home Care, Inc.

2908 Cheverny (972) 542-3797
Mckinney, TX 75070

SEE CHAPTER 1 FOR A DESCRIPTION OF IN-HOME CARE SERVICES.

### DETAILS

Years in Business: 6 months
Home Health Services Provided: No
Care Visits Provided Within a Facility: Yes
Dementia Care Provided: Yes
Will Replace Caregiver Within 48 Hours Upon Request: Yes

### CAREGIVERS

RN on Staff: No
Hiring Qualifications: DMV check, Criminal background check, CNA certification, 3 references required
Caregiver Training: Dementia, Ethics, Family communication, Grief, Patient transfers, Transition issues
Frequency of Caregiver Training: Initial formal training program, Semiannual
Language(s) Spoken: English

### AVAILABILITY

Service Availability: 24/7
On-call Supervisor Availability: 24/7

### COSTS

PRICES MAY INCREASE. PLEASE CALL FOR MOST CURRENT INFORMATION.

Rate: Call for rates
Minimum Hours per Day: None
Minimum Days per Week: None
Sliding Fee Schedule Available: Yes

### UNIQUE QUALITIES

Aunt Mae's conducts a program of assessment and ongoing communication to enable each client to live independently. The owner contacts all clients personally to make sure they are happy with the care they are receiving. Any necessary adjustments are made accordingly. The agency is Medicare and Medicaid certified.

## Care Solutions Home Health LLC

1144 North Plano Road, Suite 11 (214) 646-6275
Richardson, TX 75081

SEE CHAPTER 1 FOR A DESCRIPTION OF IN-HOME CARE SERVICES.

### DETAILS

Years in Business: 1
Home Health Services Provided: No
Care Visits Provided Within a Facility: Yes
Dementia Care Provided: No
Will Replace Caregiver Within 48 Hours Upon Request: Yes

### CAREGIVERS

RN on Staff: No
Hiring Qualifications: 1 year of experience, Criminal background check, 2 references required
Caregiver Training: Dementia, Ethics, Family communication, Grief, Patient transfers, Stress management
Frequency of Caregiver Training: Initial formal training program, Monthly
Language(s) Spoken: English, Spanish

### AVAILABILITY

Service Availability: 24/7
On-call Supervisor Availability: 24/7

### COSTS

PRICES MAY INCREASE. PLEASE CALL FOR MOST CURRENT INFORMATION.

Rate: $18–$25/hour
Live-In: $215/day
Minimum Hours per Day: 4
Minimum Days per Week: None
Sliding Fee Schedule Available: No

### UNIQUE QUALITIES

Care Solutions' management believes it is important for clients and caregivers to be compatible, so they place clients accordingly. They try to create an atmosphere of fun for their clients, and to encourage mental and physical stimulation through daily activities. Caregivers attend continuing education classes on a monthly basis.

## Comfort Home Health Care, Inc.

410 West Main Street, Suite 102 (972) 203-1010
Mesquite, TX 75149

SEE CHAPTER 1 FOR A DESCRIPTION OF IN-HOME CARE SERVICES.

### DETAILS

Years in Business: 3
Home Health Services Provided: Yes
Care Visits Provided Within a Facility: Yes
Dementia Care Provided: No
Will Replace Caregiver Within 48 Hours Upon Request: Yes

### CAREGIVERS

RN on Staff: Yes
Hiring Qualifications: 1 year of experience, Criminal background check, 2 references required
Caregiver Training: Ethics, Family communication, Grief, Patient transfers, Stress management, Transition
Frequency of Caregiver Training: Initial formal training program, Quarterly
Language(s) Spoken: English, Spanish

### AVAILABILITY

Service Availability: 24/7
On-call Supervisor Availability: 24/7

### COSTS

PRICES MAY INCREASE. PLEASE CALL FOR MOST CURRENT INFORMATION.

Rate: Call for rates
Minimum Hours per Day: None
Minimum Days per Week: None
Sliding Fee Schedule Available: No

### UNIQUE QUALITIES

Comfort Home Health has an experienced nurse on staff who handles patients' needs. The management is in constant communication with caregivers in the field. The agency accepts Medicaid and Medicare.

## Comfort Keepers

231 West FM 544, Suite A101
Murphy, TX 75094
(972) 516-0055
www.comfortkeepers.com

SEE CHAPTER 1 FOR A DESCRIPTION OF IN-HOME CARE SERVICES.

### DETAILS

Years in Business: 2
Home Health Services Provided: No
Care Visits Provided Within a Facility: Yes
Dementia Care Provided: Yes
Will Replace Caregiver Within 48 Hours Upon Request: Yes

### CAREGIVERS

RN on Staff: Yes
Hiring Qualifications: 1 year of experience, DMV check, Criminal background check, CNA certification, 6 references required
Caregiver Training: Dementia, Ethics, Patient transfers
Frequency of Caregiver Training: Initial formal training program, Quarterly, Annually
Language(s) Spoken: English, Japanese, Russian, Sign Language, Spanish

### AVAILABILITY

Service Availability: 24/7
On-call Supervisor Availability: 24/7

### COSTS

PRICES MAY INCREASE. PLEASE CALL FOR MOST CURRENT INFORMATION.

Rate: Call for rates
Minimum Hours per Day: None
Minimum Days per Week: None
Sliding Fee Schedule Available: Yes

### UNIQUE QUALITIES

Comfort Keepers is the second largest homecare agency in the U.S. To maintain clients' comfort as well as their independence, the agency finds the best match between clients and caregivers. Comfort Keepers encourages strong relationships between caregivers, clients and their families. The caregivers enhance their skills through continuing education.

## Friendship Home Health Agency

190 North Stemmons Freeway, Suite 20 (214) 682-9508
Lewisville, TX 75067

SEE CHAPTER 1 FOR A DESCRIPTION OF IN-HOME CARE SERVICES.

### DETAILS

Years in Business: 1
Home Health Services Provided: Yes
Care Visits Provided Within a Facility: Yes
Dementia Care Provided: Yes
Will Replace Caregiver Within 48 Hours Upon Request: Yes

### CAREGIVERS

RN on Staff: Yes
Hiring Qualifications: 3 years of experience, DMV check, Criminal background check, CNA certification, CPR certification, 3 references required
Caregiver Training: Dementia, Ethics, Family communication, Grief, Patient transfers, Stress management
Frequency of Caregiver Training: Initial formal training program, Annually
Language(s) Spoken: English, French, Spanish, Vietnamese

### AVAILABILITY

Service Availability: 24/7
On-call Supervisor Availability: 24/7

### COSTS

PRICES MAY INCREASE. PLEASE CALL FOR MOST CURRENT INFORMATION.

Rate: Call for rates
Minimum Hours per Day: None
Minimum Days per Week: None
Sliding Fee Schedule Available: Yes

### UNIQUE QUALITIES

Friendship Home Health treats its clients like they would family members. Caregivers and clients are carefully matched, based on each client's special needs. The owner, a RN, is neonatal certified. All Friendship Home Health employees are CPR certified.

## Grace Healthcare Services

12959 Jupiter Road, Suite 230 (214) 221-8585
Dallas, TX 75238

SEE CHAPTER 1 FOR A DESCRIPTION OF IN-HOME CARE SERVICES.

### DETAILS

Years in Business: 4
Home Health Services Provided: Yes
Care Visits Provided Within a Facility: Yes
Dementia Care Provided: Yes
Will Replace Caregiver Within 48 Hours Upon Request: Yes

### CAREGIVERS

RN on Staff: Yes
Hiring Qualifications: 2 years of experience, TB test, Criminal background check, CNA certification, 2 references required
Caregiver Training: Dementia, Ethics, Family communication, Patient transfers
Frequency of Caregiver Training: Initial formal training program, Monthly
Language(s) Spoken: English, Spanish

### AVAILABILITY

Service Availability: 24/7
On-call Supervisor Availability: 24/7

### COSTS

PRICES MAY INCREASE. PLEASE CALL FOR MOST CURRENT INFORMATION.

Rate: Call for rates
Minimum Hours per Day: None
Minimum Days per Week: None
Sliding Fee Schedule Available: No

### UNIQUE QUALITIES

Grace Healthcare Services works hard to build strong relationships with clients and their families. One of the agency's top priorities is to maintain clients' dignity. Grace Healthcare caregivers attend monthly continuing education sessions.

## Heaven At Home

1104 Dallas Drive, Suite 234 A
Denton, TX 76205

(940) 380-0500
(866) 381-0500
www.heavenathomecare.com

SEE CHAPTER I FOR A DESCRIPTION OF IN-HOME CARE SERVICES.

### DETAILS

Years in Business: Unknown
Home Health Services Provided: No
Care Visits Provided Within a Facility: Yes
Dementia Care Provided: No
Will Replace Caregiver Within 48 Hours Upon Request: Yes

### CAREGIVERS

RN on Staff: Yes
Hiring Qualifications: 3 years of experience, DMV check, TB test, Criminal background check, CNA certification, 3 references required
Caregiver Training: Dementia, Ethics, Family communication, Grief, Patient transfers, Stress management
Frequency of Caregiver Training: Initial formal training program, Monthly
Language(s) Spoken: English, Spanish

### AVAILABILITY

Service Availability: 24/7
On-call Supervisor Availability: 24/7

### COSTS

PRICES MAY INCREASE. PLEASE CALL FOR MOST CURRENT INFORMATION.

Rate: $14.95–$17.95/hour
Live-In: $175–$225/day
Sleepover: $125–$135/night
Minimum Hours per Day: 4
Minimum Days per Week: 3
Sliding Fee Schedule Available: No

### UNIQUE QUALITIES

Heaven at Home's objective is to help clients stay safely at home, thereby preserving their dignity and independence. To that end, the caregivers address the concerns of clients as well their families, and work closely with home health care and hospice services. This agency serves Collin, Cooke, Dallas, Denton, Grayson, Tarrant and Wise counties.

## Homewatch Caregivers

1700 Alma Drive, Suite 242
Plano, TX 75075

(972) 422-1156
(800) 777-9770
www.homewatchcaregivers.com

---

SEE CHAPTER 1 FOR A DESCRIPTION OF IN-HOME CARE SERVICES.

### DETAILS

Years in Business: 20
Home Health Services Provided: No
Care Visits Provided Within a Facility: Yes
Dementia Care Provided: Yes
Will Replace Caregiver Within 48 Hours Upon Request: Yes

### CAREGIVERS

RN on Staff: Yes
Hiring Qualifications: 2 years of experience, Criminal background check, 3 references required
Caregiver Training: Dementia, Ethics, Family communication, Grief, Patient transfers, Stress management
Frequency of Caregiver Training: Initial formal training program, Quarterly
Language(s) Spoken: English

### AVAILABILITY

Service Availability: 24/7
On-call Supervisor Availability: 24/7

### COSTS

PRICES MAY INCREASE. PLEASE CALL FOR MOST CURRENT INFORMATION.

Rate: Call for rates
Minimum Hours per Day: None
Minimum Days per Week: None
Sliding Fee Schedule Available: No

### UNIQUE QUALITIES

Homewatch Caregivers' excellent reputation is built on twenty years of experience. Its services include mentally stimulating activities that are designed to maintain clients' dignity and independence. The agency employs an open-door policy to promote peace of mind in clients and their families. Caregivers undergo training on a continual basis. Homewatch does not require money or deposits up front.

## Lifeline Healthcare Services

1104 Lamplightway
Allen, TX 75013
(214) 724-2866

SEE CHAPTER 1 FOR A DESCRIPTION OF IN-HOME CARE SERVICES.

### DETAILS

Years in Business: 1
Home Health Services Provided: Yes
Care Visits Provided Within a Facility: No
Dementia Care Provided: Yes
Will Replace Caregiver Within 48 Hours Upon Request: Yes

### CAREGIVERS

RN on Staff: Yes
Hiring Qualifications: 1 year of experience, DMV check, TB test, Criminal background check, CNA certification, Employee misconduct register check, 3 references required
Caregiver Training: Dementia, Ethics, Family communication, Patient transfers
Frequency of Caregiver Training: Initial formal training program, Semiannual
Language(s) Spoken: English, Mandarin, Spanish

### AVAILABILITY

Service Availability: 24/7
On-call Supervisor Availability: 24/7

### COSTS

PRICES MAY INCREASE. PLEASE CALL FOR MOST CURRENT INFORMATION.

Rate: Call for rates
Minimum Hours per Day: 4
Minimum Days per Week: None
Sliding Fee Schedule Available: Yes

### UNIQUE QUALITIES

Lifeline Healthcare Services works with low-income clients. The agency promotes healthy and caring relationships between clients, their families and caregivers. Lifeline is Medicare and Medicaid certified.

## Miracle Home Health, Inc.

810 Office Park Circle, Suite 112 (972) 436-5229
Lewisville, TX 75057

SEE CHAPTER 1 FOR A DESCRIPTION OF IN-HOME CARE SERVICES.

### DETAILS

Years in Business: 8
Home Health Services Provided: Yes
Care Visits Provided Within a Facility: Yes
Dementia Care Provided: Yes
Will Replace Caregiver Within 48 Hours Upon Request: Yes

### CAREGIVERS

RN on Staff: Yes
Hiring Qualifications: TB test, Criminal background check, 4 references required
Caregiver Training: Ethics, Stress management, Transition issues
Frequency of Caregiver Training: Initial formal training program, Monthly
Language(s) Spoken: Cantonese, Vietnamese

### AVAILABILITY

Service Availability: Based on individual need
On-call Supervisor Availability: 24/7

### COSTS

PRICES MAY INCREASE. PLEASE CALL FOR MOST CURRENT INFORMATION.

Rate: Call for rates
Minimum Hours per Day: None
Minimum Days per Week: None
Sliding Fee Schedule Available: No

### UNIQUE QUALITIES

Miracle Home Health treats clients with respect and strives to preserve each person's dignity. The staff includes nurses who are skilled in caring for dementia clients, and are very experienced with wound care. The staff doctor makes house calls. The agency's occupational therapist is available twenty-four hours a day. Miracle Home Health is Medicare certified.

## Paradigm Home Health Services

6033 Melody Lane, Suite 141 (214) 378-8484
Dallas, TX 75231

SEE CHAPTER 1 FOR A DESCRIPTION OF IN-HOME CARE SERVICES.

### DETAILS

Years in Business: 21
Home Health Services Provided: No
Care Visits Provided Within a Facility: Yes
Dementia Care Provided: Yes
Will Replace Caregiver Within 48 Hours Upon Request: Yes

### CAREGIVERS

RN on Staff: Yes
Hiring Qualifications: 1 year of experience, DMV check, TB test, Criminal background check, CNA certification, 4 references required
Caregiver Training: Dementia, Ethics, Family communication, Grief, Patient transfers, Stress management
Frequency of Caregiver Training: Initial formal training program, Monthly
Language(s) Spoken: English, French, Spanish

### AVAILABILITY

Service Availability: 24/7
On-call Supervisor Availability: 24/7

### COSTS

PRICES MAY INCREASE. PLEASE CALL FOR MOST CURRENT INFORMATION.

Rate: Call for rates
Minimum Hours per Day: None
Minimum Days per Week: None
Sliding Fee Schedule Available: No

### UNIQUE QUALITIES

Paradigm has provided homecare for over two decades. The administrator makes regular home visits to ensure that clients' needs are being met. Paradigm specializes in caring for people with dementia. The agency provides a monthly continuing education program to its caregivers.

## Primestaff Home Health Agency

3906 Lemmon Avenue, Suite 212
Dallas, TX 75219
(214) 599-9083
www.domestic-agency.com

SEE CHAPTER 1 FOR A DESCRIPTION OF IN-HOME CARE SERVICES.

### DETAILS

Years in Business: 26
Home Health Services Provided: No
Care Visits Provided Within a Facility: Yes
Dementia Care Provided: Yes
Will Replace Caregiver Within 48 Hours Upon Request: Yes

### CAREGIVERS

RN on Staff: Yes
Hiring Qualifications: 4 years of experience, DMV check, TB test, Criminal background check, CNA certification, 3 references required
Caregiver Training: Dementia, Ethics, Family communication, Grief, Patient transfers, Transition issues
Frequency of Caregiver Training: Initial formal training program
Language(s) Spoken: English, Spanish

### AVAILABILITY

Service Availability: 24/7
On-call Supervisor Availability: 24/7

### COSTS

PRICES MAY INCREASE. PLEASE CALL FOR MOST CURRENT INFORMATION.

Rate: $15.50–$18.50/hour
Live-In: $200/day
Minimum Hours per Day: 4
Minimum Days per Week: None
Sliding Fee Schedule Available: Yes

### UNIQUE QUALITIES

Primestaff has been in operation for twenty-six years. The caregivers take an individualized approach to client care. The agency offers personal assistance, home management and companionship services, and makes a concerted effort to keep its rates competitive.

## Trinity Home Health Care

400 South Zang Boulevard, Suite 610 (214) 942-3200
Dallas, TX 75208

SEE CHAPTER 1 FOR A DESCRIPTION OF IN-HOME CARE SERVICES.

### DETAILS

Years in Business: 14
Home Health Services Provided: Yes
Care Visits Provided Within a Facility: Yes
Dementia Care Provided: Yes
Will Replace Caregiver Within 48 Hours Upon Request: Yes

### CAREGIVERS

RN on Staff: Yes
Hiring Qualifications: 2 years of experience, DMV check, TB test, Criminal background check, CNA certification, 3 references required
Caregiver Training: Dementia, Ethics, Grief, Patient transfers, Stress management, Transition issues
Frequency of Caregiver Training: Initial formal training program, Quarterly
Language(s) Spoken: English, French, Hindi, Sign Language, Spanish

### AVAILABILITY

Service Availability: 24/7
On-call Supervisor Availability: 24/7

### COSTS

PRICES MAY INCREASE. PLEASE CALL FOR MOST CURRENT INFORMATION.

Rate: Call for rates
Minimum Hours per Day: None
Minimum Days per Week: None
Sliding Fee Schedule Available: No

### UNIQUE QUALITIES

Trinity boasts a neuropathy program and anodyne therapy, which is used to reduce pain and increase circulation. Trinity has extensive experience in caring for clients with congestive heart failure. The caregiving staff is impressively multilingual. Trinity is Medicare and Medicaid certified.

ADULT DAY CARE CENTERS

## Friend's Place Adult Day Services A/D

1960 Nantucket Drive
Richardson, TX 75080

(982) 437-2940
www.friendsplaceads.com

---

### GILBERT GUIDE OBSERVATIONS gggg

#### DETAILS

Owner/Affiliation: Pam Kovacs
Years in Business: Less than 1
License/Certification: Texas Department of Aging and Disability Services, Texas Department of Human Services
Business Hours: Monday–Friday, 8:00am–6:00pm
Conditions Accepted: Alzheimer's/Dementia, Incontinence, Limited mobility, Vision/Hearing impairment

#### SPECIAL

Special diets accommodated
Wheelchair accessible
Proximity to Emergency Svcs.: Under 8 miles

#### STAFF

Staff/Patient Ratio: 1:6
Criminal Background Check: Yes
Language(s) Spoken: English, Spanish

#### COSTS

Prices may increase. Please call for most current information.
Daily Costs: $45–$75 based on individual need
Reimbursement: LTCI, Private pay

#### PORTRAIT

Friend's Place serves mainly a dementia clientele. The caring owner and staff focus on developing warm relationships with the participants. A variety of stimulating activities are offered, ranging from croquet and dancing to trivia games and craft projects. Multiple activities, such as pet therapy and cooking, are directed simultaneously in different areas of the facility. The white stucco building is divided into an array of spaces, including an outdoor patio, a music room and a barbershop, as well as a number of themed rooms where participants reminisce. Some participants prefer more "useful" activities, such as watering the garden or feeding the birds.

Participants enjoy breakfast, lunch and snacks planned by the staff dietician. Lunch is a formal affair that involves several courses—even dessert! Meals take place in the dining room, which features elegant Chippendale furniture. The dietician ensures that participants follow

FRIEND'S PLACE ADULT DAY SERVICES (CONTINUED)

any special diets ordered by their doctors. The facility's nurse sees to participants' care, through services such as blood pressure monitoring and administering medications. For a nominal fee, participants may receive assistance with showering and other activities such as nail care and massage.

Friend's Place Resource Center offers support groups for caregivers and family members of individuals with dementia and related conditions. The center also educates caregivers on Alzheimer's, communication and a variety of other helpful topics.

## ADULT DAY HEALTH CARE CENTERS

### Day Stay for Adults A/D

2109 West University Drive
Denton, TX 76201

(940) 383-8371
www.daystay.org

---

**GILBERT GUIDE OVERALL OBSERVATIONS** g g g

#### DETAILS

Owner/Affiliation: Day Stay for Adults
Years in Business: 11
License/Certification: Texas Department of Aging and Disabilities
Business Hours: Monday–Friday, 7:30am–5:30pm
Conditions Accepted: Alzheimer's/Dementia, Developmental disabilities, HIV/AIDS, Incontinence, Limited mobility, Mental illness, Stroke, Traumatic brain injury, Vision/Hearing impairment

#### SPECIAL

Special diets accommodated
Wheelchair accessible
Proximity to Emergency Svcs.: Under 8 miles
Onsite Care: Nursing, Occupational therapy, Physical therapy

#### STAFF

Staff/patient ration: 1:8
Criminal Background Check: Yes
Language(s) spoken: English, Spanish

#### COSTS

PRICES MAY INCREASE. PLEASE CALL FOR MOST CURRENT INFORMATION.

Daily Costs: $40
Reimbursement: Medicaid, LTCI

### PORTRAIT

Day Stay for Adults serves ill and impaired Denton County residents who are eighteen and older. The facility enjoys a convenient location on West University Drive, a major Denton thoroughfare. Presbyterian Hospital of Denton and the University of North Texas are nearby. The wheelchair-accessible building has ample parking. Abundant windows flood the well-maintained interior with sunlight. Numerous couches, chairs and tables furnish the main room, which also features a TV.

We found Day Stay interns and direct care staff extremely friendly. A registered dietician monitors the nutritious snacks and meals served at the facility. The staff also features a licensed nurse who supervises participants' care and administers their prescriptions. Day Stay happily provides participants with transportation to medical appointments. Participants enjoy a variety of stimulating activities, including pet and music therapy, bingo, dominoes, card games, exercise and arts and crafts.

#### GERIATRIC CARE MANAGERS

## DALLAS CARE CONNECTION

Carol K. Franzen, MS, LMSW
P.O. Box 815848
Dallas, TX 75381

(972) 242-0901
cfranzen@dallascareconnection.com
www.dallascareconnection.com

SEE CHAPTER 1 FOR A DESCRIPTION OF GERIATRIC CARE MANAGER SERVICES.

### DETAILS

Years of GCM Experience: 21
Degree(s) Held: Licensed Master Social Worker
Member of National Association of Professional Geriatric Care Managers
Language(s) Spoken: English

### SERVICES

Staff on Call: 24/7
Client References Provided: Yes
Areas of Practice: Assessment, Care management, Counseling, Education, Family/Professional liaison
Assistance with Medicare/Medicaid Process: Yes

### COSTS

PRICES MAY INCREASE. PLEASE CALL FOR MOST CURRENT INFORMATION.

Assessment: Call for rates
Hourly: Call for rates

DALLAS CARE CONNECTION (CONTINUED)

### UNIQUE QUALITIES

With over twenty years of case management experience behind her, Carol K. Franzen is highly skilled in assisting seniors and people with disabilities. Carol has provided case management services in the Dallas-Fort Worth area since 1985. Not surprisingly, other local care managers have referred a number of challenging cases to Dallas Care Connection; Carol's familiarity with long-term care services in the area is a great strength.

## KAY PAGGI, LPC, NCGC, CMC

1134 Wilderness Trail
Richardson, TX 75080

(972) 839-0065
kay@kaypaggi.com
www.kaypaggi.com

SEE CHAPTER 1 FOR A DESCRIPTION OF GERIATRIC CARE MANAGER SERVICES.

### DETAILS

Years of GCM Experience: 10
Degree(s) Held: Certified Care Manager, Licensed Professional Counselor
Member of National Association of Professional Geriatric Care Managers
Language(s) Spoken: English

### SERVICES

Staff on Call: 24/7
Client References Provided: Yes
Areas of Practice: Assessment, Care management, Counseling, Education, Family/Professional liaison
Assistance with Medicare/Medicaid Process: Yes

### COSTS

PRICES MAY INCREASE. PLEASE CALL FOR MOST CURRENT INFORMATION.

Hourly: $70

### UNIQUE QUALITIES

Kay Paggi is the only National Certified Gerontological Counselor (NCGC) in the North Texas area. Her thorough care assessments include asking her elderly clients how they perceive aging, how they cared for their own parents, and what their expectations are for the final stage of life. This information guides her care recommendations. Kay counsels adult children privately and facilitates discussion and support groups for adults who are caring for their parents. Some of the topics include information on end-of-life care and purchasing long-term care insurance.

**HOSPICE PROVIDERS**

## Southern Care Denton

5800 North I-35, Suite 200
Denton, TX 76207

(940) 243-0901
www.southerncarehospice.com

SEE CHAPTER 1 FOR A DESCRIPTION OF HOSPICE SERVICES.

### DETAILS

Affiliation: None
Licensed By: Texas Department of Health Services
Medicare certified

### CARE

At-home Care Provided: Yes
Inpatient Care Provided: No
Caregivers trained, supervised, and monitored
Supervisor on call 24/7
Language(s) Spoken: English

### UNIQUE QUALITIES

Southern Care strives for excellence in all facets of client care. The driving force behind outstanding service begins with the employees; the agency recognizes the magnitude of end-of-life care and handpicks caregivers that are special in skill and personality. The agency scored 100% on its Medicare certification with the Texas Department of Health Services.

# MID-CITIES

ASSISTED LIVING FACILITIES

## Alterra Clare Bridge Cottage A/D

7520 B Glenview Drive
Richland Hills, TX 76118

(817) 589-9688
www.assisted.com

### GILBERT GUIDE OBSERVATIONS

| | | | |
|---|---|---|---|
| Administration & Staff | g g g g | Dietary & Food Selection | g g g |
| Facility Aesthetics | g g g | Activities | g g g |
| Facility Condition & Safety | g g g | Alzheimer's & Dementia Capabilities | g g g g |
| Residents | g g g | | |

### DETAILS

Year Built: 1997
Year Remodeled: 2001
Current Mgmt. Since: 1997
No. of Floors: 1
Resident Capacity: 32

### SPECIAL

Alzheimer's/Dementia Only Facility
Diets Accommodated: Diabetic, Low-fat, Low-salt
Proximity to Emergency Svcs.: Under 8 miles
Nearby shopping and entertainment
No pets allowed

### STAFF

Nurse/LVN/LPN: 40 hours/week, On-call 24/7
Caregiver Training: Dementia, Ethics, Family communication, Grief, Stress management, Transition issues, Validation therapy
Criminal Background Check: Yes
Principal Staff Language(s): English

### FACILITY FEATURES

Activities/Recreation
Beauty/Barber Shop ($)
Guest Meals ($)
Outside Patio/Gardens
Pharmaceutical Service
Private Dining Room
Separate Therapy Room
Transportation to MD Appointments, Scheduled Outings
24-hour Security

### ROOM FEATURES

Cable TV Ready ($)
Emergency Call System
Furnished
Shared & Private Bathrooms
Telephone Ready ($)
Temperature Controls

### COSTS

PRICES MAY INCREASE. PLEASE CALL FOR MOST CURRENT INFORMATION.

| | |
|---|---|
| Alzheimer's Unit | $1,995/month for shared room<br>$2,495/month for private room |
| Costs of Care | $300–$1,200/month based on individual need |
| Rate Increase | Annually; usually 2–3% |
| Reimbursement | LTCI, Private pay, Veterans |

## PORTRAIT

Alterra Clare Bridge Cottage shares an expansive, lush campus with its sister assisted living facility. Past the secured entrance, a quaint common area features a red brick fireplace flanked by built-in bookcases. Rich sofas and chairs in deep grays, maroons and greens are lovely against the subdued walls; attractive painted landscapes add the finishing touch.

Residents' semi-private rooms are spacious enough to accommodate two nightstands and twin beds. Each room features dark green carpeting and eggshell-colored walls. Residents personalize their rooms with memory box displays of personal knickknacks and memorabilia. Each hallway is painted a different color to help residents easily identify their rooms. Both dining areas (one is reserved for residents who require more assistance) are strategically located close to the activity area and center courtyard. The cozy layout gives staff a clear vantage point of residents in each area. Residents are able to wander safely within the secured courtyard. The garden features grassy lawns and many shaded spots for outdoor relaxation. Paved sections of the patio accommodate residents who use wheelchairs.

Residents enjoy a packed activities calendar. At least twice a week, residents from both the Cottage and the assisted living facility get together for shared events, allowing a change of scenery for both groups. Other scheduled activities include morning exercise, cooking pursuits and staff-chaperoned trips to plays and North East Mall. Alterra Clare Bridge residents seem very active. Staff and residents interacted comfortably with one another during our visit. When we arrived, residents were busy preparing various snacks for the holiday party scheduled that day.

# ALTERRA STERLING HOUSE OF RICHLAND HILLS

7520 A Glenview Drive
Richland Hills, TX 76118

(817) 589-8600
www.assisted.com

---

### GILBERT GUIDE OBSERVATIONS

| | | | |
|---|---|---|---|
| Administration & Staff | g g g g | Residents | g g g |
| Facility Aesthetics | g g g | Dietary & Food Selection | g g g g g |
| Facility Condition & Safety | g g g | Activities | g g g g |

## DETAILS

Year Built: 1997
Year Remodeled: 2000
Current Mgmt. Since: 1997
No. of Floors: 1
Resident Capacity: 37

## SPECIAL

Mild dementia care provided
Diets Accommodated: Diabetic, Low-fat, Low-salt
Proximity to Emergency Svcs.: Under 8 miles
Nearby shopping and entertainment
No pets allowed

ALTERRA STERLING HOUSE OF RICHLAND HILLS (CONTINUED)

### STAFF

Nurse/LVN/LPN: 40 hours/week, On-call 24/7
Caregiver Training: Dementia, Ethics, Family communication, Grief, Patient transfers, Stress management, Transition issues, Validation therapy
Criminal Background Check: Yes
Principal Staff Language(s): English

### FACILITY FEATURES

Activities/Recreation
Beauty/Barber Shop ($)
Facility Parking
Guest Meals ($)
Outside Patio/Gardens
Pharmaceutical Service
Private Dining Room
Transportation to MD Appointments, Scheduled Outings

### ROOM FEATURES

Cable TV Ready ($)
Emergency Call System
Kitchenette
Private Bathrooms
Telephone Ready ($)
Temperature Controls

### COSTS

PRICES MAY INCREASE. PLEASE CALL FOR MOST CURRENT INFORMATION.

| | |
|---|---|
| Studio Apt. | $1,995/month |
| One Bedroom Apt. | $2,195–$2,395/month |
| Costs of Care | $200–$1,800/month based on individual need |
| Rate Increase | Annually; usually 2% |
| Reimbursement | LTCI, Private pay, Veterans |

### PORTRAIT

Alterra Sterling House of Richland Hills resembles a country home with its red brick frame, white awnings and stone entryway. In the lobby, blue upholstered sofas and chairs are striking against the rich green carpeting. Next to the fireplace is a magnificent floor-to-ceiling bookcase that calls attention to the vaulted ceiling overhead. The fireplace serves as a partition, separating the lobby and TV room.

Residents' rooms receive plenty of natural light. The broad hallways are equipped with handrails and decked with photographs of the residents. The dining area doubles as the activity room. When we arrived, fragrant aromas filled the air as Chef Janet and the kitchen staff whipped up an appetizing menu of barbeque chicken, rice, oriental vegetables, creamy salad and assorted spice cakes. The center courtyard is a popular area for lounging. The shaded portion of the patio features rocking chairs and benches; in the garden, residents plant seasonal vegetables, fruits and flowers.

Residents regularly participate in outings to Wal-Mart, movie theaters and even the zoo! Crafty residents enjoy a candle-making workshop. The atmosphere at the facility is energetic and vibrant. Groups of residents and staff were hard at work making holiday decorations for the house during our visit. Pleasant conversation between the two groups could be heard throughout the facility. Many of the staff members have been with the residence for over five years. We found their eagerness to attend to residents' needs touching.

## Alterra Sterling House of Watauga

5800 North Park Drive
Watauga, Texas 76148

(817) 498-2222
www.assisted.com

---

**GILBERT GUIDE OBSERVATIONS**

| | | | |
|---|---|---|---|
| Administration & Staff | g g g | Residents | g g g |
| Facility Aesthetics | g g g | Dietary & Food Selection | g g g g |
| Facility Condition & Safety | g g g | Activities | g g g g |

### DETAILS

Year Built: 1997
Year Remodeled: 2000
Current Mgmt. Since: 1997
No. of Floors: 1
Resident Capacity: 35

### SPECIAL

Mild dementia care provided
Diets Accommodated: Diabetic, Low-fat, Low-salt
Proximity to Emergency Svcs.: Under 8 miles
Nearby shopping and entertainment
No pets allowed

### STAFF

Nurse/LVN/LPN: 40 hours/week, On-call 24/7
Caregiver Training: Dementia, Ethics, Family communication, Grief, Stress management, Transition issues, Validation therapy
Criminal Background Check: Yes
Principal Staff Language(s): English

### FACILITY FEATURES

Activities/Recreation
Beauty/Barber Shop ($)
Facility Parking
Guest Meals ($)
Outside Patio/Gardens
Pharmaceutical Service
Private Dining Room
Transportation to MD Appointments, Scheduled Outings

### ROOM FEATURES

Cable TV Ready ($)
Emergency Call System
Kitchenette
Private Bathrooms
Telephone Ready ($)
Temperature Controls

### COSTS

PRICES MAY INCREASE. PLEASE CALL FOR MOST CURRENT INFORMATION.

| | |
|---|---|
| Studio Apt. | $1,995/month |
| One Bedroom Apt. | $2,195–$2,395/month |
| Costs of Care | $200–$1,000/month based on individual need |

ALTERRA STERLING HOUSE OF WATAUGA (CONTINUED)

| | |
|---|---|
| Rate Increase | Annually; usually 2–3% |
| Reimbursement | LTCI, Private pay, Veterans |

**PORTRAIT**

Alterra Sterling House of Watauga is located in a residential area off of Highway 377. A grand portico shades the west entrance to the brick facility. Crepe myrtles and budding flowerbeds add color to the lawns, while grand oak trees line the perimeter. The interior is undeniably cozy. Pictures of residents and their families adorn the walls, adding a homey quality.

Residents' rooms are spacious and bright. Rich purple carpeting complements the oak accents in each room. The dining room flanking the lobby opens up to a comfortably furnished common area with a big-screen TV. The open layout is more reminiscent of a family home than an assisted living facility. Chef Tim and his kitchen staff prepare delicious and generously portioned meals. The appetizing aroma of pot roast, seasoned red potatoes, baby carrots and corn bread wafted from the dining area during our lunchtime visit.

The groomed courtyard in the center of the facility is a popular gathering spot for residents. The garden boasts such striking features as a pebbled walkway, a gazebo and a beautiful magnolia tree. We observed residents utilizing the furnished rest areas in the hallways for group card games and dominoes. Plenty of windows let in an abundance of natural light.

Residents at Watauga enjoy a calendar chock-full of events. From Red Hat Society functions to "boys' night out" and weekly trips to the grocery store, everyone has an opportunity to participate. At the time of our visit, residents and staff were busy decorating for the Christmas celebration, in which they hosted children from the neighboring elementary school. Residents seemed to be very much at home.

## ARDEN COURTS OF ARLINGTON A/D

1501 Northeast Green Oaks Boulevard
Arlington, TX 76006

(817) 795-1700
www.hcr-manorcare.com

**GILBERT GUIDE OBSERVATIONS**

| | | | |
|---|---|---|---|
| Administration & Staff | g g g g | Dietary & Food Selection | g g g g g |
| Facility Aesthetics | g g g g | Activities | g g g g g |
| Facility Condition & Safety | g g g g g | Alzheimer's & Dementia Capabilities | g g g g g |
| Residents | g g g g | | |

**DETAILS**

Year Built: 1999
Year Remodeled: 1999
Current Mgmt. Since:
No. of Floors: 1
Resident Capacity: 60

**SPECIAL**

Alzheimer's/Dementia Only Facility
Diets Accommodated: Diabetic, Low-fat, Low-salt, Renal
Proximity to Emergency Svcs.: Under 8 miles
Nearby shopping and entertainment
Pet visits allowed

**STAFF**

Nurse/LVN/LPN: 60 hours/week
Caregiver Training: Dementia, Ethics, Family communication, Patient transfers, Stress management, Transition issues, Validation therapy
Criminal Background Check: Yes
Principal Staff Language(s): English
Other Staff Language(s): Spanish

**FACILITY FEATURES**

Activities/Recreation
Beauty/Barber Shop
Chapel Services
Computer/Internet Access
Facility Parking
Guest Meals ($)
Outside Patio/Gardens
Pharmaceutical Service
Private Dining Room
24-hour Security

**ROOM FEATURES**

Cable TV Ready ($)
Furnished
Grab Bars
Shared & Private Bathrooms
Telephone Ready ($)
Temperature Controls

**COSTS**

PRICES MAY INCREASE. PLEASE CALL FOR MOST CURRENT INFORMATION.

| | |
|---|---|
| Alzheimer's Unit | $3,700/month for private room |
| Respite Stays | $75–$125/day for private room |
| Costs of Care | Based on individual need |
| Rate Increase | Annually |
| Reimbursement | LTCI, Private pay |

**PORTRAIT**

Arden Courts is nestled in a hilly, upscale neighborhood of Arlington. Its surrounding woodsy landscaping and quiet isolation makes for a country-like haven within the city. The interior color scheme is an attractive blend of earthy tones. A mixture of fresh and artificial flower arrangements are bright accents to the shadow box displays sitting outside residents' rooms. Comfortably furnished common areas are strategically spaced throughout the building. Residents' rooms are moderately sized, and all have windows.

The building is divided into four wings; each has its own dining and common areas, kitchen, bathroom and laundry room. The layout facilitates closeness and familiarity among neighboring residents. The secured outdoor area provides refuge as well as safety. The raised

ARDEN COURTS OF ARLINGTON (CONTINUED)

planters and gardens are designed for easy accessibility; residents are encouraged to participate in leisure gardening.

The wide hallways are free of clutter and are furnished intermittently with seating areas to encourage socializing among residents. Arden Courts residents enjoy various physical and mentally stimulating activities each month. The home offers Montesorri-based programming tailored to the needs of residents with Alzheimer's; the program focuses on individual abilities and strengths to increase participation and skill level.

## Arkansas House

1103 West Arkansas Lane
Arlington, TX 76013

(817) 861-4644

---

**GILBERT GUIDE OBSERVATIONS**

| | | | |
|---|---|---|---|
| Administration & Staff | g g g g g | Residents | g g g |
| Facility Aesthetics | g g g g | Dietary & Food Selection | g g g g |
| Facility Condition & Safety | g g g g g | Activities | g g g g |

### DETAILS

Year Built: 1985
Year Remodeled: 2005
Current Mgmt. Since: 1985
No. of Floors: 2
Resident Capacity: 75

### SPECIAL

Mild dementia care provided
Diets Accommodated: Diabetic
Proximity to Emergency Svcs.: Under 8 miles
Nearby shopping and entertainment
Pets allowed

### STAFF

Nurse/LVN/LPN: 8 hours/week
Caregiver Training: Dementia, Ethics, Family communication, Patient transfers, Transition issues
Criminal Background Check: Yes
Principal Staff Language(s): English
Other Staff Language(s): Spanish

### FACILITY FEATURES

Activities/Recreation
Beauty/Barber Shop
Chapel Services
Facility Parking
Guest Meals
Private Dining Room
Room Service
Separate Therapy Room
Transportation to MD Appointments ($), Scheduled Outings

### ROOM FEATURES

Cable TV Ready ($)
Emergency Call System
Grab Bars
Kitchenette
Shared & Private Bathrooms
Telephone Ready ($)

### COSTS

PRICES MAY INCREASE. PLEASE CALL FOR MOST CURRENT INFORMATION.

| | |
|---|---|
| One Bedroom Apt. | $1,795–$1,895/month<br>Double occupancy add $995/month |
| Two Bedroom Apt. | $2,095–$2,295/month |
| Costs of Care | Based on individual need |
| Rate Increase | Annually |
| Reimbursement | Private pay, Veterans |
| Entrance Fee | $500 |
| Security Deposit | $500 + $25/month |
| Pet Deposit | $500 |

### PORTRAIT

Arkansas House Assisted Living is part of an active Arlington neighborhood. Parking is available at the rear of the building. The attractive landscaping includes a manicured lawn with ornamental shrubs. The home was established over twenty years ago, but thanks to a recent remodel, the interior appears brand new. Residents' rooms surround the common areas, each of which is furnished to resemble a living room; all of the common areas are uniquely decorated. Residents may choose from floor plans that range from one-bedrooms to apartment-like units that feature separate living areas. Residents enjoy ample natural light and lovely views in their rooms. The wide hallways allow wheelchair users to easily navigate the facility. The building houses two dining areas, both of which are beautifully appointed and boast restaurant-style service. Fresh flowers throughout the home are bright reminders of the outdoors. The facility's grounds include an inviting wooden deck where residents may often be found visiting and enjoying the fresh air.

The relationships between residents and staff are warm and comfortable. The staff members seem well acquainted with each resident's personality and preferences. Many of the staff members have a long history working at Arkansas House—the manager has been there for twenty-eight years! The residents love to play board games and attend socials. Field trips are another favorite activity.

## AUTUMN LEAVES OF ARLINGTON A/D

514 Central Park Drive
Arlington, TX 76014

(817) 419-6700, (817) 691-6602
www.autumnleavesliving.com

---

**GILBERT GUIDE OBSERVATIONS**

| | | | |
|---|---|---|---|
| Administration & Staff | g g g g | Dietary & Food Selection | g g g |
| Facility Aesthetics | g g g g | Activities | g g g g |
| Facility Condition & Safety | g g g g | Alzheimer's & Dementia Capabilities | g g g g |
| Residents | g g g g | | |

AUTUMN LEAVES OF ARLINGTON (CONTINUED)

**DETAILS**

Year Built: 1999
Current Mgmt. Since: 1999
No. of Floors: 1
Resident Capacity: 40

**SPECIAL**

Alzheimer's/Dementia Only Facility
Diets Accommodated: Diabetic, Low-fat, Low-salt
Proximity to Emergency Svcs.: Under 8 miles
Nearby shopping and entertainment
No pets allowed

**STAFF**

Nurse/LVN/LPN: 40 hours/week, On-call 24/7
Caregiver Training: Dementia, Ethics, Family communication, Grief, Patient transfers, Stress management, Transition issues, Validation therapy
Criminal Background Check: Yes
Principal Staff Language(s): English

**FACILITY FEATURES**

Activities/Recreation
Beauty/Barber Shop ($)
Guest Meals ($)
Outside Patio/Gardens
Pharmaceutical Service
Private Dining Room
Separate Therapy Room
Transportation to MD Appointments, Scheduled Outings
24-hour Security

**ROOM FEATURES**

Cable TV Ready ($)
Emergency Call System
Furnished
Shared & Private Bathrooms
Telephone Ready ($)
Temperature Controls

**COSTS**

PRICES MAY INCREASE. PLEASE CALL FOR MOST CURRENT INFORMATION.

| | |
|---|---|
| Alzheimer's Unit | $3,550/month for shared room<br>$3,950/month for private room |
| Costs of Care | Included in monthly rate |
| Rate Increase | Annually; usually 3% |
| Reimbursement | LTCI, Private pay, SSI, Veterans |

**PORTRAIT**

The founders of Autumn Leaves of Arlington, an RN and her husband, always intended for the facility to be as homelike as possible. Thus, each of the approximately forty residents receives personalized care and attention. Oak trees, crepe myrtles and magnolia saplings thrive on the front lawn. Blue jays bathe in the fountain near the entrance to the stucco building, which features beautiful views of neighboring Vandergriff Park. We observed extensive interaction between the residents and the friendly staff. Residents' voices filled one of the activity rooms as they sang Christmas carols, led by the director. Many of the activities, including exercise, take place in any of the three secure courtyards so that residents may enjoy plants, sunlight and fresh air. Residents go on regular outings to local plays, shopping malls and farmers' markets.

Light brown walls, white baseboards and crown moldings create an elegant backdrop for the floral-accented furniture. In addition to the cozy lamp-lit seating areas, the facility boasts a library, a craft room, a game room and a kitchen therapy room where residents can often be found baking. The building has three dining rooms, including one for feeding assistance. Abundant natural light supplements the artificial light that brightens the home. Handrails and framed artwork that depicts landscapes and historical figures line the walls of the broad hallways. Separate color schemes, such as green or burgundy, in each hallway assist residents in finding their rooms. Photographs of friends and family decorate the small alcoves in residents' moderately sized rooms, further promoting the comfortable atmosphere.

## Avalon—North Country Club A/D

3400 North Country Club Road
Irving, TX 75062

(214) 752-7050
(800) 696-6536
www.avalon-care.com

---

**GILBERT GUIDE OBSERVATIONS**

| | | | |
|---|---|---|---|
| Administration & Staff | g g g g g | Dietary & Food Selection | g g g g |
| Facility Aesthetics | g g g | Activities | g g g g |
| Facility Condition & Safety | g g g | Alzheimer's & Dementia Capabilities | g g g g |
| Residents | g g g g | | |

### DETAILS

Year Built: 1991
Year Remodeled: 2000
Current Mgmt. Since: 1991
No. of Floors: 1
Resident Capacity: 46

### SPECIAL

Alzheimer's/Dementia Only Facility
Diets Accommodated: Diabetic, Low-fat, Low-salt
Proximity to Emergency Svcs.: Under 8 miles
Nearby shopping and entertainment
No pets allowed

### STAFF

Nurse/LVN/LPN: On-call 24/7
Caregiver Training: Dementia, Grief, Stress management
Criminal Background Check: Yes
Principal Staff Language(s): English
Other Staff Language(s): Spanish

### FACILITY FEATURES

Activities/Recreation
Beauty/Barber Shop ($)Guest Meals
Outside Patio/Gardens
Pharmaceutical Service
Private Dining Room
Separate Therapy Room

### ROOM FEATURES

Cable TV Ready
Emergency Call System
Grab Bars
Shared & Private Bathrooms
Telephone Ready
Temperature Controls

AVALON—NORTH COUNTRY CLUB (CONTINUED)

FACILITY FEATURES (CONTINUED)

Transportation to MD Appointments
24-hour Security

## COSTS

PRICES MAY INCREASE. PLEASE CALL FOR MOST CURRENT INFORMATION.

| | |
|---|---|
| Alzheimer's Unit | $4,774/month for shared room<br>$3,775/month for private room |
| Costs of Care | $200/month for incontinence supplies |
| Rate Increase | Annually; usually 1–2% |
| Reimbursement | LTCI, Private pay, SSI, Veterans |
| Security Deposit | $500 |

## PORTRAIT

Avalon North Country Club's staff exemplifies Southern hospitality. The high quality of care is reflected in the residents' positive attitudes. They are an active group with a busy schedule of exercise, drawing, painting, neighborhood strolls, ice cream socials, movie nights and other activities. The facility's day care program, which includes three meals and a daily snack, allows non-residents to experience Avalon for themselves.

The covered entrance to the red brick building is set back from the street between two of its wings, which are bordered by shrubs. A 7-Eleven and a middle school neighbor the facility. Irving Mall is just a few miles away. A gilt-edged mirror hangs above a glass table in the foyer. To the left of the entrance lies one of the facility's multiple common areas, furnished with brown leather couches, a TV and a piano. Bright oil paintings spice up the décor. Another common area features dark pink carpet, maroon couches and a complementary floral border on the walls. A third common room showcases an organ.

Golden fixtures illuminate the dining area, which is located near the entrance. Mahogany tables and chairs, as well as four leather recliners, provide residents with comfortable places to eat and socialize. The menu listed baked chicken, red beans and rice, and green beans followed by fruit smoothies on the day of our visit. Oil paintings of wildlife, plants and snowy cityscapes adorn the walls of the dining area and the facility's broad hallways. Frosted glass fixtures brighten the home. Neutral beige carpet complements the variety of décor and personal taste found in residents' sunny rooms. Each room boasts at least one closet and additional storage in the bathroom. A tall fence secures the paved outdoor courtyard, where residents are fond of walking. Oak trees and canopies shade the wrought iron patio furniture and barbecue.

## AVALON—SOUTH ARLINGTON A/D

7200 US Highway 287
Arlington, TX 76001

(214) 752-7050
(800) 696-6536
www.avalon-care.com

### GILBERT GUIDE OBSERVATIONS

| | | | |
|---|---|---|---|
| Administration & Staff | g g g g g | Dietary & Food Selection | g g g g g |
| Facility Aesthetics | g g g | Activities | g g g g |
| Facility Condition & Safety | g g g | Alzheimer's & Dementia Capabilities | g g g g |
| Residents | g g g g | | |

### DETAILS

Year Built: 1995
Year Remodeled: 2000
Current Mgmt. Since: 2000
No. of Floors: 1
Resident Capacity: 24

### SPECIAL

Alzheimer's/Dementia Only Facility
Diets Accommodated: Diabetic, Low-fat, Low-salt
Proximity to Emergency Svcs.: Under 8 miles
Nearby shopping and entertainment
No pets allowed

### STAFF

Nurse/LVN/LPN: On-call 24/7
Caregiver Training: Dementia, Ethics, Family communication, Grief, Patient transfers, Stress management, Transition issues, Validation therapy
Criminal Background Check: Yes
Principal Staff Language(s): English

### FACILITY FEATURES

Activities/Recreation
Beauty/Barber Shop
Chapel Services
Facility Parking
Guest Meals
Outside Patio/Gardens
Pharmaceutical Service
Private Dining Room
Transportation
24-hour Security

### ROOM FEATURES

Cable TV Ready ($)
Furnished
Grab Bars
Kitchenette
Private Bathrooms
Telephone Ready ($)

### COSTS

PRICES MAY INCREASE. PLEASE CALL FOR MOST CURRENT INFORMATION.

| | |
|---|---|
| Alzheimer's Unit | $3,875–$4,275/month for private room |
| Costs of Care | $200/month for incontinence |
| Rate Increase | Every 2–3 years; usually 2–3% |
| Reimbursement | Private pay |
| Security Deposit | $500 |

AVALON—SOUTH ARLINGTON (CONTINUED)

### PORTRAIT

The two buildings of Avalon South Arlington rest on a tranquil country road. Several tall trees punctuate the lawn between the buildings. We had the distinct impression of visiting a friend's home when we stepped inside. Softly hued paint, hanging plants and a wooden coat rack at the front door create a warm atmosphere. Residents often assist with meal preparation in the kitchen. The lunch served during our visit looked and smelled delicious. Down-home entrees such as pot roast, ham and baked chicken are among some of the mouthwatering selections. Daily snack offerings include fruit, homemade cookies and juice.

Although they were generally reserved during our visit, several residents excitedly mentioned that they enjoy frequent trips to the mall and zoo. Other favorite activities include manicures and pedicures, exercise and game hour. The staff and residents interact as though they were family. This was exemplified when, during our tour, one resident noticed our guide and ran to greet him with a hug, calling him "the nicest person in the whole world."

Residents like to watch television as they eat; the dining area and adjoining common room are conducive to this. Several recliners and sofas are arranged cozily in the common room. The house is softly lit by overhead fixtures and lamps. Due to the open design of the home there are only two short hallways. Residents decorate their large rooms with their own belongings. An attractive floral border painted between the walls and ceilings helps with depth perception and adds a homey touch to residents' rooms. A beautiful wrought iron fence secures the large outdoor area. Residents often watch the squirrels play from a covered seating area at the center of the garden patio.

## COOPER VILLA & THE COTTAGE AT COOPER VILLA A/D

1860–1950 North Cooper Street
Arlington, CA 76011

(817) 261-3601

---

**GILBERT GUIDE OBSERVATIONS**

| | | | |
|---|---|---|---|
| Administration & Staff | g g g g | Dietary & Food Selection | g g g g g |
| Facility Aesthetics | g g g g | Activities | g g g g g |
| Facility Condition & Safety | g g g g g | Alzheimer's & Dementia Capabilities | g g g g g |
| Residents | g g g g g | | |

### DETAILS

Year Built: 1988
Year Remodeled: 2005
Current Mgmt. Since: 1988

### SPECIAL

Diets Accommodated: Diabetic, Low-fat, Low-salt
Proximity to Emergency Svcs.: Under 8 miles

DETAILS (CONTINUED)
No. of Floors: 1
Resident Capacity: 80 (AL), 18 (ALZ)

SPECIAL (CONTINUED)
Nearby shopping and entertainment
Some pets allowed

## STAFF

Nurse/LVN/LPN: On-call 24/7
Caregiver Training: Dementia, Ethics, Family communication, Grief, Patient transfers, Stress management, Transition issues, Validation therapy
Criminal Background Check: Yes
Principal Staff Language(s): English
Other Staff Language(s): Spanish

## FACILITY FEATURES

Activities/Recreation
Beauty/Barber Shop ($)
Chapel Services
Computer/Internet Access
Facility Parking
Fitness Room/Gym
Guest Meals ($)
Outside Patio/Gardens
Pharmaceutical Service
Private Dining Room
Separate Therapy Room
Transportation
24-hour Security

## ROOM FEATURES

Cable TV Ready ($)
Emergency Call System
Furnished
Grab Bars
Kitchenette
Shared & Private Bathrooms
Telephone Ready ($)
Temperature Controls

## COSTS

PRICES MAY INCREASE. PLEASE CALL FOR MOST CURRENT INFORMATION.

| | |
|---|---|
| Studio Apt. | $1,618–$2,456/month |
| One Bedroom Apt. | $2,069–$2,956/month |
| Two Bedroom Apt. | $2,469–$3,356/month |
| Alzheimer's Unit | $2,500–$3,800/month for shared room<br>$3,000–$4,500/month for private room |
| Respite Stays | $95–$150/day for shared room |
| Costs of Care | Included in monthly rate |
| Rate Increase | Annually; usually 7% |
| Reimbursement | LTCI, Private pay |
| Entrance Fee | $1,000 |
| Pet Deposit | $500 |

## PORTRAIT

Cooper Villa is conveniently located in Arlington's entertainment district. The facility is close to shopping malls, the Six Flags amusement park and the Ameriquest Field ballpark, home of the Texas Rangers. The red and white brick facility is situated on well-maintained grounds of trimmed lawns and hedges. The lobby is especially bright and airy due to its skylights and high ceilings. We were greeted by the welcoming sounds of residents laughing and socializing in this warm setting.

COOPER VILLA & THE COTTAGE AT COOPER VILLA (CONTINUED)

Residents' spacious rooms all have windows. The recent remodeling of the building has upgraded its overall appearance but left all the charm and coziness of home. The Cottage's dining room is suitably sized for the residents of this unit. The main dining room, which is a bit larger, is furnished with dark tables and chairs upholstered in pretty fabrics. Residents use the common areas for scheduled activities. The building features skylights and windows throughout. Soft light radiating from glass and metal fixtures is a gentler alternative to fluorescent lighting. The wide hallways are equipped with support systems.

The well-kept outdoor area sports a large furnished patio; it is secured for added safety and comfort. Residents stroll along curved pathways and gather around the hanging birdfeeders, near the designated gardening areas. Residents benefit from the enthusiasm of three activity coordinators. Residents offer suggestions and feedback, participating in event planning on nearly every level. Activity mainstays include manicures and pedicures, dominoes, bingo, arts and crafts, and nightly movies. Residents look energetic and content. The management and staff were friendly and attentive to both residents and their guests. Heavy participation from staff and residents has created a tight-knit community.

## Eden Estates

1997 Forest Ridge Drive
Bedford, TX 76021

(817) 267-2488
www.EdenEstatesSLC.com

**GILBERT GUIDE OBSERVATIONS**

| | | | |
|---|---|---|---|
| Administration & Staff | g g g | Residents | g g g g |
| Facility Aesthetics | g g g g g | Dietary & Food Selection | g g g g g |
| Facility Condition & Safety | g g g g | Activities | g g g |

### DETAILS

Year Built: 1997
Year Remodeled: 2005
Current Mgmt. Since: 1997
No. of Floors: 2
Resident Capacity: 126

### SPECIAL

Diets Accommodated: Diabetic, Low-fat, Low-salt
Proximity to Emergency Svcs.: Under 8 miles
Nearby shopping and entertainment
Some pets allowed

### STAFF

Nurse/LVN/LPN: On-call 24/7
Caregiver Training: Dementia, Ethics, Grief, Patient transfers, Stress management, Transition issues
Criminal Background Check: Yes
Principal Staff Language(s): English

### FACILITY FEATURES

Activities/Recreation
Beauty/Barber Shop ($)
Facility Parking
Fitness Room/Gym
Guest Meals ($)
Outside Patio/Gardens
Private Dining Room
Separate Therapy Room
Transportation to MD Appointments, Scheduled Outings
24-hour Security

### ROOM FEATURES

Cable TV Ready ($)
Emergency Call System
Kitchenette
Private Bathrooms
Telephone Ready ($)
Temperature Controls

### COSTS

PRICES MAY INCREASE. PLEASE CALL FOR MOST CURRENT INFORMATION.

| | |
|---|---|
| Studio Apt. | $1,525–$2,675/month |
| One Bedroom Apt. | $3,190–$3,395/month<br>Double occupancy add $500/month |
| Two Bedroom Apt. | $3,595/month<br>Double occupancy add $500/month |
| Costs of Care | Included in monthly rate |
| Rate Increase | Annually; usually 3% |
| Reimbursement | Veterans |
| Entrance Fee | $500 |
| Pet Deposit | $300 |

### PORTRAIT

The gated community of Eden Estates is similar in appearance to a neighboring apartment complex, from the red brick exterior to the contrasting wood trim. Trees and neatly cut grass characterize the outdoor area, which features a gazebo and cement pathways. Several residents had gathered outside to chat and take advantage of the beautiful weather. Many told us that they enjoy scheduled weekly outings to shopping centers. Residents watch movies, work on puzzles and play a variety of classic games, such as dominoes, bingo and bridge in the facility's numerous common areas. The staff impressed us with their intimate knowledge of residents' lives and personalities.

Attractive, comfortable furniture contributes to the hotel-like atmosphere. The facility's hallways are wide enough to accommodate two wheelchair users abreast. Bright lighting and off-white walls enhance the spacious feel. Residents decorate their rooms to suit their tastes. The rooms are moderately sized. Each room features a spacious walk-in closet. Wheelchair users have rooms that are designed specifically to accommodate them.

Elegant Queen Anne tables furnish the sunny main dining area. The menu lists homey meals such as pot roast or chicken and dumplings, sautéed onions and carrots, mashed potatoes and buttermilk pie. Residents may choose an alternate entrée if they wish. The facility boasts a private kitchen and dining area that can seat as many as sixty people.

## The Estates at Grand Prairie

1005 Southwest Third Street
Grand Prairie, TX 75051

(972) 237-1943
www.theestatesatgp.org

### GILBERT GUIDE OBSERVATIONS

| | | | |
|---|---|---|---|
| Administration & Staff | g g g g | Residents | g g g g |
| Facility Aesthetics | g g g g | Dietary & Food Selection | g g g g |
| Facility Condition & Safety | g g g g g | Activities | g g g |

### DETAILS

Year Built: 2001
Current Mgmt. Since: 2001
No. of Floors: 1
Resident Capacity: 50

### SPECIAL

Mild dementia care provided
Diets Accommodated: Diabetic, Low-salt
Proximity to Emergency Svcs.: 9–15 Miles
No pets allowed

### STAFF

Nurse/LVN/LPN: 40 hours/week, On-call 24/7
Caregiver Training: Dementia, Ethics, Family communication, Patient transfers, Transition issues, Validation
Criminal Background Check: Yes
Principal Staff Language(s): English
Other Staff Language(s): German, Spanish

### FACILITY FEATURES

Activities/Recreation
Beauty/Barber Shop ($)
Chapel Services
Facility Parking
Outside Patio/Gardens
Overnight Guest Room ($)
Private Dining Room ($)
Separate Therapy Room
Transportation
24-hour Security

### ROOM FEATURES

Cable TV Ready ($)
Emergency Call System
Grab Bars
Private Bathrooms
Telephone Ready ($)
Temperature Controls

### COSTS

PRICES MAY INCREASE. PLEASE CALL FOR MOST CURRENT INFORMATION.

| | |
|---|---|
| Studio Apt. | $1,800/month |
| Two Bedroom Apt. | $2,700/month |
| Respite Stays | $65/day for private room |
| Costs of Care | $200–$500/month based on individual need |
| Rate Increase | Periodically |
| Reimbursement | Private pay |
| Security Deposit | $250 |

## PORTRAIT

The Estates at Grand Prairie is located in an older urban neighborhood at 3rd and Jefferson. Decorated with photos of residents and their families, and bright silk flower arrangements, the lobby is a spacious, comfortable seating area with floor-to-ceiling windows. Several residents were smiling and chatting as they relaxed in the lobby on our visit.

Residents' unfurnished rooms are moderately sized and brightened by large double windows. The facility has a dining hall, activity room and several common areas for socializing—all are spacious and bright. Restaurant-style service allows residents to order meals a day in advance. The hallways are spacious and uncluttered, leaving ample room for residents who use wheelchairs or walkers. Built-in cushioned benches in the halls provide rest stops and impromptu visiting areas. Overhead fixtures offer a gentler alternative to standard fluorescent lighting. Lovely plants line the hallways outside residents' rooms.

The secured outdoor courtyard is located in the center of the facility. Its well-maintained landscape, featuring various shrubs and mature flowering trees, is a peaceful refuge. Large umbrellas shade the comfortable patio seating. Residents and staff interacted well with one another. The staff, many of who have been in place since the facility's opening, were delighted and eager to help us get acquainted with the facility and its residents.

# Good Place Assisted Living Facility

7801 North Richland Boulevard
North Richland Hills, TX 76180

(817) 581-6310
www.thegoodplace.net

## GILBERT GUIDE OBSERVATIONS

| | | | |
|---|---|---|---|
| Administration & Staff | g g g | Residents | g g |
| Facility Aesthetics | g g g | Dietary & Food Selection | g g g |
| Facility Condition & Safety | g g g | Activities | g g |

## DETAILS

Year Built: 1997
Current Mgmt. Since: 2004
No. of Floors: 1
Resident Capacity: 80

## SPECIAL

Diets Accommodated: Diabetic, Low-fat, Low-salt
Proximity to Emergency Svcs.: Under 8 miles
Nearby shopping and entertainment
No pets allowed

## STAFF

Nurse/LVN/LPN: 40 hours/week, On-call 24/7
Caregiver Training: Ethics, Family communication, Grief, Stress management, Transition issues, Validation
Criminal Background Check: Yes

GOOD PLACE ASSISTED LIVING FACILITY (CONTINUED)

Principal Staff Language(s): English
Other Staff Language(s): Spanish

### FACILITY FEATURES

Activities/Recreation
Beauty/Barber Shop ($)
Facility Parking
Guest Meals ($)
Outside Patio/Gardens
Private Dining Room
Transportation to MD Appointments, Scheduled Outings

### ROOM FEATURES

Cable TV Ready ($)
Emergency Call System
Kitchenette
Private Bathrooms
Telephone Ready ($)
Temperature Controls

### COSTS

PRICES MAY INCREASE. PLEASE CALL FOR MOST CURRENT INFORMATION.

| | |
|---|---|
| Studio Apt. | $1,910–$2,180/month |
| One Bedroom Apt. | $3,010/month<br>Double occupancy add $400/month |
| Costs of Care | $300–$1,200/month |
| Rate Increase | Annually; usually 3% |
| Reimbursement | LTCI, Private pay, SSI, Veterans |
| Entrance Fee | $500 |

### PORTRAIT

The branches of majestic oaks soar over the landscaping surrounding Good Place. An H-shaped building of red brick houses the facility. A cheerful receptionist welcomed us as we entered the spacious foyer before resuming her conversation with a group of residents. Many residents relaxed in their rooms and several watched the big-screen TV in the common area while they enjoyed hot popcorn. A large fireplace, plush maroon couches and forest green carpet contribute to the homey atmosphere. Soothing watercolors add an artful touch to the décor. A mixture of natural and fluorescent lighting brightens the facility. Handrails line the hallways, where photographs and seasonal decorations adorn residents' doors. Maroon carpeting extends from wall to wall in the moderately sized rooms, which are sunny and feature large walk-in showers and additional storage space.

Staff members assisted residents with walking and other tasks. The chefs prepared grilled chicken and rice with vegetables on the day of our visit. Residents spice up the menu by submitting personal recipes for holidays and special events. Assorted snacks including fresh fruit are available throughout the day. A checkerboard pattern of green and white floor tiles adds color to the dining area and adjacent activities room. The dining area, situated in the hall that connects the building's two larger wings, boasts courtyard views on two sides. Residents seem to enjoy strolling along the pathways that wind through the courtyards. Bingo is a favorite activity among residents, who also engage in exercise, socials, trivia games and scenic drives. Religious activities also occupy much of the residents' time.

## Hearthstone at Arlington

4101 West Arkansas Lane
Arlington, TX 76016

(817) 469-7671
www.hearthstoneassisted.com

### GILBERT GUIDE OBSERVATIONS

| | | | |
|---|---|---|---|
| Administration & Staff | g g g | Residents | g g |
| Facility Aesthetics | g g g g | Dietary & Food Selection | g g g g g |
| Facility Condition & Safety | g g g g | Activities | g g g |

### DETAILS

Year Built: 1998
Current Mgmt. Since: 1998
No. of Floors: 1
Resident Capacity: 119

### SPECIAL

Mild dementia care provided
Diets Accommodated: Low-fat, Low-salt
Proximity to Emergency Svcs.: Under 8 miles
Nearby shopping and entertainment
Pets allowed

### STAFF

Nurse/LVN/LPN: None on staff
Caregiver Training: Dementia, Ethics, Stress management
Criminal Background Check: Yes
Principal Staff Language(s): English
Other Staff Language(s): Spanish

### FACILITY FEATURES

Activities/Recreation
Beauty/Barber Shop ($)
Facility Parking
Guest Meals ($)
Outside Patio/Gardens
Overnight Guest Room ($)
Private Dining Room
Transportation to MD Appointments, Scheduled Outings
24-hour Security

### ROOM FEATURES

Cable TV Ready ($)
Emergency Call System
Grab Bars
Kitchenette
Shared & Private Bathrooms
Telephone Ready ($)
Temperature Controls

### COSTS

PRICES MAY INCREASE. PLEASE CALL FOR MOST CURRENT INFORMATION.

| | |
|---|---|
| Studio Apt. | $2,095–$4,600/month |
| One Bedroom Apt. | Up to $4,600/month |
| Two Bedroom Apt. | Up to $4,600/month |
| Respite Stays | $100–$125/day for shared/private room |
| Costs of Care | Based on individual assessment |
| Rate Increase | Periodically |
| Reimbursement | Private pay |
| Pet Deposit | $250 |

HEARTHSTONE AT ARLINGTON (CONTINUED)

### PORTRAIT

Hearthstone at Arlington sits on lovely West Arkansas Lane in an upscale neighborhood. Trees shelter the pristine building. Earth tones and comfortable furniture mark the elegant décor. The broad hallways are lined with handrails. A combination of natural and artificial light brightens the facility. Residents' moderately sized rooms boast views of the landscaped grounds. Pathways that curve past colorful flowerbeds in the manicured outdoor area are an attractive spot for an afternoon stroll. We observed one resident enjoying sunshine on the patio.

Staff members raved to us about the facility's mouthwatering meals. Breakfast is a hearty affair that involves eggs, bacon, sausages, pancakes and biscuits and gravy. Hearthstone's chefs regularly make delicious soups from scratch. The reigning favorite seems to be chicken and dumplings. The friendly activities director arranges a full calendar of events each month. Residents enjoy Bible study and religious services. At Christmas, residents decorate coffee tins to fill with fudge and give as presents. Outings to movie theaters, shopping malls and Wal-Mart are popular. Outside entertainers frequently delight the residents with their performances—especially the musicians!

## HEARTHSTONE AT BEDFORD

3800 Central Drive
Bedford, TX 76021

(817) 283-6604, (817) 637-6953
www.hearthstoneassisted.com

---

**GILBERT GUIDE OBSERVATIONS**

| | | | |
|---|---|---|---|
| Administration & Staff | g g g | Residents | g g g g |
| Facility Aesthetics | g g g g | Dietary & Food Selection | g g g g |
| Facility Condition & Safety | g g g | Activities | g g g |

### DETAILS

Year Built: 2000
Year Remodeled: 2000
Current Mgmt. Since: 2002
No. of Floors: 1
Resident Capacity: 90

### SPECIAL

Mild dementia care provided
Diets Accommodated: Diabetic, Low-fat, Low-salt
Proximity to Emergency Svcs.: Under 8 miles
Nearby shopping and entertainment

### STAFF

Nurse/LVN/LPN: 40 hours/week
Caregiver Training: Dementia, Ethics, Family communication, Grief, Patient transfers, Stress management, Transition issues, Validation therapy
Criminal Background Check: Yes
Principal Staff Language(s): English
Other Staff Language(s): Sign Language, Spanish

### FACILITY FEATURES

Activities/Recreation
Beauty/Barber Shop ($)
Facility Parking
Guest Meals ($)
Outside Patio/Gardens
Pharmaceutical Service ($)
Separate Therapy Room
Transportation to MD Appointments, Scheduled Outings
24-hour Security

### ROOM FEATURES

Cable TV Ready ($)
Emergency Call System
Kitchenette
Shared & Private Bathrooms
Telephone Ready ($)
Temperature Controls

### COSTS

PRICES MAY INCREASE. PLEASE CALL FOR MOST CURRENT INFORMATION.

| | |
|---|---|
| Studio Apt. | $3,295/month |
| One Bedroom Apt. | $3,645/month |
| Two Bedroom Apt. | $4,890/month |
| Costs of Care | $175–$1,600/month based on individual need |
| Rate Increase | Annually; usually 3% |
| Reimbursement | LTCI, Private pay, SSI, Veterans |
| Entrance Fee | $500 |
| Pet Deposit | $200 |

### PORTRAIT

Hearthstone at Bedford is ensconced between a daycare center and a Baptist church on Central Drive. Ferns and shrubs border its emerald lawn. Gray bricks strewn across the building's red exterior match the shingled roof. A large portico shelters rocking chairs, potted flowers and a cherrywood front door. The reception desk shares space in the lobby with three seating areas formed by off-white sofas. China cabinets display delicate pottery. The forest green carpet complements the lobby's white baseboards and tan walls, and extends throughout the facility. Sunlight streams in from numerous windows. White handrails offer support in the broad hallways, which also feature seating areas. Nightlights glow near the doors and in the spacious bathrooms of residents' rooms. The windows in residents' rooms frame lovely views of the garden. Walkways lead to shrubs and perennial plants at the center of the inner courtyard.

Three chandeliers hang from the high ceiling in the vast dining area. White tablecloths dress the tables, where residents ate chef salads while we visited. The kitchen staff's monthly "Tour of the World" features cuisines from different countries. Residents enjoy a healthy mid-afternoon snack in addition to a variety of drinks from the 24-hour beverage bar. Large tables furnish the activity room, which houses an extensive selection of board games. We observed a group of lively residents power-walking through the halls, led by a staff member. Other residents chatted and played cards in the common area. Residents regularly partake in scenic drives and shopping trips—and they love to visit the children at the daycare next door.

## Heartland

2001 Forest Ridge Drive
Bedford, TX 76021

(817) 571-6804
www.hcr-manorcare.com

---

| GILBERT GUIDE OBSERVATIONS | | | |
|---|---|---|---|
| Administration & Staff | g g g g | Residents | g g g |
| Facility Aesthetics | g g g | Dietary & Food Selection | g g g |
| Facility Condition & Safety | g g g | Activities | g g g |

### DETAILS

Year Built: 1988
Year Remodeled: 1996
Current Mgmt. Since: 2003
No. of Floors: 2
Resident Capacity: 120

### SPECIAL

Mild dementia care provided
Diets Accommodated: Diabetic, Low-fat, Low-salt, Renal
Proximity to Emergency Svcs.: Under 8 miles
Nearby shopping and entertainment
Pets allowed

### STAFF

Nurse/LVN/LPN: Onsite 24/7
Caregiver Training: Dementia, Ethics, Family communication, Grief, Patient transfers, Stress management, Transition issues, Validation therapy
Criminal Background Check: Yes
Principal Staff Language(s): English

### FACILITY FEATURES

Activities/Recreation
Chapel Services
Guest Meals
Outside Patio/Gardens
Pharmaceutical Service
Separate Therapy Room
Transportation to MD Appointments, Scheduled Outings
24-hour Security

### ROOM FEATURES

Cable TV Ready ($)
Emergency Call System
Grab Bars
Private Bathrooms
Telephone Ready ($)
Temperature Controls

### COSTS

PRICES MAY INCREASE. PLEASE CALL FOR MOST CURRENT INFORMATION.

| | |
|---|---|
| Studio Apt. | $2,215–$2,326/month |
| Costs of Care | $150–$800/month based on individual need |
| Rate Increase | Annually; usually 3% |
| Reimbursement | LTCI, Private pay, SSI, Veterans |
| Entrance Fee | $2,000 |
| Security Deposit | $500 |

## PORTRAIT

Heartland's pentagonal shape of red brick evokes an old Texan schoolhouse. The facility is located near Highway 183. Floral-patterned sofas and Queen Anne chairs furnish the spacious entry room. Light green carpet contrasts attractively with maroon wallpaper. A combination of sunlight and fluorescent light brightens the facility. Maroon carpet covers the floors of the wide hallways, which have wooden handrails. Residents decorate tables next to their doors; one resident changes the attire of a porcelain duck to reflect the season. Some residents' rooms boast sliding doors that open to the inner courtyard. Others have windows and are more spacious. All of the bathrooms have sit-in showers.

Concrete paths crisscross the lawn in the inner courtyard, where residents grow flowers and ferns. Maple trees shade the benches and iron patio furniture. Decorative shrubs and small trees add elements of green to the mostly paved area.

Residents and their guests occupy plush sofas while they chat and watch the children on the nearby playground through floor-to-ceiling windows. The dining areas double as activity areas. The lunch menu featured grilled chicken breast with zucchini, macaroni and cheese, and lemon chess pie when we visited. The desserts were autumn-themed and included pumpkin pie and candy apples. Fresh fruit, muffins and crackers are available all day. Residents make weekly trips to restaurants and shopping centers, including Wal-Mart. Other activities include daily exercise, beading and jewelry repair. We noted the attentiveness of the staff, who smiled as they saw to residents' needs.

# Holiday Lane Estates

6155 Holiday Lane
North Richland Hills, TX 76180

(817) 427-0275
www.holidaylanealf.com

## GILBERT GUIDE OBSERVATIONS

| | | | |
|---|---|---|---|
| Administration & Staff | g g g | Residents | g g g |
| Facility Aesthetics | g g g | Dietary & Food Selection | g g g |
| Facility Condition & Safety | g g g g | Activities | g g g |

## DETAILS

Year Built: 2000
Year Remodeled: Ongoing
Current Mgmt. Since: 2000
No. of Floors: 1
Resident Capacity: 50

## SPECIAL

Mild dementia care provided
Diets Accommodated: Diabetic, Low-fat, Low-salt, Renal
Proximity to Emergency Svcs.: Under 8 miles
Nearby shopping and entertainment
Some pets allowed

HOLIDAY LANE ESTATES (CONTINUED)

## STAFF

Nurse/LVN/LPN: 40 hours/week, On-call 24/7
Caregiver Training: Dementia, Ethics, Grief, Patient transfers, Stress management
Criminal Background Check: Yes
Principal Staff Language(s): English
Other Staff Language(s): Spanish

## FACILITY FEATURES

Activities/Recreation
Beauty/Barber Shop
Chapel Services
Facility Parking
Guest Meals ($)
Outside Patio/Gardens
Pharmaceutical Service ($)
Private Dining Room
Room Service ($)
Transportation to MD Appointments, Personal Outings
24-hour Security

## ROOM FEATURES

Cable TV Ready ($)
Emergency Call System
Grab Bars
Kitchenette
Private Bathrooms
Telephone Ready ($)
Temperature Controls

## COSTS

PRICES MAY INCREASE. PLEASE CALL FOR MOST CURRENT INFORMATION.

| | |
|---|---|
| Studio Apt. | $2,355/month |
| One Bedroom Apt. | $2,655/month<br>Double occupancy add $500/month |
| Costs of Care | $300–$1,200/month based on individual need |
| Rate Increase | Annually; usually 1–5% |
| Reimbursement | LTCI, Private pay |
| Pet Deposit | $500 |

## PORTRAIT

Holiday Lane Estates is a modern facility in a quiet residential area. During our visit, we heard the children from the neighboring elementary school playing and laughing. The well-groomed entrance is lined with young trees that provide plentiful shade. The front of the facility features a comfortable seating area with a stone fireplace, which is a popular spot for residents to gather. Beautiful tropical fish in the aquarium brighten the room.

Residents' moderately sized rooms all have roomy closets. Wallpapered in green and neutral colors, each room is adorned with hanging prints of landscapes and decorative urns. The dining room has green carpeting and is furnished with dark wood tables and chairs. The menu features appetizing selections such as meatloaf, mashed potatoes and gravy, buttered carrots and angel food cake. Residents enjoy walking their dogs in the outdoor courtyard. The garden was bare due to the winter climate, but residents use their green thumbs in warmer weather. The atmosphere at Holiday Lane is comfortable. The spacious hallways are adorned with artwork in homey wooden frames. Soft artificial lighting radiates from pretty glass and metal sconces.

The tireless event coordinator organizes fitness classes, musical entertainment, arts and crafts, baking, ceramics, movie nights, bingo, gardening, field trips and church services. At the time of our visit, most of the residents were out on a scheduled activity. Although we didn't see too many residents out and about, the staff at Holiday Lane seems well prepared to accommodate residents' needs.

## Merrill Gardens at Grand Prairie

335 West Westchester Parkway
Grand Prairie, TX 75052

(972) 263-3663
www.merrillgardens.com

### GILBERT GUIDE OBSERVATIONS

| | | | |
|---|---|---|---|
| Administration & Staff | g g g | Residents | g g g g |
| Facility Aesthetics | g g g g | Dietary & Food Selection | g g g g g |
| Facility Condition & Safety | g g g g g | Activities | g g g g |

### DETAILS

Year Built: 1996
Current Mgmt. Since: 1996
No. of Floors: 2
Resident Capacity: 85

### SPECIAL

Mild dementia care provided
Diets Accommodated: Diabetic, Low-fat, Low-salt
Proximity to Emergency Svcs.: Under 8 miles
Nearby shopping and entertainment
Pets allowed

### STAFF

Nurse/LVN/LPN: 40 hours/week, On-call 24/7
Caregiver Training: Dementia, Ethics, Family communication, Grief, Patient transfers, Stress management, Transition issues, Validation therapy
Criminal Background Check: Yes
Principal Staff Language(s): English
Other Staff Language(s): Spanish

### FACILITY FEATURES

Activities/Recreation
Beauty/Barber Shop
Chapel Services
Facility Parking
Fitness Room/Gym
Guest Meals ($)
Outside Patio/Gardens
Overnight Guest Room ($)
Pharmaceutical Service

### ROOM FEATURES

Cable TV Ready
Emergency Call System
Grab Bars
Kitchenette
Private Bathrooms
Temperature Controls

MERRILL GARDENS AT GRAND PRAIRIE (CONTINUED)

**FACILITY FEATURES (CONTINUED)**

Private Dining Room
Room Service ($)
Transportation to MD Appointments, Scheduled Outings
24-hour Security

## COSTS

PRICES MAY INCREASE. PLEASE CALL FOR MOST CURRENT INFORMATION.

| | |
|---|---|
| Studio Apt. | $1,495–$1,745/month |
| One Bedroom Apt. | $2,350/month |
| Two Bedroom Apt. | $2,450/month<br>Double occupancy add $500/month |
| Respite Stays | Call for rates for private room |
| Costs of Care | $500–$1,200/month based on individual need |
| Rate Increase | Annually; usually 3–5% |
| Reimbursement | LTCI, Private pay, Veterans |
| Entrance Fee | $500 |
| Pet Deposit | $500 |

## PORTRAIT

Merrill Gardens is located in Westchester, minutes away from shopping, restaurants, medical offices and wooded walking trails. A large white portico supported by brick columns and backed by floor-to-ceiling windows is the attractive entrance to this well-maintained building. Residents relax in rocking chairs on the porch.

The lobby, which doubles as the common area, is comfortably furnished with maroon lounge chairs. The room is carpeted in shades of green and features decorative knickknacks and an elegant stone fireplace. Residents' rooms vary in size. Each has extra storage space. Residents decorate the rooms to suit their tastes.

The dining room is open from morning until evening, which affords residents the luxury of choosing their own dining schedule. During our visit, the kitchen staff prepared an appetizing selection of homestyle and deli meals. Residents may reserve the private dining room for special events. The hallways are spacious and equipped with handrails. The building is brightened by a combination of artificial and natural light.

The outdoor area is an inviting setting with posh patio furniture. Residents are welcome to garden. The activity room hosts bingo and dominoes. The event calendar was chock-full of social events such as shopping trips and Sunday drives. The staff encourages residents to exercise for thirty minutes daily. During our visit, residents seemed content, visiting among themselves, while the staff was busy at work.

## Merrill Gardens at North Richland Hills

8500 Emerald Hills Way
North Richland Hills, TX 76180

(817) 577-3337
www.merrillgardens.com

### GILBERT GUIDE OBSERVATIONS

| | | | |
|---|---|---|---|
| Administration & Staff | g g g g g | Residents | g g g g g |
| Facility Aesthetics | g g g g | Dietary & Food Selection | g g g |
| Facility Condition & Safety | g g g g g | Activities | g g g g |

### DETAILS

Year Built: 1998
Year Remodeled: Ongoing
Current Mgmt. Since: 1999
No. of Floors: 2
Resident Capacity: 110

### SPECIAL

Diets Accommodated: Diabetic, Low-fat, Low-salt, Renal
Proximity to Emergency Svcs.: Under 8 miles
Nearby shopping and entertainment
Some pets allowed

### STAFF

Nurse/LVN/LPN: 40 hours/week, On-call 24/7
Caregiver Training: Ethics, Family communication, Grief, Stress management, Transition issues
Criminal Background Check: Yes
Principal Staff Language(s): English
Other Staff Language(s): Spanish

### FACILITY FEATURES

Activities/Recreation
Beauty/Barber Shop ($)
Chapel Services
Computer/Internet Access
Facility Parking
Guest Meals ($)
Outside Patio/Gardens
Overnight Guest Room ($)
Pharmaceutical Service ($)
Private Dining Room
Room Service ($)
Separate Therapy Room
Transportation
24-hour Security

### ROOM FEATURES

Cable TV Ready
Emergency Call System
Grab Bars
Kitchenette
Private Bathrooms
Telephone Ready ($)
Temperature Controls

### COSTS

PRICES MAY INCREASE. PLEASE CALL FOR MOST CURRENT INFORMATION.

| | |
|---|---|
| Studio Apt. | $1,595–$1,825/month |
| One Bedroom Apt. | $2,160–$2,260/month |
| | Double occupancy add $550/month |

MERRILL GARDENS AT NORTH RICHLAND HILLS (CONTINUED)

| | |
|---|---|
| Two Bedroom Apt. | $2,525/month |
| Costs of Care | $500–$1,200/month based on individual need |
| Rate Increase | Annually; usually 2–5% |
| Reimbursement | LTCI, Private pay, Veterans |
| Entrance Fee | $500 |
| Pet Deposit | $500 |

### PORTRAIT

A stately building, set well back from the street, houses Merrill Gardens at North Richland Hills. A grand covered entrance supported by four brick columns greets visitors. Young oaks grow on the front lawn. Residents preparing for the daily exercise filled the great room when we began our tour. We overhead one resident suggest poetry readings as a possible activity to a staff member. The staff member agreed and designated that resident as poetry reading organizer. The facility's monthly newsletter lists activities which include computer time, ceramics, bridge, shopping and excursions to nearby casinos in Oklahoma.

The facility is divided into neighborhoods; each neighborhood has a separate living room for residents of that area. Elegant dark wood furnishings complement the wood paneling on the walls throughout the facility. Attractive glass and brass sconces provide fluorescent lighting throughout the building. The exceptionally wide hallways are carpeted in forest green and lined with benches. Residents' rooms are small and each features a spacious walk-in closet. Some have bay windows. Dark wood chairs and tables furnish the dining area. Residents lunched on barbecued pork sandwiches, potatoes, broccoli and fruit, and enjoyed a view of the patio area when we visited. The back patio features a plush lawn and numerous potted plants, which are tended by residents.

## OAK HOLLOW ALZHEIMER'S SPECIAL CARE CENTER A/D

2016 L. Don Dodson Parkway
Bedford, TX 76021

(817) 267-6200
www.jeaseniorliving.com

---

### GILBERT GUIDE OBSERVATIONS

| | | | |
|---|---|---|---|
| Administration & Staff | g g g g | Dietary & Food Selection | g g g g |
| Facility Aesthetics | g g g g | Activities | g g g g g |
| Facility Condition & Safety | g g g g g | Alzheimer's & Dementia Capabilities | g g g g g |
| Residents | g g g g g | | |

## DETAILS

Year Built: 1999
Current Mgmt. Since: 2000
No. of Floors: 1
Resident Capacity: 56

## SPECIAL

Alzheimer's/Dementia Only Facility
Diets Accommodated: Diabetic, Low-fat, Low-salt, Renal
Proximity to Emergency Svcs.: Under 8 miles
Nearby shopping and entertainment
No pets allowed

## STAFF

Nurse/LVN/LPN: Onsite 24/7
Caregiver Training: Dementia, Ethics, Family communication, Grief, Patient transfers, Stress management, Transition issues, Validation therapy
Criminal Background Check: Yes
Principal Staff Language(s): English

## FACILITY FEATURES

Activities/Recreation
Beauty/Barber Shop ($)
Computer/Internet Access
Facility Parking
Guest Meals
Outside Patio/Gardens
Pharmaceutical Service
Private Dining Room
Transportation to MD Appointments, Scheduled Outings
24-hour Security

## ROOM FEATURES

Cable TV Ready ($)
Emergency Call System
Shared Bathrooms
Telephone Ready ($)
Temperature Controls

## COSTS

PRICES MAY INCREASE. PLEASE CALL FOR MOST CURRENT INFORMATION.

| | |
|---|---|
| Alzheimer's Unit | $3,450–$4,760/month for shared room |
| Costs of Care | $300–$1,000/month based on individual need |
| Rate Increase | Annually; usually 3–5% |
| Reimbursement | Private pay, SSI, Veterans |
| Entrance Fee | $650 |

## PORTRAIT

A verdant lawn and abundant parking lay before Oak Hollow, a pinkish brick building marked by a covered entrance and black shingled roof. Pastel color schemes and plush furniture accented with pillows decorate the common areas. A wood-burning fireplace flanked by bookcases warms residents as they read on a comfortable couch in one of the common rooms. Patterned pink wallpaper and shelves of knickknacks create a country-like atmosphere in the dining room. Residents enjoyed a delicious meal of fried chicken, mashed potatoes, green beans and Jell-O during our visit. Homemade apple pie with hot apple cider were recent Halloween goodies. The snack table is laden with nutritious offerings including

OAK HOLLOW ALZHEIMER'S SPECIAL CARE CENTER (CONTINUED)

bananas, apples and crackers. Natural and fluorescent lights illuminate the facility. The wide hallways feature several large signs to direct residents and guests. Bay windows flood a hallway seating area with light.

Baseboards line the white walls of residents' large, sunny rooms. Some of the rooms boast individual closets. Chairs in the walk-in showers provide a practical touch.

Staff members encourage residents to spend time outside of their rooms socializing. Oak Hollow's management runs a tight ship to ensure the facility is tidy and the residents are comfortable. The varied activities scheduled on the facility's calendar impressed us—it is one of the most diverse we have ever seen! Activities range from cooking therapy to seasonal parties. Residents perform regular mental exercises, such as playing trivia games, as well as a variety of physical activities. They also attend festivals and weekly restaurant outings. Residents often opt to spend time in the building's inner courtyard, where an awning shades black wrought iron furniture. Walkways cut a path through the lawn and shrubbery to a lovely area decorated with pansies, trees and a fountain.

## PARKWOOD A/D

2600 Parkview Lane
Bedford, TX 76022

(817) 267-7373

---

**GILBERT GUIDE OBSERVATIONS**

| | | | |
|---|---|---|---|
| Administration & Staff | g g g g | Dietary & Food Selection | g g g g |
| Facility Aesthetics | g g g g | Activities | g g g |
| Facility Condition & Safety | g g g g | Alzheimer's & Dementia Capabilities | g g g g g |
| Residents | g g g g g | | |

### DETAILS

Year Built: 1996
Current Mgmt. Since: 2003
No. of Floors: 1
Resident Capacity: 120 (AL), 40 (ALZ)

### SPECIAL

Diets Accommodated: Diabetic
Proximity to Emergency Svcs.: Under 8 miles
Nearby shopping and entertainment
Pet visits allowed

### STAFF

Nurse/LVN/LPN: Onsite 24/7
Caregiver Training: Dementia, Ethics, Family communication, Grief, Patient transfers, Stress management, Transition issues, Validation therapy
Criminal Background Check: Yes
Principal Staff Language(s): English
Other Staff Language(s): Spanish

### FACILITY FEATURES

Activities/Recreation
Beauty/Barber Shop ($)
Chapel Services
Facility Parking
Guest Meals ($)
Outside Patio/Gardens
Pharmaceutical Service
Transportation to MD Appointments, Scheduled Outings

### ROOM FEATURES

Cable TV Ready ($)
Emergency Call System
Grab Bars
Shared & Private Bathrooms
Telephone Ready ($)
Temperature Controls

### COSTS

PRICES MAY INCREASE. PLEASE CALL FOR MOST CURRENT INFORMATION.

| | |
|---|---|
| Studio Apt. | $2,380–$3,100/month |
| One Bedroom Apt. | $3,475–$3,875/month<br>Double occupancy add $550/month |
| Alzheimer's Unit | $2,910–$4,415/month for shared room |
| Costs of Care | $400–$500/month based on individual need; call for Alzheimer's rates |
| Rate Increase | Annually; usually 3% |
| Reimbursement | LTCI, Private pay, SSI, Veterans |
| Security Deposit | $500 |

### PORTRAIT

A large brick building with black shingles houses Parkwood and its sister Alzheimer's unit. An undeveloped portion of land covered with trees surrounds the facility. Oaks and maples shade the expanse of lawn fronting Parkwood, which is just a block from Harris Methodist HEB Hospital. A reception desk furnishes the stately foyer. Patterned rugs reflect the vivid hues of the floral lithographs hanging on the walls.

The building features high ceilings, fluorescent lighting and expansive windows. The hallways are exceptionally broad. The facility boasts several common areas; in one, a wooden grandfather clock and a baby grand sit near a fireplace and leather couches. An indoor courtyard-provides a gathering spot for residents. Several residents and staff members cheerfully bustled about the facility during our tour as they prepared for a Halloween party. Residents enjoy exercising twice a day. Other popular pastimes include puzzles and board games, as well as trips to a local library and nearby malls and restaurants.

Cream-colored walls, white baseboards and beige carpet lend an airy feel to residents' sunny rooms. In the Mayfair, the facility's Alzheimer's unit, residents' rooms feature pink privacy curtains that match the curtains on the expansive windows. Marble-patterned linoleum floors and white walls brighten the rooms. All bathrooms have spacious walk-in showers with seats. On the day of our tour, the menu listed a hearty breakfast of ham and eggs with toast. Pumpkin pie and cinnamon apples provided fall-themed desserts. The special snack of the day was rice krispies, which were available in each of the activity rooms.

## St. Joseph Village Assisted Living

1201 East Sandy Lake Road
Coppell, TX 75019

(972) 304-0300
www.stjosephvillage.org

### GILBERT GUIDE OBSERVATIONS

| | | | |
|---|---|---|---|
| Administration & Staff | g g g g | Residents | g g g g g |
| Facility Aesthetics | g g g g g | Dietary & Food Selection | g g g g g |
| Facility Condition & Safety | g g g g g | Activities | g g g g |

### DETAILS

Year Built: 2003
Year Remodeled: 2003
Current Mgmt. Since: 2003
No. of Floors: 3
Resident Capacity: 48

### SPECIAL

Diets Accommodated: Diabetic, Low-fat, Low-salt
Proximity to Emergency Svcs.: Under 8 miles
Nearby shopping and entertainment
Some pets allowed

### STAFF

Nurse/LVN/LPN: Onsite 24/7, On-call 24/7
Caregiver Training: Ethics, Family communication, Grief
Criminal Background Check: Yes
Principal Staff Language(s): English

### FACILITY FEATURES

Activities/Recreation
Beauty/Barber Shop ($)
Chapel Services
Computer/Internet Access
Facility Parking
Fitness Room/Gym
Guest Meals ($)
Outside Patio/Gardens
Private Dining Room
Room Service
Separate Therapy Room
Transportation
24-hour Security

### ROOM FEATURES

Cable TV Ready ($)
Emergency Call System
Kitchenette
Private Bathrooms
Telephone Ready ($)
Temperature Controls

### COSTS

PRICES MAY INCREASE. PLEASE CALL FOR MOST CURRENT INFORMATION.

| | |
|---|---|
| One Bedroom Apt. | $2,700–$3,100/month |
| Two Bedroom Apt. | $3,800/month |
| Costs of Care | Included in monthly rate |
| Rate Increase | Annually; usually 3% |
| Reimbursement | Private pay |
| Security Deposit | $300 |

## PORTRAIT

Picturesque fields of tall grass surround St. Joseph Village, a Catholic-based facility located in a developing area of Coppell. An unusual V-shaped building houses the main facility, which is encircled by a fence with an elegant iron gate. Ample parking is available. Walkways flanked with saplings, among the property's grassy knolls, provide a lovely area for an afternoon stroll. Benches offer a view of a small pond where ducks swim among the lilypads.

Inviting sofas sit upon marble floors in the living room, which also features white stone fireplaces against dramatic crimson walls. Arched ceilings soar above the wide hallways. Sconces and lighting concealed by crown molding illuminate the handrail-equipped halls. Carpeted sitting rooms feature comfortable blue couches, brown leather chairs and maple tables. Residents' spacious apartments have plush carpet, oak cabinets, walk-in closets and spacious bathrooms with sit-down showers. Windows let in plentiful sunlight. Residents are welcome to paint their rooms if they wish. Black laquered tables and chairs furnish the dining areas. Daily snacks include cookies, fruit, crackers and cheese.

We witnessed residents and their families exercising in the spacious workout room, as others engaged in water aerobics in the large indoor pool. Activities include daily outings, Catholic mass, Protestant mass, card games such as bridge and pinochle, happy hour, music appreciation, jewelry repair and tea socials. We also noticed extensive interaction between the staff, residents and their families. The staff wears scrubs, which is somewhat out of keeping with the facility's luxurious ambiance.

# SUMMERVILLE AT IRVING

820 North Britain Road
Irving, TX 75061

(972) 721-1500
www.sslusa.com

---

## GILBERT GUIDE OBSERVATIONS

| | | | |
|---|---|---|---|
| Administration & Staff | g g g g g | Residents | g g g |
| Facility Aesthetics | g g g g | Dietary & Food Selection | g g g |
| Facility Condition & Safety | g g g g g | Activities | g g g g |

## DETAILS

Year Built: 1996
Year Remodeled: 2004
Current Mgmt. Since: 2002
No. of Floors: 1
Resident Capacity: 64

## SPECIAL

Mild dementia care provided
Diets Accommodated: Diabetic, Low-fat, Low-salt, Renal
Proximity to Emergency Svcs.: Under 8 miles
Nearby shopping and entertainment
Pets allowed

SUMMERVILLE AT IRVING (CONTINUED)

### STAFF

Nurse/LVN/LPN: 60 hours/week, On-call 24/7
Caregiver Training: Dementia, Ethics, Family communication, Grief, Patient transfers, Stress management, Transition issues, Validation therapy
Criminal Background Check: Yes
Principal Staff Language(s): English
Other Staff Language(s): Spanish

### FACILITY FEATURES

Activities/Recreation
Beauty/Barber Shop
Chapel Services
Computer/Internet Access
Facility Parking
Fitness Room/Gym
Guest Meals
Outside Patio/Gardens
Pharmaceutical Service
Private Dining Room
Room Service
Separate Therapy Room
Transportation

### ROOM FEATURES

Cable TV Ready ($)
Emergency Call System
Grab Bars
Kitchenette
Shared & Private Bathrooms
Telephone Ready ($)
Temperature Controls

### COSTS

PRICES MAY INCREASE. PLEASE CALL FOR MOST CURRENT INFORMATION.

| | |
|---|---|
| Studio Apt. | $2,195–$2,845/month |
| One Bedroom Apt. | $2,695–$3,345/month<br>Double occupancy add $350/month |
| Costs of Care | Included in monthly rate |
| Rate Increase | Annually |
| Reimbursement | Private pay, Veterans |
| Entrance Fee | $500 |
| Security Deposit | $500 |
| Pet Deposit | $250 |

### PORTRAIT

Don't be fooled by the institutional look and busy location of Summerville at Irving; the affectionate staff members make this facility a true home. Special touches including a classic popcorn machine, colorful aquariums and comfortable furniture are found just inside. The wide hallways are clean and feature safety handrails as well as several convenient sitting areas. Residents' rooms are modestly sized but large windows let in sunlight and create a more spacious feel. The food selection is appetizing, although somewhat limited. Residents enjoy snacking on fresh, hot popcorn or the occasional treat from the facility's ice cream and cappuccino bar.

During our visit we were impressed by the staff's superior service. Every member of management greeted us and several staff members introduced themselves. The staff knew each resident by name and genuinely seemed to be having fun as they socialized with one another. Over 100 well-organized activities are held each month, including ice cream socials, and field trips to shopping malls and casinos.

## Valley Ranch Deluxe

8855 West Valley Ranch Parkway
Irving, TX 75063

(972) 831-8200

---

**GILBERT GUIDE OBSERVATIONS**

| | | | |
|---|---|---|---|
| Administration & Staff | g g g | Residents | g g g g |
| Facility Aesthetics | g g g g | Dietary & Food Selection | g g g |
| Facility Condition & Safety | g g g | Activities | g g g |

### DETAILS

Year Built: 2001
Year Remodeled: 2003
Current Mgmt. Since: 2001
No. of Floors: 1
Resident Capacity: 52

### SPECIAL

Mild dementia care provided
Diets Accommodated: Diabetic, Low-fat, Low-salt, Renal
Proximity to Emergency Svcs.: Under 8 miles
Nearby shopping and entertainment
Some pets allowed

### STAFF

Nurse/LVN/LPN: Onsite 24/7
Caregiver Training: Dementia, Ethics, Patient transfers, Transition issues
Criminal Background Check: Yes
Principal Staff Language(s): English
Other Staff Language(s): Cantonese, Hindi, Mandarin, Spanish, Tagalog

### FACILITY FEATURES

Activities/Recreation
Beauty/Barber Shop
Chapel Services
Computer/Internet Access
Facility Parking
Fitness Room/Gym
Guest Meals
Outside Patio/Gardens
Overnight Guest Room
Pharmaceutical Service
Private Dining Room
Room Service
Separate Therapy Room
Transportation

### ROOM FEATURES

Cable TV Ready ($)
Emergency Call System
Furnished
Grab Bars
Shared Bathrooms
Telephone Ready ($)
Temperature Controls

VALLEY RANCH DELUXE (CONTINUED)

## COSTS

PRICES MAY INCREASE. PLEASE CALL FOR MOST CURRENT INFORMATION.

| | |
|---|---|
| Studio Apt. | $2,500–$5,200/month |
| Costs of Care | $500–$1,000/month based on individual need |
| Rate Increase | Periodically |
| Reimbursement | Private pay |
| Security Deposit | $500 (refundable) |
| Pet Deposit | $500 (refundable) |

## PORTRAIT

Valley Ranch Deluxe is a luxurious ranch home nestled in the hills. The well-maintained lawn is the fresh face of this village motif; the interior is modeled after a town square. Decorative awnings hang over the office doors and windows throughout the building resemble storefronts. Benches and antique lampposts add authenticity to this charming atmosphere.

Residents' rooms are cozy and in excellent condition. New carpeting and freshly painted walls complement residents' decorative personal displays. The common areas are furnished with lounge chairs and sofas. The dining room is a snug arrangement of tables and chairs. Residents enjoy the independence of cafeteria-style dining. The staff hosts a weekly ice cream social. Residents attended a watermelon social the weekend before our visit. The outdoor seating area is surrounded by pruned landscapes. Residents do not have to go outside to bask in the sunlight; an abundance of windows bathe the facility in natural light.

The busy event calendar includes bingo, board games and religious activities. The environment at Valley Ranch was playful and welcoming. During our visit, we observed a group of residents watching a caregiver and resident dancing together.

SKILLED NURSING FACILITIES

## Arbrook Plaza

401 West Arbrook Boulevard
Arlington, TX 76014

(817) 466-3094, (817) 467-1400
www.apsnf.com

**GOVERNMENT DEFICIENCIES: 3**

Reviewed on: October 14, 2005

| Mistreatment | Quality Care | Resident Assessment |
|---|---|---|
| 1 | 1 | 1 |

*IMPORTANT: REVIEW DETAILS OF EACH DEFICIENCY AT WWW.MEDICARE.GOV

**GILBERT GUIDE OBSERVATIONS**

| | | | |
|---|---|---|---|
| Administration & Staff | g g g | Dietary & Food Selection | g g g g |
| Facility Aesthetics | g g g | Activities | g g g |
| Facility Condition & Safety | g g g | Medical Care | g g g g |
| Residents | g g g | | |

### DETAILS

Year Built: 2001
Current Mgmt. Since: 2001
No. of Floors: 1
Resident Capacity: 120
Facility Type: Long-term care, Short-term rehab

### SPECIAL

Special diets accommodated
Proximity to Emergency Svcs.: Under 8 miles

### STAFF

Caregiver Training: Ethics, Family communication, Pain management, Patient transfers, Stress management, Transition issues, Universal Precautions, Wound Care
Criminal Background Check: Yes
Principal Staff Language(s): English
Other Staff Language(s): Spanish

### FACILITY FEATURES

Activities/Recreation
Beauty/Barber Shop ($)
Guest Meals ($)
Separate Therapy Room
Whirlpool Baths

### ROOM FEATURES

Cable TV Ready
Space for personal items
Shared & Private Bathrooms
Telephone Ready

### COSTS

PRICES MAY INCREASE. PLEASE CALL FOR MOST CURRENT INFORMATION.

| | |
|---|---|
| Shared Room | $115/day |
| Private Room | $175/day |
| Respite Stays | $115/day for shared room, $175/day for private room |

ARBROOK PLAZA (CONTINUED)

| | |
|---|---|
| Rate Increase | Annually; usually 3% |
| Reimbursement | Medicare, Medicaid, LTCI, HMO, Private pay, SSI, Veterans |

**PORTRAIT**

Arbrook is situated on a bustling boulevard of the same name. Flowers trace the small lawn before the red brick building, which is flanked by trees. Residents observe neighborhood activity from any of the numerous rocking chairs on the front patio. A glass chandelier illuminates mahogany coffee tables and floral upholstered chairs in the foyer. The dining room is used for all types of activities from bingo to religious services. Fluorescent lighting brightens the nursing station, which sits at the confluence of four residential wings. Dark green carpeting extends into residents' rooms, all of which have small windows. A curtain separates the hospital beds and nightstands in the semi-private rooms. The hallways are broad enough to allow two hospital beds to pass each other, but are somewhat dim. Walk-in showers with handrails are featured in two of the halls.

The busy staff accommodates a variety of medical needs, including intravenous therapy, wound care, respite and hospice care. Arbrook has a quiet atmosphere; many of the residents were napping in their rooms or quietly watching television in the common area when we visited.

## Bishop Davies Nursing Center

2712 North Hurstview Drive
Hurst, TX 76054

(817) 281-6707, (817) 498-2390
www.bishopdaviescenter.com

**GOVERNMENT DEFICIENCIES: 4** Reviewed on: October 20, 2005

| Administration | Pharmacy Service | Quality Care |
|---|---|---|
| 1 | 2 | 1 |

*IMPORTANT: REVIEW DETAILS OF EACH DEFICIENCY AT WWW.MEDICARE.GOV

**GILBERT GUIDE OBSERVATIONS**

| | | | |
|---|---|---|---|
| Administration & Staff | g g g | Dietary & Food Selection | g g g |
| Facility Aesthetics | g g g | Activities | g g g |
| Facility Condition & Safety | g g g | Access to Medical Care | g g g |
| Residents | g g g | | |

**DETAILS**

Year Built: 1973
Year Remodeled: 1997
Current Mgmt. Since: 1996

**SPECIAL**

Special diets accommodated
Proximity to Emergency Svcs.: Under 8 miles

DETAILS (CONTINUED)

No. of Floors: 1
Resident Capacity: 160
Facility Type: Long-term care, Short-term rehab

## STAFF

Caregiver Training: Dementia, Ethics, Family communication, Grief, Pain management, Patient transfers, Stress management, Transition issues, Universal precautions, Validation therapy, Wound care
Criminal Background Check: Yes
Principal Staff Language(s): English
Other Staff Language(s): Spanish

## FACILITY FEATURES

Activities/Recreation
Beauty/Barber Shop ($)
Chapel Services
Guest Meals ($)
Outside Patio/Gardens
Separate Therapy Room
24-hour Security
Wanderguard
Whirlpool Baths

## ROOM FEATURES

Cable TV Ready ($)
Space for personal items
Shared & Private Bathrooms
Telephone Ready ($)

## COSTS

PRICES MAY INCREASE. PLEASE CALL FOR MOST CURRENT INFORMATION.

| | |
|---|---|
| Shared Room | $115–$135/day |
| Private Room | $135–$165/day |
| Respite Stays | $115–$135/day for shared room<br>$135–$165/day for private room |
| Rate Increase | Annually; usually 3% |
| Reimbursement | Medicare, Medicaid, LTCI, HMO, Private pay, SSI, Veterans |

## PORTRAIT

Bishop Davies Nursing Center is harbored in a placid area of Hurst. A shopping center and grocery store are conveniently located across the street. The white awning and covered entrance add shade and protection from inclement weather. Beams of sunlight brighten the entrance through overhead skylights.

Sky blue and crimson carpet complement the home's contemporary furnishings. Oak crown moldings and cream-colored walls provide a soothing backdrop for the seating areas, which are comprised of comfortable chairs with floral upholstery. The fluorescent lighting tends to be somewhat harsh. Nursing stations are located at the confluence of the generously sized hallways, which have wooden handrails and convenient seating areas. The windows in residents' moderately sized rooms allow generous light to shine through. Oak baseboards and crown moldings add texture and interest to the walls. Each room features

BISHOP DAVIES NURSING CENTER (CONTINUED)

a vanity and additional space for residents' belongings. Most residents relaxed and watched TV in their rooms during our tour, while others moved about the facility with assistance from staff members. Residents and staff conversed comfortably with one another as they went about their day.

A skylight in the dining room floods the spacious area with light. The layout of the dining room reminded us of a cozy restaurant with numerous oak tables for two accompanied by baby blue chairs. Artificial trees bring touches of green to the predominantly white space. Expansive windows showcase views of the central courtyard, where a quaint wooden bench surrounded by leafy plants invites residents to enjoy the fresh air and sunshine. The facility boasts additional patio areas in the backyard; pathways wind across the grassy area beneath the shade of oak trees, and residents are fond of watching birds congregate at the birdbath.

## HEARTLAND NURSING FACILITY

2001 Forest Ridge Drive
Bedford, TX 76021

(817) 571-6804
www.hcr-manorcare.com

**GOVERNMENT DEFICIENCIES: 16** — Reviewed on: November 3, 2004

| Administration | Environmental | Nutrition & Dietary | Pharmacy Service |
|---|---|---|---|
| 3 | 3 | 2 | 2 |
| **Quality Care** | **Resident Assessment** | **Resident Rights** | |
| 3 | 1 | 2 | |

*IMPORTANT: REVIEW DETAILS OF EACH DEFICIENCY AT WWW.MEDICARE.GOV

**GILBERT GUIDE OBSERVATIONS**

| Category | Rating | Category | Rating |
|---|---|---|---|
| Administration & Staff | g g g g g | Dietary & Food Selection | g g g |
| Facility Aesthetics | g g g g | Activities | g g g g |
| Facility Condition & Safety | g g g | Access to Medical Care | g g g g g |
| Residents | g g g | | |

### DETAILS

Year Built: 1988
Current Mgmt. Since: 1988
No. of Floors: 2
Resident Capacity: 120
Facility Type: Long-term care, Short-term rehab

### SPECIAL

Special diets accommodated
Proximity to Emergency Svcs.: Under 8 miles

## STAFF

Caregiver Training: Dementia, Ethics, Family communication, Grief, Pain management, Patient transfers, Stress management, Transition issues, Universal precautions, Validation therapy, Wound care
Criminal Background Check: Yes
Principal Staff Language(s): English

## FACILITY FEATURES

Activities/Recreation
Beauty/Barber Shop ($)
Guest Meals ($)
Outside Patio/Gardens
Separate Therapy Room ($)
24-hour Security
Wanderguard
Whirlpool Baths

## ROOM FEATURES

Cable TV Ready ($)
Space for personal items
Shared Bathrooms
Telephone Ready ($)

## COSTS

PRICES MAY INCREASE. PLEASE CALL FOR MOST CURRENT INFORMATION.

| | |
|---|---|
| Shared Room | $114/day |
| Rate Increase | Annually; usually 3% |
| Reimbursement | Medicare, Medicaid, LTCI, HMO, Private pay, SSI, Veterans |

## PORTRAIT

Heartland is conveniently located less than a mile from various restaurants and shopping centers, off of Highway 183. The impressive pentagon-shaped building, reminiscent of an old schoolhouse, neighbors a newly built playground, where we observed many children playing. Residents gather in the well-furnished lobby. The rich green carpeting, complemented by cream-colored sofas, Victorian chairs, wooden tables and porcelain decorations, creates an altogether homey atmosphere.

Residents' rooms are spacious enough to accommodate a queen-size bed and two accent pieces. The dining room doubles as an activity space. Residents often gather in the common area that boasts the best view of the playground. For outdoor leisure, residents get plenty of fresh air and sunlight in the courtyard. They stroll the crisscrossing garden paths, lounge under the shade of maple trees or rest on benches that line the lush grassy area. A few of the residents have personalized the garden with their own potted ferns and flowers. Soft fluorescent lighting prevails throughout the building. Maroon berber carpeting lines the wide hallways of the building. Residents keep decorative tables outside their doors to showcase seasonal decorations. One resident dresses a porcelain duck in the appropriate seasonal garb.

Management and staff emphasize efficiency without compromising the quality of care. Although the staff was busy tending to residents' needs on our visit, they were always smiling and pleasant.

## La Dora

1960 Bedford Road
Bedford, TX 76021

(817) 283-4771
www.eldercare.bz

**GOVERNMENT DEFICIENCIES: 5** Reviewed on: December 9, 2004

| Administration | Mistreatment | Quality Care |
|---|---|---|
| 1 | 1 | 3 |

*IMPORTANT: REVIEW DETAILS OF EACH DEFICIENCY AT WWW.MEDICARE.GOV

**GILBERT GUIDE OBSERVATIONS**

| | | | |
|---|---|---|---|
| Administration & Staff | g g g g g | Dietary & Food Selection | g g g |
| Facility Aesthetics | g g | Activities | g g g |
| Facility Condition & Safety | g g g | Access to Medical Care | g g g |
| Residents | g g g | | |

### DETAILS

Year Built: 1962
Year Remodeled: 2002
Current Mgmt. Since: 1989
No. of Floors: 1
Resident Capacity: 66
Facility Type: Long-term care, Short-term rehab

### SPECIAL

Special diets accommodated
Proximity to Emergency Svcs.: Under 8 miles

### STAFF

Caregiver Training: Dementia, Ethics, Family communication, Grief, Pain management, Patient transfers, Stress management, Transition issues, Universal precautions, Validation therapy, Wound care
Criminal Background Check: Yes
Principal Staff Language(s): English
Other Staff Language(s): Spanish

### FACILITY FEATURES

Activities/Recreation
Outside Patio/Gardens
24-hour Security
Whirlpool Baths

### ROOM FEATURES

Space for personal items
Shared & Private Bathrooms
Telephone Ready ($)

### COSTS

PRICES MAY INCREASE. PLEASE CALL FOR MOST CURRENT INFORMATION.

| | |
|---|---|
| Shared Room | $99–$155/day |
| Private Room | $171–$269/day |
| Rate Increase | Annually; usually 3.5% |
| Reimbursement | Medicare, Medicaid, LTCI, HMO, Private pay, SSI, Veterans |

## PORTRAIT

A dog and two cats rescued from an animal shelter freely roam La Dora. We noted residents glowing with affection as they cuddled the animals. Residents interact comfortably with each other and staff members. One staff member who has worked at La Dora for seventeen years and still "loves it." Others have been there nearly as long.

The administrator informed us that plans to remodel the facility were in the works. Off-white walls, large windows and fluorescent lighting brighten the interior. Comfortable high-backed chairs and a stone fireplace in the foyer evoke a rustic lodge, a nice touch for a SNF. Residents enjoy gathering to eat meals, watch TV and take part in activities in the expansive dining room. Floral arrangements top the numerous long tables, which are reminiscent of a school cafeteria. Couches and tables furnish the library, a favorite place for residents to read and play card games. Paintings depicting nature scenes adorn the narrow hallways, which are lined with handrails. Lamps and windows light residents' small rooms. Each room features a closet and some rooms have additional storage space. Bluebonnets and sunflowers grace the building's exterior. Residents exercise in the patio area on the lawn, which is shaded by tall oak trees. La Dora blends in well in its tranquil residential neighborhood.

# TOWN HALL ESTATES OF ARLINGTON

824 West Mayfield Road (817) 465-2222
Arlington, TX 76015

---

**GOVERNMENT DEFICIENCIES: 10** Reviewed on: December 16, 2004

| Administration | Mistreatment | Nutrition and Dietary | Quality Care |
|---|---|---|---|
| 2 | 3 | 1 | 2 |
| **Resident Assessment** | **Resident Rights** | | |
| 1 | 1 | | |

*IMPORTANT: REVIEW DETAILS OF EACH DEFICIENCY AT WWW.MEDICARE.GOV

**GILBERT GUIDE OBSERVATIONS**

| | | | |
|---|---|---|---|
| Administration & Staff | g g g g | Dietary & Food Selection | g g g |
| Facility Aesthetics | g g g g g | Activities | g g g g |
| Facility Condition & Safety | g g g g | Access to Medical Care | g g g g g |
| Residents | g g g g g | | |

## DETAILS

Year Built: 1993
Year Remodeled: 2003
Current Mgmt. Since: 1996

## SPECIAL

Special diets accommodated
Proximity to Emergency Svcs.: Under 8 miles

TOWN HALL ESTATES OF ARLINGTON (CONTINUED)

DETAILS (CONTINUED)
No. of Floors: 1
Resident Capacity: 116
Facility Type: Long-term care

## STAFF

Caregiver Training: Ethics, Family communication, Grief, Pain management, Patient transfers
Criminal Background Check: Yes
Principal Staff Language(s): English
Other Staff Language(s): Spanish

## FACILITY FEATURES

Activities/Recreation
Beauty/Barber Shop ($)
Chapel Services
Facility Parking
Guest Meals
Outside Patio/Gardens
Private Dining Room
Private Visiting Room
Separate Therapy Room
24-hour Security
Whirlpool Baths

## ROOM FEATURES

Cable TV Ready ($)
Space for personal items
Shared & Private Bathrooms
Telephone Ready

## COSTS

PRICES MAY INCREASE. PLEASE CALL FOR MOST CURRENT INFORMATION.

| | |
|---|---|
| Shared Room | $94–$99/day |
| Private Room | $129–$139/day |
| Rate Increase | Annually; usually 1–2.5% |
| Reimbursement | Private pay |

## PORTRAIT

Town Hall Estates of Arlington rests on Mayfield Road, a mere two blocks from Arlington Memorial Hospital. White trim neatly outlines the red brick façade. Upon entering the facility, we were greeted by one resident's performance on the grand piano; a group of residents raised their voices in accompaniment. A generous seating area comprised of dark green and maroon furnishings, lies beyond the musical group. Garden paintings complement the rose and beige carpet. Nearby, two striking stained glass windows fill the home's beautiful chapel with richly colored rays of light. Pews line the tranquil room, in which residents enjoy their devotions.

We observed several animated residents who challenged friendly staff members to games of chess in the activity room, where they also play cards, bingo and dominoes. A sea of tables draped in white stretches across the spacious dining area. Mellow sunlight and fluorescent lighting brighten the home. Nursing stations sit at the junctures of the hallways, which are amply sized to accommodate residents in hospital beds and wheelchairs. Painted depictions of gardens add an artful touch to the handrail-lined hallways. Nightstands, entertainment centers and beds furnish residents' spacious, sunny rooms. Closets provide additional storage space. The large bathrooms feature raised sinks and toilets as well as walk-in showers. The home boasts a beautiful central patio that is verdant with plants grown by residents. A stately gazebo provides plenty of seating when residents gather outdoors. Wide pathways invite residents to walk beneath a canopy of oak and maple boughs.

## IN-HOME CARE PROVIDERS

## Angels of Hands Home Health Agency

630 Blue Creek Drive
Cedar Hill, TX 75104

(972) 230-2828

SEE CHAPTER 1 FOR A DESCRIPTION OF IN-HOME CARE SERVICES.

### DETAILS

Years in Business: 2
Home Health Services Provided: Yes
Care Visits Provided Within a Facility: Yes
Dementia Care Provided: No
Will Replace Caregiver Within 48 Hours Upon Request: Yes

### CAREGIVERS

RN on Staff: Yes
Hiring Qualifications: 6 months of experience, DMV check, TB test, Criminal background check, CNA certification, 1 reference required
Caregiver Training: Dementia, Ethics, Family communication, Grief, Patient transfers, Stress management
Frequency of Caregiver Training: Initial formal training program, Monthly
Language(s) Spoken: English, Sign Language, Spanish

### AVAILABILITY

Service Availability: 24/7
On-call Supervisor Availability: 24/7

### COSTS

PRICES MAY INCREASE. PLEASE CALL FOR MOST CURRENT INFORMATION.

Rate: Call for rates
Minimum Hours per Day: None
Minimum Days per Week: None
Sliding Fee Schedule Available: No

### UNIQUE QUALITIES

The owner of this agency, an experienced nurse, treats clients as if they were family. The staff of skilled caregivers focuses on prolonging clients' independence so that they may continue to stay with their loved ones rather than move to a long-term care facility.

## Aspen Home Care

1000 Nora Lane
Desoto, TX 75115
(214) 500-6009

SEE CHAPTER I FOR A DESCRIPTION OF IN-HOME CARE SERVICES.

### DETAILS

Years in Business: 1
Home Health Services Provided: Yes
Care Visits Provided Within a Facility: Yes
Dementia Care Provided: No
Will Replace Caregiver Within 48 Hours Upon Request: Yes

### CAREGIVERS

RN on Staff: Yes
Hiring Qualifications: 2 years of experience, TB test, Criminal background check, CNA certification, 3 references required
Caregiver Training: Dementia, Ethics, Family communication, Grief, Patient transfers, Stress management
Frequency of Caregiver Training: Initial formal training program, Semiannual
Language(s) Spoken: English, Spanish

### AVAILABILITY

Service Availability: 24/7
On-call Supervisor Availability: 24/7

### COSTS

PRICES MAY INCREASE. PLEASE CALL FOR MOST CURRENT INFORMATION.

Rate: Call for rates
Minimum Hours per Day: None
Minimum Days per Week: None
Sliding Fee Schedule Available: No

### UNIQUE QUALITIES

Aspen Home Care fights to prolong the independence of its clients. The caregivers strive to provide compassionate, nonintrusive care. An experienced nurse supervises the care. The agency accepts Medicare and Medicaid.

## Beacon Home Health Services

1000 Nora Lane
Desoto, TX 75115
(972) 223-0074

SEE CHAPTER 1 FOR A DESCRIPTION OF IN-HOME CARE SERVICES.

### DETAILS

Years in Business: 9
Home Health Services Provided: No
Care Visits Provided Within a Facility: Yes
Dementia Care Provided: No
Will Replace Caregiver Within 48 Hours Upon Request: Yes

### CAREGIVERS

RN on Staff: Yes
Hiring Qualifications: 2 years of experience, TB test, Criminal background check, CNA certification, 3 references required
Caregiver Training: Dementia, Ethics, Family communication, Grief, Patient transfers, Stress management
Frequency of Caregiver Training: Initial formal training program, Semiannual
Language(s) Spoken: English, Spanish

### AVAILABILITY

Service Availability: 24/7
On-call Supervisor Availability: 24/7

### COSTS

PRICES MAY INCREASE. PLEASE CALL FOR MOST CURRENT INFORMATION.

Rate: $15.50/hour
Live-In: $372/day
Sleepover: $186/night
Minimum Hours per Day: 4
Minimum Days per Week: None
Sliding Fee Schedule Available: No

### UNIQUE QUALITIES

The goal of Beacon Home is to provide excellent care at a cost that is lower than average. The agency's management and caregivers listen carefully to clients' needs, to maximize their independence and comfort. Beacon Home works hard to establish trust and friendship between clients and caregivers.

## Home Health Specialties

4239 Road to the Mall (817) 496-5400
North Richland Hills, TX 76180

SEE CHAPTER 1 FOR A DESCRIPTION OF IN-HOME CARE SERVICES.

### DETAILS

Years in Business: 30
Home Health Services Provided: Yes
Care Visits Provided Within a Facility: Yes
Dementia Care Provided: Yes
Will Replace Caregiver Within 48 Hours Upon Request: Yes

### CAREGIVERS

RN on Staff: Yes
Hiring Qualifications: 1 year of experience, TB test, Criminal background check, CNA certification, 2 references required
Caregiver Training: Dementia, Ethics, Family communication, Grief, Patient transfers, Transition issues
Frequency of Caregiver Training: Initial formal training program, Monthly, Annually
Language(s) Spoken: English, Spanish

### AVAILABILITY

Service Availability: 24/7
On-call Supervisor Availability: 24/7

### COSTS

PRICES MAY INCREASE. PLEASE CALL FOR MOST CURRENT INFORMATION.

Rate: Call for rates
Minimum Hours per Day: None
Minimum Days per Week: None
Sliding Fee Schedule Available: Yes

### UNIQUE QUALITIES

Home Health Specialties boasts thirty years of homecare experience in the Dallas area. The agency offers services that range from pediatrics to geriatrics. The therapy program is staffed by full-time professionals who specialize in speech, physical and occupational therapies. They pride themselves on smoothly transitioning clients from one program to another as necessary.

## In Home Care

8700 North Stemmons Freeway, Suite 4070 (214) 920-9296
Dallas, TX 75247

SEE CHAPTER 1 FOR A DESCRIPTION OF IN-HOME CARE SERVICES.

### DETAILS

Years in Business: 18
Home Health Services Provided: Yes
Care Visits Provided Within a Facility: Yes
Dementia Care Provided: No
Will Replace Caregiver Within 48 Hours Upon Request: Yes

### CAREGIVERS

RN on Staff: Yes
Hiring Qualifications: 5 months of experience, DMV check, TB test, Criminal background check, CNA certification, 4 references required
Caregiver Training: Dementia, Ethics, Family communication, Grief, Patient transfers, Stress management
Frequency of Caregiver Training: Initial formal training program, Monthly
Language(s) Spoken: English, Spanish

### AVAILABILITY

Service Availability: 24/7
On-call Supervisor Availability: 24/7

### COSTS

PRICES MAY INCREASE. PLEASE CALL FOR MOST CURRENT INFORMATION.

Rate: Call for rates
Minimum Hours per Day: None
Minimum Days per Week: None
Sliding Fee Schedule Available: No

### UNIQUE QUALITIES

In Home Care believes in educating their clients in addition to caring for them. The agency conducts evaluations to assess clients' needs and recommends other services they might find beneficial. In Home Care offers its caregivers a monthly continuing education program. This agency is Medicare and Medicaid certified.

## Primestaff Home Health Agency

3906 Lemmon Avenue, Suite 212
Dallas, TX 75219

(214) 599-9083
www.domestic-agency.com

SEE CHAPTER 1 FOR A DESCRIPTION OF IN-HOME CARE SERVICES.

### DETAILS

Years in Business: 26
Home Health Services Provided: No
Care Visits Provided Within a Facility: Yes
Dementia Care Provided: Yes
Will Replace Caregiver Within 48 Hours Upon Request: Yes

### CAREGIVERS

RN on Staff: Yes
Hiring Qualifications: 4 years of experience, DMV check, TB test, Criminal background check, CNA certification, 3 references required
Caregiver Training: Dementia, Ethics, Family communication, Grief, Patient transfers, Transition issues
Frequency of Caregiver Training: Initial formal training program
Language(s) Spoken: English, Spanish

### AVAILABILITY

Service Availability: 24/7
On-call Supervisor Availability: 24/7

### COSTS

PRICES MAY INCREASE. PLEASE CALL FOR MOST CURRENT INFORMATION.

Rate: $15.50–$18.50/hour
Live-In: $200/day
Minimum Hours per Day: 4
Minimum Days per Week: None
Sliding Fee Schedule Available: Yes

### UNIQUE QUALITIES

Primestaff has been in operation for twenty-six years. The caregivers take an individualized approach to client care. The agency offers personal assistance, home management and companionship services, and makes a concerted effort to keep its rates competitive.

### ADULT DAY CARE & HEALTH CARE CENTERS

## Arlington Adult Day Health Care A/D

2117-B Roosevelt
Arlington, TX 76013

(817) 795-8066

**GILBERT GUIDE OBSERVATIONS** gggg

## DETAILS

Owner/Affiliation: Cliff Haven
Years in Business: 10
License/Certification: Texas Department of Human Services
Business Hours: Monday–Friday, 7:30am–5:30pm
Conditions Accepted: Alzheimer's/Dementia, Developmental disabilities, Incontinence, Limited mobility, Mental illness, Stroke, Vision/Hearing impairment

## SPECIAL

Special diets accommodated
Wheelchair accessible
Proximity to Emergency Svcs.: 9–15 Miles
Onsite Care: Nursing,

## STAFF

Staff/patient ration: 1:8
Criminal Background Check: Yes
Language(s) spoken: English, Spanish

## COSTS

Prices may increase. Please call for most current information.
Daily Costs: $25–$35; $600/month
Reimbursement: Medicaid, Private pay, Veterans

## PORTRAIT

Arlington offers both adult day and adult day health care. The institutional stucco exterior of the facility disguises the wonderful programming and people inside. Staff members conduct activities in a large room furnished with recliners. The facility also boasts a kitchen and office, in addition to a designated "napping" room for participants who need to rest for a bit. Staff members tailor the daily programming to address participants' varying needs. The seniors eagerly take part in Arlington's activities, which include crafts, games, exercise and spiritual programs. Participants also enjoy meals at the center. Volunteers, a mix of adults and schoolchildren, entertain participants on Cinco de Mayo, Christmas and a number of other holidays.

The staff's great affection for participants was evident in the friendly conversations we observed between them. The director has been with Arlington since its opening. Other staff members have worked there for nearly as long. The RN who dispenses participants' medications also performs blood pressure and insulin checks. The director told us a touching story of two participants, who were relatives who had lost touch with one another, but were recently reunited at the day care.

## GERIATRIC CARE MANAGERS

### DALLAS CARE CONNECTION

Carol K. Franzen, MS, LMSW
P.O. Box 815848
Dallas, TX 75381

(972) 242-0901
cfranzen@dallascareconnection.com
www.dallascareconnection.com

SEE CHAPTER 1 FOR A DESCRIPTION OF GERIATRIC CARE MANAGER SERVICES.

#### DETAILS

Years of GCM Experience: 21
Degree(s) Held: Licensed Master Social Worker
Member of National Association of Professional Geriatric Care Managers
Language(s) Spoken: English

#### SERVICES

Staff on Call: 24/7
Client References Provided: Yes
Areas of Practice: Assessment, Care management, Counseling, Education, Family/Professional liaison
Assistance with Medicare/Medicaid Process: Yes

#### COSTS

PRICES MAY INCREASE. PLEASE CALL FOR MOST CURRENT INFORMATION.

Assessment: Call for rates
Hourly: Call for rates

#### UNIQUE QUALITIES

With over twenty years of case management experience behind her, Carol K. Franzen is highly skilled in assisting seniors and people with disabilities. Carol has provided case management services in the Dallas-Fort Worth area since 1985. Not surprisingly, other local care managers have referred a number of challenging cases to Dallas Care Connection; Carol's familiarity with long-term care services in the area is a great strength.

## HOSPICE PROVIDERS

### ANOINTED CHILD

2510 Texas Drive, Suite 100
Irving, TX 75062

(972) 261-5500

SEE CHAPTER 1 FOR A DESCRIPTION OF HOSPICE SERVICES.

#### DETAILS

Affiliation: None
Licensed By: Texas Department of Health Services
Medicare certified

### CARE

At-home Care Provided: Yes
Inpatient Care Provided: Yes
Caregivers trained, supervised, and monitored
Supervisor on call 24/7
Language(s) Spoken: English, Spanish

### UNIQUE QUALITIES

Anointed Child is locally owned and operated. Management's philosophy is that superior service and care begins with one-on-one attention. Staffed by veteran caregivers, the organization's mission is to provide the best end-of-life care possible. By managing patients' pain, Anointed Child strives to bring dignity and peace to this final stage. When it comes to making a decision about care, patients and their families depend on the organization's commitment to timely responses and active resolutions.

## Libbys Hospice

6633 Grapevine Highway
North Richland Hills, TX 76180
(817) 498-7733

SEE CHAPTER 1 FOR A DESCRIPTION OF HOSPICE SERVICES.

### DETAILS

Affiliation: None
Licensed By: Texas Department of Health Services
Medicare certified

### CARE

At-home Care Provided: Yes
Inpatient Care Provided: No
Caregivers trained, supervised, and monitored
Supervisor on call 24/7
Language(s) Spoken: English, Hindi, Spanish

### UNIQUE QUALITIES

Libbys Hospice is a fairly new, privately owned agency in North Richland Hills. The owner, Molly Zacharia, ensures her personal involvement in all clients' end-of-life care.

## Samaritan Care Hospice North Richland Hills

7001 Grapevine Highway, Suite 500
North Richland Hills, TX 76180
(817) 590-9623
www.samaritancarehospice.com

SEE CHAPTER 1 FOR A DESCRIPTION OF HOSPICE SERVICES.

### DETAILS

Affiliation: Trans-Health Care
Licensed By: Texas Department of Health Services
Medicare certified

SAMARITAN CARE HOSPICE NORTH RICHLAND HILLS (CONTINUED)

## CARE

At-home Care Provided: Yes
Inpatient Care Provided: Yes
Caregivers trained, supervised, and monitored
Supervisor on call 24/7
Language(s) Spoken: English, Hindi, Spanish

## UNIQUE QUALITIES

Samaritan Care Hospice promises its patients two things: first, neither pain nor illness will lessen the quality of one's remaining days; and second, patients and their loved ones will not be alone at a time when emotional support means so much. Samaritan Care in North Richland Hills is committed to remaining a small organization so that individualized care is never compromised. This agency has a decade of experience providing hospice care within the community; the majority of staff has been with Samaritan for over five years.

# GEMS

• Little-known resources that make a BIG difference

- Animal Therapy
- Arts
- Caregiver Resources
- Counseling and Support Groups
- Dentists
- Estate Sales and Liquidation
- Financial Management
- Fitness
- General Senior Services
- Hearing
- Home Design and Modifications
- Independent Living Facilities and Services
- In-Home Specialty Services
- Library on Wheels
- Living Will
- Meal Delivery
- Medical Supplies and Specialty Items
- Movers
- Pharmacies
- Real Estate
- Transportation

## Animal Therapy

### All Star Equestrian Foundation

P.O. Box 892/6601 FM 2738
Mansfield, TX 76063

(817) 477-1437
allstar892@juno.com
www.allstarfoundation.org

AREAS SERVED: Mid-Cities

Affiliation/Owner: North American Riding for the Handicapped Association
Nonprofit Organization
Business Hours: Monday–Friday, 9:00am–5:00pm

The All Star Equestrian Foundation offers horseback riding as a therapeutic form of mental, physical and emotional fitness. Participants enjoy a wealth of benefits, including improved motor skills and balance. All Star's team of certified instructors emphasize riding and various horse-related activities for individuals with cerebral palsy, stroke injuries, autism and other conditions, to foster participants' independence and well-being.

### K-9 FRIENDS Visiting Therapy Dogs of GTDOG

1931 Pin Oak Drive
Flower Mound, TX 75028

(800) 730-4925
hohenstauffen@peoplepc.com
www.gtdog.org

AREAS SERVED: North Dallas

Nonprofit Organization
Business Hours: Monday–Friday, 9:00am–5:00pm

Dog-lovers in the Visiting Therapy Dogs group unite in support of a wonderful cause. By sponsoring weekly pet visits to local long-term care facilities, the group facilitates the primary tenet of its mission statement: everyone should have an opportunity to enjoy the unconditional love and friendship of their K-9 Friends!

### SPCA: Compassion Connection

362 South Industrial Boulevard
Dallas, TX 75207

(214) 651-9611
spca@spca.org
www.spca.org

AREAS SERVED: Dallas, North Dallas

Affiliation/Owner: Science Diet, VCA Animal Hospital
Nonprofit Organization
Business Hours: Monday–Friday, 12:00pm–6:00pm; Saturday, 10:00am–6:00pm; Sunday, 12:00pm–6:00pm

The SPCA of Texas' Compassion Connection brings the healing presence of animals to people in health care facilities. Society volunteers take their own pets on the visits: dogs, rabbits, birds—even cats.

## Arts

### A.R.T.S. (Artistic, Recreational, Therapeutic Services) for People

2525 Ross Avenue
Dallas, TX 75201

(214) 841-9200
rwilliams@artsforpeople.org
www.artsforpeople.org

AREAS SERVED: Dallas County

Nonprofit Organization
Business Hours: Monday–Friday, 9:00am–5:00pm

A.R.T.S. for People is an alliance of artists, therapists and healthcare workers. Guided by the conviction that well-being is greatly improved through positive social interaction and self-expression, A.R.T.S. for People employs music, dance, expressive therapies and other recreational activities to engage clients and promote wellness. The exciting programming includes drama, creative movement and fine art. Clients benefit by improving their communication skills and building self-esteem. Other benefits include physical and emotional release. A.R.T.S. for People welcomes clients of all ages.

### ArtReach-Dallas, Inc.

2801 Swiss Avenue, Suite 120
Dallas, TX 75204

(214) 827-1025

AREAS SERVED: Dallas

Affiliation/Owner: City of Dallas
Nonprofit Organization
Business Hours: Monday–Friday, 9:00am–5:00pm

For over two decades, Artreach-Dallas has provided over 200,000 low-income, disabled and elderly participants with access to artistic and cultural events each year. Participants in the Community Events program attend symphonies, movie screenings, ballet performances and other events free of charge. A number of senior centers in the Dallas area host the popular Senior Theatre Arts program, in which participants enjoy weaving, sculpture, and creative writing, drawing and painting classes, among other activities. In the past, seniors have joined forces with playwrights, directors and other theater professionals to produce plays based on their individual histories—and performed them for standing-room-only crowds.

### Arts for Children and Adults at Risk (ACAR)

2000 West Airport Freeway
Irving, TX 75015

(972) 721-2488, (972) 721-8063
info@irvingart.org
www.irvingart.org

AREAS SERVED: Irving

Affiliation/Owner: City of Irving, Dayspring Counseling, Irving Art Association
Nonprofit Organization
Business Hours: Monday–Friday, 9:00am–5:00pm

The ACAR advocates the therapeutic benefits of the arts. The program serves as a creative outlet for persons living with learning and physical disabilities, chronic illnesses, depression, and other challenges. The agency's art therapy classes are free to the public and run for nine to twelve months, depending on individual needs. Regularly scheduled workshops include composition and painting; all materials are provided by ACAR.

## Caregiver Resources

### La Voz del Anciano

3316 Sylvan Avenue
Dallas, TX 75212

(214) 741-5700
lavoz@sbcglobal.net
www.lavozdelanciano.org

AREAS SERVED: Dallas County

Affiliation/Owner: Dallas Area Agency on Aging, Department On Aging, National Hispanic Association Disability Services
Nonprofit Organization
Business Hours: Monday–Friday, 9:00am–4:00pm

La Voz del Anciano, a long-standing organization of nearly three decades, helps Dallas County's Hispanic seniors locate and obtain social services and community resources. La Voz employs a number of activities to educate Hispanic seniors, their families and caregivers. These include training seminars, health fairs and study circles. La Voz also promotes seniors' health by offering three-kilometer walks for the elderly.

### MedicalView

www.MedicalView.com

AREAS SERVED: Nationwide

Affiliation/Owner: Visual Data Corporation

The MedicalView website provides links to interactive programs that address a wealth of medical issues, including cancer, multiple sclerosis and heart attacks. The site offers a comprehensive list of short, informational programs that answers questions pertaining to specific medical conditions. Web audiences click on the queries to receive detailed, accurate responses from medical specialists.

## Counseling and Support Groups

### Heritage Outpatient for Senior Adults

3500 Interstate 30
Mesquite, TX 75150

(972) 682-4260, (972) 698-3300
susan.blankenship@mch.hma-corp.com
www.mchtx.com

AREAS SERVED: Mesquite

Affiliation/Owner: Mesquite Community Hospital
Nonprofit Organization
Business Hours: Monday–Friday, 9:00am–5:00pm

The Heritage Outpatient Program for Senior Adults provides mental health intervention to seniors, who are referred to the program by concerned individuals—which may include friends, family or members of the clergy. Participants undergo a free clinical assessment. Individual and group counseling are both available. A licensed staff comprised of counselors, RNs and social workers, who are supervised by psychiatrists, provide treatment for dealing with depression, anxiety, isolation, grief, anger and other mental health issues. Participants receive free transportation to the program via wheelchair-accessible vans. Heritage is Medicare certified.

## Dentists

### Community Dental Care

1440 West Mockingbird, Suite 120
Dallas, TX 75247

(214) 630-7080
phoffmann@communitydentalcare.org
www.communitydentalcare.org

AREAS SERVED: Dallas

Affiliation/Owner: Dallas County Dental Society, United Way
Nonprofit Organization
Business Hours: Monday–Friday, 8:00am–4:30pm

Community Dental Care, formerly Dental Health Programs, was founded over four decades ago. Today, the nonprofit organization operates nine clinics throughout Dallas and Collin counties that offer preventative care such as X-rays, cleanings and fluoride treatments, and routine dental care that ranges from fillings to oral surgery. Community Dental Care primarily serves a low-income population, in addition to individuals with HIV/AIDS. Some centers provide dentures. Patients who require periodontal work and other special procedures may be referred to Parkland Oral Surgery and Baylor College of Dentistry. Community Dental Care also educates the public on oral hygiene and proper nutrition at Dallas County health fairs.

## Estate Sales and Liquidation

### Millchell Estate Sales, Inc.

2112 Lipscomb Street
Fort Worth, TX 76110

(817) 923-3274
www.millchell.com

AREAS SERVED: Fort Worth

Business Hours: Monday–Friday, 9:00am–5:00pm

Millchell Estates Sales, Inc. provides its clients with various estate liquidation services. Experienced, certified appraisers manage every step of the process—initial consultation, preparing inventories, advertising, final sale and post-sale clean-ups. Whether clients are selling their homes or relocating, Millchell's aims to make this transition seamless.

## Financial Management

### Griffin Financial Mortgage, LLC

1701 River Run, Suite 308
Fort Worth, TX 76107

(888) 415-1955
loaninfo@griffinloans.com
www.griffinloans.com

AREAS SERVED: Fort Worth

Business Hours: Monday–Friday, 9:00am–5:00pm

Griffin Financial Mortgage specializes in reverse mortgages, a process that helps homeowners over the age of sixty-two generate income, helping to preserve their financial freedom and independence. Homeowners retain the title and can choose from several payment options ranging from a line of credit to a lump sum or monthly payments. The money is non-taxable and does not affect Social Security or Medicare benefits. Borrowers do not need to worry about making monthly payments, since none are required for the term of the loan.

### Reliance Mortgage Company

8115 Preston Road, Suite 800
Dallas, TX 75225

(214) 346-5210, (214) 360-9000
jchase@reliancemortgage.com
www.reliancemortgage.com

AREAS SERVED: Dallas

Business Hours: Monday–Friday, 9:00am–5:00pm

Reliance Mortgage Company specializes in reverse mortgages, a process that helps homeowners over the age of sixty-two generate income, helping to preserve their financial freedom and independence. Homeowners retain the title and can choose from different payment options, including a lump sum or monthly payments. The money is non-taxable and does not affect Social Security or Medicare benefits. Borrowers do not need to worry about making monthly payments, since none are required for the term of the loan.

## Fitness

### Texercise

210 East Ninth Street
Fort Worth, TX 76102

(817) 258-8081
www.dads.state.tx.us

AREAS SERVED: Fort Worth

Affiliation/Owner: Area Agency on Aging of Tarrant County, Department of Aging & Disability Services
Nonprofit Organization
Business Hours: Monday–Friday, 8:30am–5:00pm

Statewide program Texercise encourages healthy eating habits and regular physical activity among seniors and their families. It also promotes participation in recreational programs such as the Texas Senior Volleyball Association, an organization for men and women who are fifty or older. Additionally, Texercise works with senior centers and communities to organize new fitness programs. The agency's website features helpful logs to monitor physical fitness and activity. It promotes healthy nutrition by educating seniors about the MyPyramid food guide, which has replaced the traditional Food Guide Pyramid.

## General Senior Services

### Bedford Hurst Senior Citizen Center

2817 R D Hurst Parkway
Bedford, TX 76021

(817) 952-2325, (817) 952-2329
vchamblee@ci.bedford.tx.us
www.ci.bedford.tx.us

AREAS SERVED: Bedford, Hurst and surrounding cities

Affiliation/Owner: City of Bedford
Nonprofit Organization
Business Hours: Monday–Friday, 8:00am–5:00pm

For over twenty years, the Bedford-Hurst Center has provided an array of services and activities to vibrant seniors in both cities. For a dollar, members enjoy a full year of community fun! The event calendar, brimming with activities, includes weekly dances, tai chi instruction, line and tap dance classes, ceramics, china painting workshops, needlecraft and quilting groups, bridge games and AARP meetings. Bedford-Hurst's staff organizes field trips and group travel as well.

### Geriatric Wellness Center of Collin County

401 West 16th Street, Suite 600
Plano, TX 75075

(972) 941-7335
www.gwccc.org

AREAS SERVED: Collin County and surrounding areas

Affiliation/Owner: United Way
Nonprofit Organization
Business Hours: Monday–Friday, 9:00am–5:00pm

The Geriatric Wellness Center of Collin County offers services to residents fifty-five years and older, as well as their loved ones and caregivers. The Center is a one-stop facility for: routine health screenings such as physicals, lab work and blood pressure checks; support groups that educate members on diabetes, Alzheimer's, hearing loss and other medical issues; resource referrals that pertain to housing, transportation and nutrition; and senior network groups. Members may borrow medical equipment such as wheelchairs, canes and walkers from the Center free of charge.

### Jewish Community Center of Dallas

7900 Northaven Road
Dallas, TX 75230

(214) 739-2737
info@jccdallas.org
www.jccdallas.org

AREAS SERVED: Dallas County

Affiliation/Owner: Jewish Federation of Greater Dallas, United Way of Metropolitan Dallas
Nonprofit Organization
Business Hours: Monday–Thursday, 6:00am–10:00pm; Friday, 6:00am–5:00pm; Saturday and Sunday, 7:00am–6:00pm

The Jewish Community Center of Dallas is at the heart of the Jewish community. People of all ages and religious affiliations are welcome, and participants are accepted regardless of their financial situation. The programs include cultural, recreational, social, and educational offerings. The center hosts art exhibits and a periodic lecture series for the enjoyment and enrichment of its members. Senior-specific activities and nutritional programs are also available. The center boasts a health club, a swimming pool, a tennis court, and athletic fields as well as youth and adult sports leagues.

### Lake Worth Senior Citizens Center

3501 Roberts Cutoff Road
Fort Worth, TX 76114

(817) 237-3281

AREAS SERVED: Tarrant County

Affiliation/Owner: City of Lake Worth
Nonprofit Organization
Business Hours: Monday, Wednesday, Thursday, Friday, 9:00am–3:00pm; Tuesday, 9:00am–4:00pm

Lake Worth Senior Citizens Center offers several wonderful activities that satisfy a wide range of interests. Active seniors enjoy ballroom dance and country western dance; those who prefer quieter pursuits enjoy ceramics, quilting, oil painting and crochet. Bingo, bridge, and other games provide a little friendly competition. There are even computer classes for the technologically inclined. Lake Worth hosts a half-day social every Tuesday, and a daylong social featuring games and food every Friday.

### Lighthouse for the Blind of Fort Worth

912 West Broadway
Fort Worth, TX 76104
(817) 332-3341
www.lighhousefw.org

4245 Office Parkway
Dallas, TX 75204
(214) 821-2375

AREAS SERVED: Tarrant County

Affiliation/Owner: City of Fort Worth
Nonprofit Organization
Business Hours: Monday–Friday, 8:00am–5:00pm

Lighthouse for the Blind has been serving the visually-impaired communities of Forth Worth and Dallas for over sixty years. The nonprofit organization offers a broad range of programs that provides assistance through education, training, skills enhancement and job placement. Lighthouse for the Blind operates an online retail store, Servmart, that distributes specialized office products and supplies to employers of visually-impaired and disabled persons.

### Retired and Senior Volunteer Program (RSVP)

1400 Crescent, Suite 3
Denton, TX 76201
(940) 383-1508
dmcorona@rsvpdentoncounty.org
www.rsvpserves.org

Lewisville Office
217 South Stemmons, Suite 202
Lewisville, TX 75067
(972) 221-9663
dynatron@rsvpdentoncounty.org

AREAS SERVED: Denton County

Affiliation/Owner: Corporation for National & Community Service, Cities of Denton and Lewisville
Nonprofit Organization
Business Hours: Monday–Friday, 8:30am–5:00pm

RSVP places adults, age fifty-five and older, in volunteer positions with local nonprofit organizations. Volunteers serve within a variety of settings, including churches, nursing homes, public schools and Habitat for Humanity. RSVP offers five programs of its own. Childhood Immunization volunteers visit hospitals to educate new mothers on childhood immunizations. The Rockin' Readers program sends volunteers to kindergarten and first grade classes, where they read to students weekly. The Senior Environmental Corps addresses environmental issues; for example, volunteers lead approximately 15,000 schoolchildren, annually, through the Elm Fork Environmental Education Center. Participants in Grand Connections, a mix of grandparents raising grandchildren and other nontraditional families, engage in support groups and other programs that address their special needs. At the Learning Center, RSVP staff and volunteers attend educational seminars on running nonprofit agencies. RSVP also hosts senior-specific seminars that focus on topics like identity theft prevention and personal safety.

### Wesley Rankin Community Center

3100 Crossman
Dallas, TX 75212

(214) 742-6674
stacy@wesleyrankin.org
www.wesleyrankin.org

AREAS SERVED: Dallas County

Affiliation/Owner: Area Methodist Churches
Nonprofit Organization
Business Hours: Monday–Friday, 9:00am–5:00pm

Wesley-Rankin Community Center, a Christian-based organization, has been serving West Dallas residents since 1902. The Senior Citizen program is the center's fastest growing program. Seniors receive complimentary transportation to the center, where they enjoy nutritious lunches, companionship and activities such as bingo. Participants also receive transportation to medical appointments and community center-sponsored outings. The seniors create decorative heart-shaped pillows for heart surgery patients at the Veteran's Administration Hospital of Dallas. Many also take part in free sewing classes, where they make items such as clothing and curtains. The Senior Citizen program takes place on weekdays.

## Hearing

### Deaf Action Center Texas

3115 Crestview Drive
Dallas, TX 75235

(214) 521-0407 TTY
seniorcitizens@deafactioncentertexas.org
www.deafactioncentertexas.org

AREAS SERVED: North Texas

Affiliation/Owner: Dallas Council for the Deaf
Nonprofit Organization

Deaf Action Center, a nonprofit, provides a multitude of services to assist individuals who are deaf or hard of hearing to maintain their independence and improve their quality of life. The center's interpreters help individuals to communicate in job interviews, theatrical performances and numerous other situations. American Sign Language lessons are offered at the center, as is counseling for conditions that range from anger and depression to employment and adjustment issues. Home visits may be arranged to assist individuals who need help coping with hearing loss and want to learn how to use assistive devices. Seniors enjoy meals, field trips and other activities, as well as helpful services such as casework, health screenings and benefits counseling—all available through the Senior Center. The Deaf Action Center runs a forty-unit apartment building specifically designed to accommodate individuals and families who are deaf or hard of hearing.

### Goodrich Center for the Deaf and Hard of Hearing

2500 Lipscomb Street
Fort Worth, TX 76110

(817) 926-5305
(817) 926-4101 TTY
interpreting@goodrichcenter.org
www.goodrichcenter.org

AREAS SERVED: DALLAS, Fort Worth

Affiliation/Owner: Alcon, Cash America, Charter Communication, Coors Light, Neiman Marcus, Omni American, Pier 1, Star Telegram, Texas Rangers
Nonprofit Organization
Business Hours: Monday–Friday, 8:30am–5:30pm

Goodrich Center is a nonprofit communication center for the deaf and hard of hearing in Tarrant County. For thirty-five years, the organization has been bringing the deaf, hearing impaired and hearing communities together. Goodrich case managers conduct needs assessments and advocate on behalf of clients. The center also provides around-the-clock interpreters for legal and medical emergencies. The Deaf Senior Citizen Program is for people who are sixty years of age or older who communicate mainly through sign language. Participants meet twice a week at the center, and also undertake visits to homebound or hospitalized individuals.

### Richardson Senior Center: Older Adult Program

820 West Arapaho
Richardson, TX 75080

(972) 231-4798
www.cor.net/seniorresources

AREAS SERVED: Richardson

Affiliation/Owner: City of Richardson
Nonprofit Organization
Business Hours: Monday, Tuesday, Thursday, 9:00am–9:00pm; Wednesday, Friday, 9:00am–5:00pm; Saturday, 1:00pm–5:00pm
Years in Business: 25

Richardson Senior Center serves adults who are fifty-five or older. The Center's monthly newsletter details the activities that are offered. A sampling of activities includes hatha yoga, pool tournaments, golf lessons, line dancing, voice lessons and scenic trips. The Center also

RICHARDSON SENIOR CENTER: OLDER ADULT PROGRAM (CONTINUED)

provides regular blood pressure screenings. Lunch, snacks and beverages are available daily for a small charge.

Trained volunteers answer questions about eligibility for public health benefits, such as Medicare and Medicaid. They also educate seniors about important issues like living wills and supplemental health insurance.

### Senior Adult Services

1111 West Beltline Road, Suite 110
Carrollton, TX 75006
(972) 242-4464
www.senioradultservices.org

AREAS SERVED: Addison, Carrollton, Coppell, Farmers Branch

Affiliation/Owner: Cities of Addison, Carrollton, Coppell and Farmers Branch, Metrocrest Medical Foundation, United Way of Metropolitan Dallas
Nonprofit Organization
Business Hours: Monday–Friday, 8:00am–12:00pm, 1:00pm–5:00pm
Years in Business: 25

Senior Adult Services aids seniors, their families, and caregivers in many ways. Case managers conduct needs assessments to determine participants' needs. Seniors may borrow walkers, wheelchairs and other medical equipment free of charge. Support and educational groups meet regularly. Volunteers deliver hot lunches to participants. The organization's monthly newsletter shares information on helpful resources and upcoming activities.

Participants in the Tel-A-Friend program call daily to check on each other. The Friendly Visitor program provides visitors to homebound seniors. Participants who own their homes have access to the Home Repair program. Volunteers perform functions such as painting, replacing broken windows, doing minor electrical work and installing wheelchair ramps. Senior Adult Services volunteers install grab bars and handrails in homes, regardless of homeowners' ability to pay. Volunteers also provide seniors with transportation to medical appointments and other necessary errands.

## Home Design and Modifications

### Arlington Neighborhood Services: Housing Modifications Program

201 East Abram
Arlington, TX 76010
(817) 459-6777, (817) 276-6707
powella@ci.arlington.tx.us
www.ci.arlington.tx.us/neighborhoodservices/grants/housing_modifications.html

AREAS SERVED: Arlington

Affiliation/Owner: City of Arlington
Nonprofit Organization
Business Hours: Monday–Friday, 8:00am–5:00pm

The Housing Modifications program is part of Arlington's Community Development plan. It is designed to assist low-income individuals and families modify their homes to accommodate elderly or disabled family members. City-approved repairs range from electrical to structural—heating, plumbing, door and porch adjustments and ramp installations are among the most common requests. The program's beneficiaries must meet eligibility requirements, due to limited grant funding.

### Premier Bathrooms

(888) 596-4904
www.premier-bathrooms.com

AREAS SERVED: Nationwide

Premier Bathrooms transforms bathrooms for elderly, frail and disabled individuals, making bathing easier, so they can comfortably maintain their independence. The products range from walk-in showers and baths, to seated bath options, grab bars and hydrotherapy tubs. Premier Bathrooms can advise its customers on the best options for their lifestyles and representatives provide a full demonstration of their products.

## Independent Living Facilities and Services

### Arlington New Beginnings, Inc.

311 North L Robinson Court
Arlington, TX 76011
(817) 860-6763

AREAS SERVED: Tarrant County

Affiliation/Owner: City of Arlington, Mount Olive Baptist Church
Nonprofit Organization
Business Hours: Monday–Friday, 8:30am–5:00pm

Arlington New Beginnings Inc is an affordable housing development for seniors. The facility has fourteen two-bedroom units spacious enough to room one senior as well as personal caregiver. The agency hosts educational seminars featuring groups such as the Alzheimer's Society and the Diabetic Society. It organizes health and nutrition focus groups to educate its residents on proper hygiene, diets and medical issues. Residents participate in various activities including bingo, Scrabble and other board games.

### Catherine Booth Friendship House

1901 East Seminary Drive
Fort Worth, TX 76119
(817) 531-2923
www.uss.salvationarmy.org/fortworth

AREAS SERVED: DALLAS, Fort Worth

Affiliation/Owner: The Salvation Army
Nonprofit Organization
Business Hours: Monday–Friday, 8:00am–6:00pm

CATHERINE BOOTH FRIENDSHIP HOUSE (CONTINUED)

The Salvation Army runs Catherine Booth Friendship House, which allows low-income residents to enjoy safe and affordable housing. The facility features nearly a hundred apartments for seniors age sixty-two and older. Single and married residents can both be accommodated.

### Dickinson Place

911 St. Joseph Street
Dallas, TX 75246

(214) 821-5390
dickinsonplace@earthlink.net
www.dickinsonplace.org

AREAS SERVED: Dallas County

Affiliation/Owner: Highland Park United Methodist Church
Nonprofit Organization
Business Hours: Monday–Friday, 8:30am–4:00pm

Dickinson Place offers affordable housing accommodations for adults age sixty-two and older. The apartments come with slight modifications—emergency pull stations and grab bars in the bathrooms—to allow easy mobility for residents with physical disabilities. Rents are based on a sliding scale and can be partially subsidized by the Department of Housing and Urban Development. Residents experience the perks of hotel conveniences such as paid utilities, grounds and building upkeep, laundry rooms, common areas and meal plans. A geriatric medical center is available on-site.

### McFadden Hall

1331 East Lancaster
Fort Worth, TX 76102

(817) 332-7747
ugm1@uniongospelmissionftw.org
www.uniongospelmissionftw.org

AREAS SERVED: Tarrant County

Affiliation/Owner: Union Gospel Mission
Nonprofit Organization
Business Hours: Monday–Friday, 9:00am–5:00pm

Union Gospel Mission operates McFadden Hall, Tarrant County's first residence for low-income senior women. Potential residents must submit an application in order to secure one of the facility's sixteen apartments. The building features handicap-accessible rooms as well as one private suite. The apartments are furnished and feature shared bathrooms. The facility boasts a kitchen and a laundry room. Residents enjoy the piano and the computer in the large common area, and attend Bible study and social events. A fence encloses the facility, which is monitored around the clock. McFadden Hall has a sliding scale of fees based on residents' income levels.

## In-Home Specialty Services

### Merry Maids

www.merrymaids.com

AREAS SERVED: Arlington, Bedford, Burleson, Carrollton, Colleyville, Dallas, Deer Park, Denton, Flower Mound, Fort Worth, Garland, Grand Prairie, Grapevine, Irving, North Richland Hills, Richardson, The Colony

Merry Maids' clients enjoy professional housecleaning that ranges from light housekeeping services such as dusting and vacuuming to more involved tasks like oven cleaning and washing the walls. Potential customers receive a cost estimate based on their particular cleaning needs. Services are rendered on a regular basis, according to clients' preferences. One-time services are also available. Visit Merry Maids' website to locate an office in your area.

### NFB Newsline

(888) 882-1629
(866) 504-7300
www.nfb.org/newsline1.htm

AREAS SERVED: Nationwide

Pioneered to assist people with visual impairments, National Federation for the Blind's Newsline is a toll-free news hotline. Gathering news bytes from over two hundred media affiliates, including giants such as USA Today, the Washington Post and Wall Street Journal and prominent magazines such as The Economist and AARP, subscribers receive their news at the touch of button. NFB-Newsline gives its "readers" access to local, national and world news twenty-four hours a day, seven days a week.

### NSeam Living At Home/Block Nurse Program

1150 South Freeway, Room 130 (817) 338-2958
Fort Worth, TX 76104

AREAS SERVED: Morningside, Near South East

Affiliation/Owner: City of Fort Worth
Nonprofit Organization
Business Hours: Monday–Friday, 8:00am–4:00pm

Since 1996, NSEAM has enabled seniors to maintain their independence. The nonprofit organization serves seniors in the 76104 zip code, also known as the Near Southeast and Morningside community. NSEAM volunteers provide companionship to seniors through phone calls and visits and aid seniors at home by doing light chores and preparing meals, as well as performing yard maintenance and minor home repairs. Volunteers also provide transportation and assist with grocery shopping. In addition, staff members help seniors make use of local resources, including food banks and Meals-On-Wheels.

## Library on Wheels

### GP Memorial Library Bookmobile

901 Conover Drive
Grand Prairie, TX 75051

(972) 237-5741
infodesk@gptx.org
www.gptx.org/Library

AREAS SERVED: City of Grand Prairie

Affiliation/Owner: Public Library of Grand Prairie
Nonprofit Organization
Business Hours: Monday–Tuesday, Thursday, 10:00am–9:00pm; Wednesday, 10:00am–6:00pm; Friday–Saturday, 9:00am–6:00pm; Sunday, 1:00pm–5:00pm

The Grand Prairie Memorial Library is on wheels! Library card in hand, book lovers may choose their favorite read from the traveling library's plentiful selection. The bookmobile makes scheduled stops at Terry's Supermarket and the Prairie Estates Apartments for local convenience.

### Irving Bookmobile

801 West Irving Boulevard
Irving, TX 75060

(972) 721-4868
www.irvinglibrary.org

AREAS SERVED: Irving

Affiliation/Owner: City of Irving
Nonprofit Organization
Business Hours: Monday–Thursday, 10:00am–9:00pm; Friday–Saturday, 10:00am–6:00pm; Sunday, 1:00pm–5:00pm

The Irving bookmobile service makes bimonthly book drop-offs to nursing homes, apartment complexes, retirement homes, assisted living residences, and local churches and schools. Book selections may be ordered through the Irving Public Library's comprehensive online catalog or from the bookmobile itself; the schedule is posted on its website.

### Library on Wheels (LOW)

1515 Young Street
Dallas, TX 75201

(214) 670-1708, (214) 670-1400
libraryonwheels@dallaslibrary.org
www.dallaslibrary.org

AREAS SERVED: Dallas

Affiliation/Owner: City of Dallas
Nonprofit Organization
Business Hours: Monday–Wednesday, 11:00am–9:00pm; Friday, 10:00am–5:00pm; Saturday, 11:00am–5:00pm; Sunday, 1:00pm–5:00pm

Library on Wheels, a program of Dallas Public Library, offers older adults the opportunity to borrow, return and reserve materials without having to visit the library. The wheelchair-accessible bookmobile makes approximately thirty stops per month throughout Dallas. In addition to print materials, seniors may borrow audio books, movies and music, and can even obtain a library card through the bookmobile if they do not already have one.

## Living Will

### Five Wishes

(888) 594-7437
www.agingwithdignity.org
AREAS SERVED: Nationwide
Affiliation/Owner: Aging with Dignity
Nonprofit Organization

Five Wishes is a living will that allows individuals to choose how they are treated if they become incapacitated. The twelve-page health directive addresses five important issues: (1) naming a health care agent to make decisions on the individual's behalf; (2) the type of medical treatment preferred if one experiences a catastrophic health event; (3) how comfortable one chooses to be, regarding pain and medication; (4) how one would like to be treated by family, friends and medical staff; and (5) what the individual wants loved ones to know (e.g., funeral arrangements). The document is easy to use and, unlike other living wills, addresses concerns beyond the scope of medical treatment, such as the spiritual well-being of the individual.

## Meal Delivery

### Meals on Wheels Inc. of Tarrant County

320 South Freeway
Fort Worth, TX 76104
(817) 336-0912
info@mealsonwheel.org
www.mealsonwheels.org

AREAS SERVED: Tarrant County
Affiliation/Owner: Meals on Wheels Association of America
Nonprofit Organization
Business Hours: Monday–Friday, 8:30am–4:30pm

Meals on Wheels of Tarrant County delivers nutritious meals to needy homebound individuals. Clients are accepted regardless of age, income level or how long they will be homebound; the main criteria is that they do not have regular access to balanced meals. The menu changes seasonally and encompasses clients' preferences and dietary needs.

Meals on Wheels case managers meet with clients on a quarterly basis to determine their needs and how to address them; for example, they process applications that allow low-income participants to receive financial help with their utility bills, and work with organizations to allow participants to borrow walkers, bath rails and other necessities free of charge. After discovering that clients were sharing their meals with their pets, the agency began working with a local animal welfare agency to provide free pet food to those with cats and dogs. The program also provides items such as blankets, fans, air conditioners and microwaves.

### Metroport Meals on Wheels, Inc.

428 North Highway 377
Roanoke, TX 76262

(817) 491-1141
bbudarf@metroportmow.org
www.metroportmow.org

AREAS SERVED: Northeast Tarrant and South Denton Counties

Affiliation/Owner: Meals on Wheels Association of America
Nonprofit Organization
Business Hours: Monday–Friday, 9:00am–5:00pm

Volunteers from Metroport Meals on Wheels deliver hot lunches to participants' homes on weekdays. Participants range from needy, homebound individuals to those recovering from surgery. The duration of meal delivery may be short- or long-term. The organization is able to deliver meals immediately to new participants. Services are available regardless of participants' ability to pay. The organization also offers lunches and activities programs within six different senior centers. Metroport Meals on Wheels serves the following communities: Argyle, Bedford, Colleyville, Grapevine, Haslet, Justin, Keller, Marshall Creek, North Richland Hills, Roanoke, Southlake, Trophy Club and Westlake.

### Traveling Chefs

(972) 248-0402

AREAS SERVED: Collin and Dallas Counties

Traveling Chefs provides full-service catering for its clients. The service includes shopping, cooking and kitchen cleanup. Experienced chefs prepare appetizing entrées from a menu with over four hundred selections, all in the comfort of your own home. Whether you're planning a party, an intimate meal or are simply too busy to prepare dinner for the family, Traveling Chefs eliminates the fuss, making mealtime a relaxing and enjoyable experience. Their "Jumpstart to Health" package is a great gift idea for someone who is interested in healthy dieting; the package includes a nutrition consultation, a customized menu and an entire month of service. Some packages include the cost of food for added convenience.

## Medical Supplies and Specialty Items

### AMS Medical Supply

911 North Beltline Road
Mesquite, TX 75149

(972) 216-7700
Info@amsmedicalsupply.com
www.amsmedicalsupply.com

AREAS SERVED: Dallas

Business Hours: Monday–Friday, 8:30am–5:00pm

AMS Medical Supply is an online retailer of affordable medical equipment and supplies that range from hospital beds and wheelchairs, to syringes and blood glucose monitors. AMS honors manufacturers' warranties.

### Body Care Boutique, Inc.

Dallas, TX

(972) 617-6646
ppage@bodycareboutique.com
www.bodycareboutique.com

AREAS SERVED: Dallas

Business Hours: Monday–Friday, 9:00am–5:00pm

Cancer survivor Peggy Page founded Body Care Boutique, an online retailer of medical garments and specialty items that range from wigs to incontinence supplies, because she personally faced the difficulty of locating such items in a single place. The website also features mastectomy garments, including bras and swimwear. Customers receive their orders in discreet packaging.

### Clothing Solutions

(800) 336-2660
www.clothingsolutions.com

AREAS SERVED: Nationwide

Clothing Solutions offers attire for people who require full or partial assistance in dressing. With a varied population in mind—from individuals with limited mobility, to those who may attempt to undress themselves at inappropriate moments, to those who are incontinent—Clothing Solutions manufactures pieces to suit individuals in various scenarios. The designs include features such as zip-fronts, inseams secured by snaps, pullover styling, rear seat panels and back openings. All of these features are disguised to promote the wearer's dignity as well as their comfort.

### E-Pill

(800) 549-0095
(781) 239-8255
www.epill.com

AREAS SERVED: Nationwide

E-Pill is an online store that offers a plethora of medication-reminder merchandise. Alarms, vibrating timers, watches and pagers, pill organizers and identifiers—all are technological solutions to the often hard-to-remember and easy-to-forget problems with tracking daily medication schedules. E-pill provides a money-back guarantee for all its products.

### Gold Violin

(877) 648-8400
www.goldviolin.com

AREAS SERVED: Nationwide

Gold Violin offers its clients nifty gadgets and support products to enhance independent living. The Gold Violin online catalogue is replete with merchandise for seniors with physical and cognitive conditions that may hinder daily routines; memory enhancing products such as photo phones and day-of-the-week clocks are as handy as they are helpful. Many of the products are specifically designed for people with arthritis, dementia or visual impairments.

### Home Delivery Incontinence Supplies (HDIS)

(800) 269-4663
www.hdis.com

AREAS SERVED: Nationwide

HDIS offers a full range of incontinence supplies. HDIS representatives answer questions and provide advice. The online catalog is extensive and all orders are delivered in discreet packaging.

### Lifeline

(800) 380-3111
www.lifelinesys.com

AREAS SERVED: Nationwide

Lifeline is an affordable, easy-to-use medical alarm that promotes the independence of seniors, individuals with disabilities, and the chronically ill by helping them to stay safely at home.

### MediKeeper

(866) 231-6007
www.medikeeper.com

AREAS SERVED: Nationwide

MediKeeper is an online record-keeping service that aids seniors, their caregivers and physicians in keeping track of important health-related information. MediKeeper's features include MediKost, which uses personal information to help seniors choose the most appropriate pharmacy and Medicare prescription discount card; MediKabinet, which tracks subscribers' medications and related information including dosage, side effects and drug interactions; MediTracker, which logs personal health markers like weight, cholesterol and blood pressure, and MediForms, which enables subscribers to avoid completing medical forms repeatedly. A phone call to MediKeeper during an emergency quickly provides medical personnel with subscribers' medical information.

### Multi-Medical, Inc.

2313 8th Avenue
Fort Worth, TX 76110

(817) 514-9403
info@multi-medicalinc.com
www.multi-medicalinc.com

AREAS SERVED: Dallas, Fort Worth, Mid-Cities, North Dallas

Business Hours: Monday–Friday, 8:00am–5:00pm

Multi-Medical, Inc. sells medical and mobility equipment. The staff is comprised of licensed therapists (fluent in Spanish and sign language), equipment specialists and service technicians who are certified by the equipments' manufacturer. The company's primary goal is to provide its clients with state-of-the-art equipment that enhances their mobility and independence.

## Movers

### Senior Moving Company

2621 Nova Drive
Dallas, TX 75229

(972) 488-1700
(877) 372-1700
phyllis.seniormove@sbcglobal.net
www.seniormovingcompany.com

AREAS SERVED: Dallas

Business Hours: Monday–Friday, 9:00am–5:00pm

Senior Moving Company specializes in helping seniors move. A company representative visits customers in their homes to provide free estimates. Available services include packing and unpacking, moving, storage and shipping. Customers may purchase packing materials from the company. Senior Moving Company also refers customers to businesses that handle estate sales.

## Pharmacies

### Mason's Pharmacy

2101 West Airport Freeway
Irving, TX 75602

(972) 252-8644
scott@masonspharmacy.com
www.masonspharmacy.com

AREAS SERVED: Irving
Business Hours: Monday–Friday, 8:30am–6:00pm; Saturday, 9:00am–2:00pm

Mason's Pharmacy has been a staple in Irving for over thirty years. Unlike pharmacy chains, Mason's is locally owned and operated, and staffed with members of the community that people know and trust. Customers depend on Mason's accurate, prompt and caring service.

### Midway Park Pharmacy

2700 West Pleasant Run Road
Lancaster, TX 75146

(972) 223-2623, (972) 223-3677
pharmacist@midwayparkpharmacy.net
www.midwayparkpharmacy.net

AREAS SERVED: Lancaster
Business Hours: Monday–Friday, 8:30am–6:00pm; Saturday 9:00am–1:00pm

Midway Park Pharmacy has served the community of Lancaster since 1983. The staff performs a variety of services for their customers, which includes educating them on medications and related contraindications and side effects. The pharmacy allows customers to use in-house charge accounts. Midway Park Pharmacy also delivers prescription medications to customers in the Lancaster and DeSoto areas.

## Real Estate

### Seniors Real Estate Specialists (SRES)

(800) 500-4564
www.seniorsrealestate.com/sarec/servlet/home
AREAS SERVED: Nationwide
Business Hours: Monday–Friday, 9:00am–5:00pm

Seniors Real Estate Specialists realtors have received a special education from the Senior Advantage Real Estate Council so they can effectively assist seniors with major decisions such as selling their home or refinancing. These specialists are equipped to counsel seniors on topics which include relocating and purchasing property. Clients receive pertinent information on the real estate market as well as referrals to attorneys and other professionals who focus on senior-related issues.

### Vintage Living

15851 Dallas Parkway, Suite 600
Addison, TX 75080

(214) 561-8611
blyle@vintageliving.net
www.vintageliving.net

AREAS SERVED: Dallas, North Dallas

Business Hours: Monday–Friday, 9:00am–5:00pm

Vintage Living is staffed by experienced Seniors Real Estate Specialists (SRES). Vintage realtors act as consultants and advocates for clients who want to refinance, rent, lease, purchase or sell their homes. The agency provides free consultations with licensed realtors to develop specialized plans for their clients, as well as vital information about community resources for seniors, moving and relocation services and home improvement.

## Transportation

### Call A Ride of Southlake (CARS)

P.O. Box 92683
Southlake, TX 76092

(817) 416-9757

AREAS SERVED: City of Southlake

Affiliation/Owner: Southlake
Nonprofit Organization
Business Hours: Monday–Friday, 8:00am–5:00pm

Call A Ride of Southlake provides non-emergency transportation for senior and disabled persons. CARS travels within a twenty-five mile radius—including Dallas, Fort Worth, Irving and Arlington—to attend to participants' medical needs, and within seven miles of Southlake to assist with shopping, errands and social events. Transportation runs Monday through Friday between the hours of 8:00am and 5:00pm.

### Dallas Area Rapid Transit (DART)

1401 Pacific Avenue
Dallas, TX 75202

(214) 515-7272, (214) 979-1111
www.dart.org

AREAS SERVED: Dallas, Carrolton

Affiliation/Owner: Cities of Carrollton, Dallas, Farmers Branch, Garland, Irving, Plano
Nonprofit Organization
Business Hours: Monday–Friday, 8:00am–5:00pm

DART's Paratransit is a specialized transportation service for people whose disabilities or health-related conditions prevent them from independently using fixed-route public transit. It is provided by public transportation systems as part of the requirements of the Americans with Disabilities Act (ADA). Each county has different service providers and different operating hours. Individuals must first qualify before they can participate.

### Grand Connection

1821 West Freeway
Grand Prairie, TX 75050

(972) 237-8545
aflowers@gptx.org
www.gptx.org

AREAS SERVED: Grand Prairie

Affiliation/Owner: City of Grand Prairie
Nonprofit Organization
Business Hours: Monday–Friday, 8:00am–5:00pm

Grand Connection provides transportation to Grand Prairie residents who are at least sixty years of age or are mentally or physically disabled. Participants receive transportation to and from school, work, grocery shopping, medical and dental appointments, and the Dallas County Health and Human Services Nutrition Program appointments. Transportation requests are subject to availability. Trips are either free or subject to a small fee of $1.00 each way depending on the destination.

### Handitran

501 West Sanford
Arlington, TX 76004

(817) 569-5390
publicworks@ci.arlington.tx.us
www.ci.arlington.tx.us

AREAS SERVED: Arlington, Pantego

Affiliation/Owner: City of Arlington
Nonprofit Organization
Business Hours: Monday–Friday, 8:00am–5:00pm

Handitran provides seniors and people with disabilities with transportation anywhere within Arlington and Pantego. Passengers use the service to get to and from work, medical appointments, recreational and personal activities. Public school trips are not allowed. Mini-buses equipped with wheelchair lifts and taxicabs transport passengers. Passengers who do not have their fare can still ride, but the fare must be repaid within two weeks, at twice the rate.

### Mid-Cities Care Corps

745 West Pipeline
Hurst, TX 76053

(817) 282-0531, (817) 280-0969

AREAS SERVED: Mid-Cities

Affiliation/Owner: St. Philip Presbyterian Church
Nonprofit Organization
Business Hours: Monday–Friday, 9:00am–12:00pm

Mid-Cities Care Corps offers several indispensable services to seniors. The organization's volunteers transport seniors to and from medical and dental appointments and personal errands, such as grocery shopping. Volunteers also assist participants with housekeeping.

Homeowner participants may have a variety of work done on their homes, ranging from minor plumbing to wheelchair ramp installation. Adopt-A-Lawn volunteers perform lawn maintenance for seniors on a bi-weekly basis. Participants must be at least sixty years of age and live in one of the following communities: Bedford, Colleyville, Euless, Grapevine, Haltom City, Hurst, Keller, North Richland Hills, Richland Hills, Southlake, Watauga or Fort Worth's Central Hospital District.

### Mobility Impaired Transportation (MITS)

1600 East Lancaster
Fort Worth, TX 76102

(817) 332-4444, (817) 215-8600
kvijil@the-t.com
www.the-t.com

AREAS SERVED: City limits of Fort Worth, Richland Hills and Blue Mound

Affiliation/Owner: Fort Worth Transportation Authority
Nonprofit Organization
Business Hours: Monday–Friday, 8:00am–5:00pm
Years in Business: 25

MITS provides door-to-door transportation for disabled individuals who cannot utilize regular buses. Passengers pay $2.50 per ride and can order tickets online or via mail. Passengers' caregivers ride free of charge. Other guests may accompany passengers when space permits. Service animals and pets may also ride if they are on a leash or in a pet carrier. MITS operates Monday through Saturday from 5:00am to 12:00am, and Sunday from 6:00am to 10:00pm. The service area includes Fort Worth, Richland Hills and Blue Mound.

### Northeast Transportation Service (NETS)

1515 South Sylvania
Fort Worth, TX 76111

(817) 336-8714, (817) 335-9137
http://chisholmtrail.redcross.org

AREAS SERVED: Fort Worth

Affiliation/Owner: American Red Cross
Nonprofit Organization
Business Hours: Monday–Friday, 7:00am–6:00pm

NETS provides transportation to seniors and the disabled who are residents of Bedford, Euless, Grapevine, Haltom City, Hurst, Keller or North Richland Hills. Passengers are driven from their homes to a variety of destinations, including medical and dental appointments, places of employment and education, and even grocery shopping. The fee is $1.50 per ride. NETS operates from 7:00am to 6:00pm, Monday through Friday. Passengers must schedule their trips in advance

# HELPFUL ORGANIZATIONS

- Organizations that really DO help

## 2-1-1

210 East Ninth Street
Fort Worth, TX 76102
2-1-1
(817) 258-8100
www.unitedwaytarrant.org

Affiliation/Owner: Texas Health and Human Services, United Way of Tarrant County
Nonprofit Organization
Business Hours: 24/7
Years in Business: 80

United Way's 2-1-1 Texas is a non-emergency, 24-hour hotline is manned by trained referral specialists that provide statewide information on topics that include housing, health services, financial assistance, transportation, recreation, support groups, caregiver issues and much more. Seniors and their caregivers use this information to decide the best, most inclusive care plan for them.

---

## AARP Senior Community Service Employment Program

1625 West Mockingbird, Suite 108
Dallas, TX 75235
(214) 741-0200
www.aarp.org

Affiliation/Owner: AARP
Nonprofit Organization
Business Hours: Monday–Friday, 9:00am–4:00pm
Years in Business: 30

AARP's Senior Community Service Employment Program (SCSEP) is designed to assist persons fifty-five years and older re-enter the job field. SCSEP staff organizes a personal employment plan that corresponds with applicants' skills and goals. The agency provides temporary job placements with "host" agencies such as libraries, food banks, hospitals, nonprofits or social services, while continuing to research permanent positions in the job market. Through the program, seniors receive tips for interviewing and résumé writing; specialized training; on-the-job experience; and employment referrals. Eligibility is based on age, residency, income and employment status.

---

## Administration on Aging (AOA) & Area Agencies on Aging (AAA)

1349 Empire Central Drive, Suite 400
Dallas, TX
(214) 871-5065
(214) 379-4636
www.ccgd.org

Affiliation/Owner: US Administration on Aging
Nonprofit Organization
Business Hours: Monday–Friday, 8:00am–5:00pm

AOA is a federal advocate agency for seniors that not only educates caregivers and seniors about important benefits and resources, but also teaches government agencies, private groups and the public about the importance of seniors and how society may best serve them. On the local level, the state and Area Agencies on Aging are devoted to delivering direct services such as: adult day care; adult protective services; case management; in-home assistance; public guardianship; representative payee services; and contracted services which handle employment, home modification, legal assistance, nutrition, transportation and more.

---

## Alliance for Retired Americans

(202) 974-8222
(800) 333-7212 Membership
www.retiredamericans.org

Alliance for Retired Americans rallies retired seniors and various community activist groups to voice the discrepancies in public policy that affect the general senior population. The agency organizes advocate groups to lobby on key legislative issues including Social Security, Medicare, long-term care insurance reform plans and affordable housing benefits. The Alliance's main goal is to give seniors a reputable voice at the national level, as well as within their respective communities.

---

## Alzheimer's Association of Greater Dallas

4144 North Central Expressway, Suite 750
Dallas, TX 75204
(214) 827-0062
(800) 272-3900
www.alzdallas.org

### Trinity Medical Center—Carrollton

4323 North Josey Lane
Carrollton, TX 75010
(214) 454-0855
Tiffany.Willis@Alz.org

### Day Stay for Adults—Denton

2109 West University
Denton, TX 76201
(940) 380-9200
(214) 454-0855
Tiffany.Willis@Alz.org

ALZHEIMER'S ASSOCIATION OF GREATER DALLAS (CONTINUED)

**Baylor Medical Center at Waxahachie**
1405 West Jefferson
Waxahachie, TX 75165
(972) 923-8081
(214) 868-0990
April.Dansby@Alz.org

Affiliation/Owner: National Alzheimer's Association
Nonprofit Organization
Business Hours: Monday–Friday, 9:00am–5:00pm
Years in Business: 20

For over twenty-five years, the Alzheimer's Association has spearheaded Alzheimer's research, influenced public policy, furthered understanding of the disease through community outreach, and provided caregiver support. One of the association's highly regarded programs, Safe Return, protects individuals who wander. The association's Green-Field Library is the largest resource center in the U.S. dedicated to the topic of dementia. Materials may be checked out through local chapters of the Alzheimer's Association.

---

## Alzheimer's Association—North Central Texas

101 Summit Avenue, Suite 300
Fort Worth, TX 76102
(817) 336-4949
(800) 272-3900
www.alz.org/northcentraltexas

**Arlington Office**
401 Sanford, Suite 200
Arlington, TX 76011
(817) 460-7001
(800) 272-3900

Affiliation/Owner: National Alzheimer's Association
Nonprofit Organization
Business Hours: Monday–Friday, 9:00am–5:00pm
Years in Business: 23

For over twenty-five years, the Alzheimer's Association has spearheaded Alzheimer's research, influenced public policy, furthered understanding of the disease through community outreach, and provided caregiver support. One of the association's highly regarded programs, Safe Return, protects individuals who wander. The association's Green-Field Library is the largest resource center in the U.S. dedicated to the topic of dementia. Materials may be checked out through local chapters of the Alzheimer's Association.

## Alzheimer's Disease Center (ADC)

5303 Harry Hines Boulevard
Dallas, TX 75235
(214) 648-3198
(214) 648-3239
www2.swmed.edu/alzheimer

Affiliation/Owner: National Institute of Aging, Southwestern Medical Center
Nonprofit Organization
Business Hours: Monday–Friday, 8:30am–5:00pm
Years in Business: 20

The Alzheimer's Disease Center at UT Southwestern Medical Center employs a number of specialists in various fields to study the disease in order to determine its cause and find a cure. The research team also tries to find ways to refine and improve diagnoses. Individuals undergo a complete memory assessment and may take part in clinical research to help improve the care and medical treatment of individuals with Alzheimer's.

---

## American Association for Geriatric Psychiatry (AAGP)

www.aagpa.org
www.gmhfonline.org (Psychiatrist locator)

AAGP is dedicated to the care and treatment of seniors' mental health. The AAGP Geriatric Mental Health Foundation offers an online geriatric psychiatrist locator.

---

## American Association for Homecare

(703) 836-6263
www.aahomecare.org

American Association for Homecare represents every line of service in the homecare community. Included in the provider listings are: home health and home medical equipment providers; hospice services; rehab and assistive technology; respiratory and infusion therapy; and telemedicine. Its online search service allows users to find providers across the U.S. within their 3,000+ membership.

---

## American Association of Retired Persons (AARP)

(888) 687-2277
www.aarp.org

Several AARP chapters are located throughout the Dallas-Fort Worth area. A variety of member benefits and services are available, including discounts on credit, health care, insurance and travel, as well as a subscription to AARP Magazine. To locate a chapter, contact AARP by web or phone. AARP volunteer groups donate time for projects such as Meals on Wheels, friendly visiting and senior advocacy.

## American Cancer Society

(800) ACS-2345
(866) 228-4327 TTY
www.cancer.org

The American Cancer Society is an unparalleled resource for individuals with cancer, their families and caregivers, and health care professionals. The interactive website connects users with treatment centers and other local resources. The Cancer Society offers excellent programs, some examples of which are: I Can Cope, a cancer education program for patients and their families; Look Good Feel Better, a free service provided by certified cosmetologists that teaches cosmetic techniques to patients to help them cope with appearance-related side effects from chemotherapy and radiation treatments; Man to Man, a support and education program for individuals affected by prostate cancer; and Road to Recovery, which provides ambulatory patients with ground transportation to and from cancer treatment.

---

## American Chronic Pain Association (ACPA)

(800) 533-3231
www.theacpa.org

ACPA educates professionals and the general public about chronic pain issues and offers a peer support program as well. Family members learn how to help their loved ones live more complete lives through pain monitoring techniques.

---

## American Heart Association

2401 Scott Avenue
Fort Worth, TX 76103
(817) 315-5000
(800) 242-8721
www.americanheart.org

### Dallas Office

1615 Stemmons Freeway
Dallas, TX 75207
(214) 748-7212
info@americanheart.org

Nonprofit Organization
Business Hours: Monday–Friday, 8:30am–5:00pm
Years in Business: 15

The American Heart Association has been informing the public about heart disease and stroke for over fifty years. Founded by professional caregivers, the agency provides educational literature on topics including CPR, nutrition and exercise, warning signs and stress control. The association has established nationwide support and educational groups such as the Mended Hearts Club and Stroke Club. The overarching goal of the American Heart Association is to lessen the number of deaths and disabilities caused by heart ailments.

## The Arc of the United States

(301) 565-3842
www.thearc.org

Nonprofit Organization

The Arc of the United States serves children and adults with developmental and cognitive deficits, ensuring that the services they require are available within their communities. The Arc's Optimal Wellness and Health Project helps older adults secure rehabilitation services and assistive devices.

---

## Area Agency on Aging (AAA)—Tarrant County

210 East Ninth Street
Fort Worth, TX 76102
(817) 258-8081
(877) 886-4833
www.aaatc.org

Affiliation/Owner: Texas Department of Aging and Disability, United Way of Tarrant County
Nonprofit Organization
Business Hours: Monday–Friday, 8:30am–5:00pm
Years in Business: 80

AAA is a leading advocate for the rights of Tarrant County citizens sixty and older. Its mission is to provide seniors the access and opportunity to continue living independently. Through the Access and Assistance program, seniors obtain benefit counseling on Social Security, Medicare and Medicaid, HMOs and supplemental insurance, long-term care insurance, veterans' benefits, legal documentation and public programs. The WHEELS program provides seniors and persons with disabilities with transportation to medical facilities, pharmacies and doctor's appointments.

---

## Assistance League (AL)

(818) 846-3777
www.assistanceleague.org

Assistance League maintains chapters throughout the U.S. Their members serve seniors in a variety of volunteer roles. Some of these include: coordinating housing for family members of patients undergoing emergency or ongoing medical treatment; maintaining a volunteer visiting program and taking personal care items to residents of retirement communities; coordinating fashion shows that tour senior centers and residences; organizing bingo parties in a variety of senior settings; providing a social connection to homebound seniors; arranging shopping and visiting services for seniors; and fundraising for assorted charitable works.

## Bread Basket Ministries

2809 Mansfield Highway
Fort Worth, TX 76119
(817) 535-2323
www.breadbasketministries.org

Affiliation/Owner: Amon G. Carter Foundation, City of Fort Worth
Nonprofit Organization
Business Hours: Tuesday–Thursday, 9:00am–4:00pm
Years in Business: 22

Bread Basket Ministries is an emergency assistance and faith outreach group that was founded by a local pastor and his wife in 1983. The volunteers and staff provide needy families with staples including food, clothing and monetary aid. With help from the community, the group distributes hundreds of toys during the holidays, bringing cheer to many children.

---

## Case Management Society of America (CMSA)

(501) 225-2229
www.cmsa.org

Nonprofit Organization
Years in Business: 16

CMSA is a nonprofit organization committed to the education and public awareness of case management as an integral part of the health care profession. CMSA spearheads annual education conferences, legislative lobbying and networking forums in an effort to standardize the case management practice and advocate for the rights of patients. CMSA provides current information about past and present health services, enabling patients to make informed decisions about their health care options.

---

## Catholic Charities

1731 King Street
Alexandria, VA 22314
(703) 549-1390
www.catholiccharitiesusa.org

Nonprofit Organization

Catholic Charities provides an assortment of services, which include: caregiver support groups; case management; multilingual senior programs; health clinics; in-home companion support; legal and financial assistance; respite programs; senior recreation services; senior nutrition; refugee programs and more.

## Collin County Committee on Aging

6001 North Tennessee
McKinney, TX 75069
(972) 562-6996
(972) 562-4275
www.cccoaweb.org

Affiliation/Owner: Area Agency on Aging of North Central Texas, City of Plano, City of McKinney, Collin County United Way
Nonprofit Organization
Business Hours: Monday–Friday, 8:00am–5:00pm
Years in Business: 29

When CCCOA was founded in 1976, its primary goal was to encourage adults over sixty to make health-conscious diet choices. Since then, the organization has broadened its scope of senior services. The "Meals on Wheels" program delivers nutritious meals to homebound seniors; the staff even prepares meals on Thanksgiving and Christmas. CCART is a "door-to-door" transportation service that is fully equipped to accommodate seniors who use wheelchairs or walkers.

---

## Dallas County Older Adult Services Program

2377 Stemmons, 2nd floor
Dallas, TX 75207
(214) 819-1860

Affiliation/Owner: County of Dallas
Nonprofit Organization
Business Hours: Monday–Friday, 8:00am–5:00pm
Years in Business: 25

Dallas County Older Adult Services Program operates thirteen senior centers in Dallas, and one each in Richardson, Lancaster, Hutchins and Grand Prairie. The program boasts over 10,000 participants. Seniors enjoy healthy lunches in between recreational activities like dances. Outings to local tourist attractions are popular among participants, as are special events such as concerts. The program promotes participants' health by offering health screenings and exercise, including low-impact water aerobics. Computer classes and other educational opportunities are also available. Seniors participate free of charge, but are encouraged to donate to the program if they are able.

---

## Dallas Legal Hospice

3626 North Hall, Suite 820
Dallas, TX 75219
(214) 521-6622
www.dlh.org

DALLAS LEGAL HOSPICE (CONTINUED)

Affiliation/Owner: Federal Ryan White/C.A.R.E. Act, Texas Department of Health, Texas Equal Access to Justice Foundation
Nonprofit Organization
Business Hours: Monday–Friday, 9:00am–5:00pm
Years in Business: 16

Dallas Legal Hospice has fifteen years of experience providing free legal assistance to terminally ill residents of north central Texas. The agency renders legal services in several areas, including insurance, housing, employment, debt counseling, family law, and public benefits. To qualify, clients must have a terminal diagnosis or be HIV-positive, face legal difficulties related to their health issues; and meet certain financial requirements.

---

## Dallas Life Foundation—Senior Citizen Program

1100 Cadiz Street
Dallas, TX 75221
(214) 421-1380
www.dallaslife.org

Affiliation/Owner: The First Baptist Church of Dallas
Nonprofit Organization
Business Hours: Monday–Friday, 9:00am–5:00pm
Years in Business: 51

Dallas Life Foundation is the largest homeless shelter in North Texas. For over fifty years, it has served the homeless in the DFW Metroplex. The Senior Citizen Program was created due to the growing number of seniors living in the shelter. Caseworkers meet regularly with these residents to help them find affordable housing and file for Social Security benefits. The program also holds activities to promote socialization between participants. The foundation provides residents with three nutritious meals a day, a place to live, clothing, religious services, spiritual counseling and Bible study.

---

## Family Caregiver Alliance (FCA)

(800) 445-8106
www.caregiver.org

Nonprofit Organization

Family Caregiver Alliance is a clearinghouse of local, state and national resources for caregivers of those with Alzheimer's and other adult-onset brain impairments. FCA's newsletter, fact sheets and reading lists can be viewed online or ordered directly. The services provided by FCA include: case management; educational workshops; legal and financial advice; policy updates; respite opportunities and support groups.

## Growth House

www.growthhouse.org

Nonprofit Organization

Growth House is a website that provides resources for life-threatening illnesses and end-of-life care. Its mission is to improve the quality of information and resources for this population. Growth House's network serves an international consortium of health organizations, which hosts a discussion forum for over 18,000 professionals. The website explains major issues in hospice and home care, pain management, grief and death with dignity. It also offers disease-specific interviews and guides, and maintains an online bookstore. Growth House Radio is a unique online entertainment service that offers a unique mix of music and educational features on end-of-life care.

---

## Huguley Plus Senior Services

11801 South Freeway
Fort Worth, TX 76115
(817) 551-2652, (817) 293-9110
www.huguley.org

Affiliation/Owner: Huguley Medical Center
Nonprofit Organization
Business Hours: Monday–Friday, 9:00am–4:00pm
Years in Business: 25

HuguleyPlus Senior Services seeks to enrich the lives of its members, who total over 9,000. Members enjoy a range of benefits, including social activities, flu shots and health screenings. The organization's newsletter features helpful articles on arthritis and other senior-related issues. HuguleyPlus Senior Services accepts people who are sixty-five or older.

---

## Jewish Family Service of Greater Dallas

5402 Arapaho Road
Dallas, TX 75248
(972) 437-9950
www.jfsdallas.org

Affiliation/Owner: Conference on Jewish Material Claims Against Germany, Congregation Tiferet Isarel Tsedakah fund, Episcopal Diocese of Dallas, Federal Emergency Management Agency, Hebrew Immigrant Aid Society, Hillcrest Foundation, Jewish Federation of Greater Dallas, Kosher Chili Cookoff, Sylvan T. Baer Trust/Bank of America Citigroup Foundation
Nonprofit Organization
Business Hours: Monday–Wednesday, 8:30am–8:30pm; Thursday–Friday, 8:30am–5:00pm
Years in Business: 55

Jewish Family Service of Greater Dallas has promoted the social and mental well-being of greater Dallas area residents since 1950. Seniors benefit from needs assessments and case

JEWISH FAMILY SERVICE OF GREATER DALLAS (CONTINUED)

management services, mental health counseling and financial assistance with prescription drugs. Jewish Family Service is qualified to act as the legal guardian of individuals who can no longer perform that service for themselves and who do not have family to assist them. Holocaust survivors have access to transportation services, counseling and assistance to help them preserve their independence. Homebound seniors enjoy kosher meal delivery. Participants in the Friendly Visitors program receive regular volunteer visits. Phone Pals volunteers perform a similar service, calling seniors to chat. In addition, Jewish Family Service provides counseling and a free support group for adult children of seniors to help them understand and cope with their parents' changing abilities and needs. Participants of all services are charged based on a sliding scale.

---

## The Legal Hotline for Older Texans

(800) 622-2520
(512) 477-3950
www.tlsc.org/hotline.html

Affiliation/Owner: Texas Department on Aging, Texas Department of Insurance, State Bar of Texas Equal Access to Justice Foundation
Nonprofit Organization

The Legal Hotline for Older Texans employs knowledgeable staff and volunteer attorneys to advise Texans sixty and older on estate planning, powers-of-attorney, housing issues, debt collection and numerous other legal matters. In coordination with several local attorneys, Hotline clients are able to receive legal assistance at a reduced cost. Seniors also contact the Hotline to receive publications on various topics, including health care rights and public benefits.

---

## Mental Health Outreach Service

2601 Tandy
Fort Worth, TX 76103
(817) 531-8330

Nonprofit Organization
Business Hours: Monday–Friday, 8:00am–6:00pm
Years in Business: 15

Mental Health Outreach Services employs five licensed psychotherapists who provide counseling in clients' homes. The therapists address a variety of mental illnesses, including dementia, schizophrenia, major depression and transitional depression. The organization also offers family therapy. In addition, Mental Health Outreach Services educates staff members of long-term care facilities on numerous issues, such as bereavement and transitions. This organization is Medicaid and Medicare certified.

## National Alliance for Caregiving

(301) 718-8444
info@caregiving.org
www.caregiving.org

Nonprofit Organization

The National Alliance for Caregiving is a consortium of national organizations and corporations with an interest in serving caregivers through research, analysis of public policy and program development. The Alliance's online Family Care Resource Collection rates and reviews websites, reading materials and videos of interest to caregivers and the professionals who serve them.

---

## National Association for Elder Law Attorneys (NAELA)

(520) 881-4005
www.naela.com

Nonprofit Organization

NAHC represents a group of entities that believes families should remain together in the home rather than institutionalizing ill, disabled or elderly individuals. NAHC creates a united front to promote health care services in the home. The association encourages public awareness, provides professional advice, and advocates better industry regulation. The trade association is comprised of hospices, home care agencies, medical equipment suppliers and home care aide organizations. Concerned individuals may also join.

---

## National Association of Home Care and Hospice (NAHC)

(202) 547-7424
www.nahc.org

Nonprofit Organization

NAHC represents a group of entities that believes families should remain together in the home rather than institutionalizing ill, disabled or elderly individuals. NAHC creates a united front to promote health care services in the home. The association encourages public awareness, provides professional advice, and advocates better industry regulation. The trade association is comprised of hospices, home care agencies, medical equipment suppliers and home care aide organizations. Concerned individuals may also join.

---

## The National Citizens' Coalition for Nursing Home Reform (NCCNHR)

(202) 332-2276
www.nccnhr.org

THE NATIONAL CITIZENS' COALITION FOR NURSING HOME REFORM (NCCNHR) (CONTINUED)

Nonprofit Organization
Years in Business: 31

NCCNHR's primary goal is to voice public concern about substandard conditions in nursing homes and various other long-term care facilities in an effort to impact public policy and legislation. NCCNHR is a grassroots organization with members from citizen action groups, nursing home employees' unions, state and local ombudsmen agencies, religious affiliates and long-term care clients and their families. NCCNHR is vested in ongoing federal and state legislative lobbying on fundamental issues that include insufficient staffing in nursing homes, improved conditions and increased wages and benefits for long-term care employees, residents' rights and family representation in development councils.

---

## National Council on the Aging (NCOA)

(202) 479-1200
(202) 479-6674 TDD
www.ncoa.org

Nonprofit Organization
Years in Business: 56

Through public policy advocacy and programming, NCOA promotes healthy aging, as well as recognition of the needs and contributions of older adults. NCOA programs and services include: the Center for Healthy Aging, a resource for aging service providers as well as the general public; Family Friends, which matches at-risk youth with senior companions; RespectAbility, a program which places seniors with volunteer work and employment opportunities; BenefitsCheckUp, an online screening tool that determines one's eligibility for benefits programs; an online reverse mortgage tool; and many other services.

---

## National Hospice and Palliative Care Organization (NHPCO)

(800) 646-6460
(703) 837-1500
www.nhpco.org

Nonprofit Organization
Years in Business: 28

NHPCO promotes access to end-of-life care and recognition of the importance of pain management throughout all stages of illness for individuals and their loved ones. The organization uses advocacy, education, research and outreach to improve and increase the availability of hospice and palliative care. NHPCO's membership is comprised of hospice and palliative care organizations and workers.

## National Long-term Care Ombudsman Resource Center

(212) 332-2275
www.ltcombudsman.org

### Dallas County

1215 Skiles Street
Dallas, TX 75232
(972)572-6330
www.theseniorsource.org

### Tarrant County

3136 West 4th Street
Fort Worth, TX 76107
(817) 335-5405

Affiliation/Owner: Administration on Aging (AoA), National Citizens' Coalition for Nursing Home Reform (NCCNHR), National Association of State Units on Aging (NASUA)
Nonprofit Organization

Ombudsman volunteers are trained advocates for high-quality care within long-term care facilities. They monitor and resolve complaints, review facilities, and provide consumers and professionals with facility information and referrals. The volunteers also support research and public education projects. Ombudsmen regularly visit long-term care facilities to ensure that residents are treated well. When residents and their families have complaints, the ombudsman will intercede when they do not want to deal directly with facility or when their previous efforts have been unsuccessful. If ombudsmen note any problems during their facility visits, they point them out to the facility staff or to the appropriate regulatory agency.

---

## Network of Community Ministries— the Seniors' Net

741 South Sherman Street
Richardson, TX 75081
(972) 234-8880
www.thenetwork.org

Affiliation/Owner: A.A.R.P, Boys & Girls Clubs of Greater Dallas, area churches
Nonprofit Organization
Business Hours: Monday–Friday, 9:00am–6:00pm
Years in Business: 13

The Seniors' Net offers an assortment of services to seniors who live in the Richardson Independent School District. These services include financial counseling and transportation to medical appointments. The Seniors' Net Loaves of Love program provides participants with free baked goods at the Network of Community Ministry. Volunteers replace smoke detector batteries and install smoke detectors in participants' homes. Participants may also

NETWORK OF COMMUNITY MINISTRIES—THE SENIORS' NET (CONTINUED)

have grab bars installed in their showers. During the summer, volunteers do yard work for elderly and disabled participants in the Hearts & Helpers program. The Seniors' Net accepts contributions toward labor and materials, but participants are not required to pay.

---

## Salvation Army Northside Corps Community Center

3023 NW 24th Street
Fort Worth, TX 76106
(817) 624-3111
(817) 624-3112
www.uss.salvationarmy.org/fortworth

Affiliation/Owner: The Salvation Army
Nonprofit Organization
Business Hours: Monday–Friday, 8:30am–6:00pm
Years in Business: 115

The Salvation Army's Northside Corps Community Center provides a weekly senior program every Thursday from 9:00 am to 11:00 am. Each participant receives a nutritious lunch for one dollar. Participants engage in activities, which include quilting, bingo, dominoes and occasional outings. The Community Center also provides spiritual enrichment through daily devotion and Bible study. The program can support 160 seniors.

---

## Senior Citizen Services of Greater Tarrant County

1000 Macon Street
Fort Worth, TX 76102
(817) 338-4433
www.scstc.org

Affiliation/Owner: Area Agency on Aging, United Way
Nonprofit Organization
Business Hours: Monday–Friday, 8:00am–5:00pm
Years in Business: 36

Senior Citizen Services of Greater Tarrant County has operated senior centers for thirty-six years. Participating seniors enjoy healthful benefits, including hot lunches, physical fitness classes, health screenings and nutritional education. Participants have access to legal clinics and case managers, who address numerous needs, such as prescription assistance and financial assistance. Many seniors also take advantage of opportunities to serve in the community. Rock 'n' Read is a program in which volunteers help schoolchildren improve their reading skills. Participants in another program, Seniors and Volunteers for Childhood Immunization, educate new mothers in hospitals on the importance of childhood immunizations. The centers also offer recreational activities—computer classes are among the most popular.

## Senior Source

1215 Skiles
Dallas, TX 75204
(214) 823-5700
www.theseniorsource.org

Affiliation/Owner: Dallas Area Agency on Aging, United Way
Nonprofit Organization
Business Hours: Monday–Friday, 8:30am–5:00pm
Years in Business: 40

Senior Source addresses the needs of the elderly through invaluable services and volunteer opportunities. The organization offers many programs to residents of the greater Dallas area who are at least fifty-five years of age. Eldercare specialists in the Elder Support program support caregivers through education. The Senior Prescription Assistance program helps low-income participants obtain free and low-cost medication. Participants in the Senior Employment Source receive job leads and sharpen their job search skills through seminars and other educational opportunities. Money Management volunteers help low-income participants to effectively manage their money. Volunteer opportunities abound for Senior Source participants. The Foster Grandparent program links low-income seniors with children who are troubled, hospitalized or disabled. The seniors receive a small stipend for participating. The Senior Companion program is similar; it pairs low-income participants with seniors who need extra help to remain independent.

---

## Services Program for Aging Needs (S.P.A.N.)

1800 Malone
Denton, TX 76201
(940) 382-2224
(940) 243-8620
www.span-transit.org

Affiliation/Owner: United Way of Denton County
Nonprofit Organization
Business Hours: Monday–Friday, 8:00am–5:00pm
Years in Business: 31

Through a variety of useful programs, SPAN improves the quality of life for its participants, who range from seniors to disabled individuals. From counseling seniors on public benefits including Medicaid, Medicare and Social Security, to delivering lunches to Denton County's homebound and helping seniors run errands, SPAN volunteers are a tireless bunch. Through the program, lonely seniors are provided with callers and visitors, and support groups are offered to caregivers. SPAN employs twenty vehicles equipped with wheelchair lifts to provide transportation to participants throughout Denton County. The organization also provides free transportation to SPAN Congregate Meal Programs, where seniors enjoy lunches and companionship at local senior centers. S.P.A.N. also transports participants to shopping centers, recreational activities, and places of education and employment.

## Visiting Nurses Association (VNA)

1400 West Mockingbird Lane
Dallas, TX 75247
(214) 689-0000
(800) 442-4490
www.vnatexas.org

### Kaufman Office

102 West Grove
Kaufman, TX 75142
(972) 287-5322
(800) 345-0576
kaufmaninfo@vnatexas.org

### Fort Worth Office

6300 Ridglea Place, Suite 801
Fort Worth, TX 76116
(817) 654-4494
(800) 824-6264
tarrantinfo@vnatexas.org

### McKinney Office

2414 West University Drive, Suite 200
McKinney, TX 75071
(972) 562-0140
(800) 942-9586
collininfo@vnatexas.org

Affiliation/Owner: Texas Department of Health, Texas Department of Human Services, United Way
Nonprofit Organization
Business Hours: Monday–Friday, 8:30am–5:00pm
Years in Business: 71

VNA offers a range of care options, ranging from respite to hospice care, to seniors and caregivers of North Central Texas. VNA Hospice has provided in-home pain management, counseling, and medical equipment longer than any other hospice in Texas. The Wellness program conducts clinics for organizations such as churches and community centers, in which participants receive immunizations, cholesterol screenings, TB testing and blood pressure checks. Volunteers in the Eldercare program provide transportation and companionship to participants. VNA sends nurses and health aides as well as occupational, physical and speech therapists to the homes of participants in the Home Health Care program. These professionals are available twenty-four hours a day. The organization also provides long-term care in the home for ill or disabled individuals.